T0215331

Sustaining Social Inclusion

Sustaining Social Inclusion is the third book in a series on social exclusion and social inclusion. It explores what different understandings of sustainability mean in respect of social inclusion in the variety of fields that deal with human health and well-being. The book is global in its scope, with chapters relating to socially inclusive health and social welfare practice internationally.

This book is divided into seven parts:

- Introduction;
- Sustainable policies for promoting social inclusion;
- Sustaining programmes which support social inclusion;
- Sustaining organisations which promote social inclusion;
- Sustainable social inclusion outcomes;
- Sustainable social development; and
- Conclusions.

It examines how social inclusion can be sustained in the long-term when funding tends to be time-limited.

This research-based book is relevant to a wide range of different readerships globally. It addresses issues of concern for those engaged in debates about the provision of health, social welfare, and other public services. *Sustaining Social Inclusion* will be of interest to academics, policy makers, and practitioners in a wide range of fields, including public health, health promotion, health sciences, history, medicine, philosophy, disability studies, social work, social policy, sociology, and urban planning.

Beth R. Crisp is Professor and Discipline Lead in Social Work, Deakin University, Australia, and a member of the Centre for Health through Action on Social Exclusion (CHASE).

Ann Taket held the Chair in Health and Social Exclusion and was Director of CHASE, Deakin University, Australia until her retirement at the end of 2019.

Sustaining Social Inclusion

Edited by
Beth R. Crisp and Ann Taket

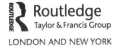
Routledge
Taylor & Francis Group

LONDON AND NEW YORK

First published 2020
by Routledge
2 Park Square, Milton Park, Abingdon, Oxon OX14 4RN

and by Routledge
605 Third Avenue, New York, NY 10017

First issued in paperback 2021

Routledge is an imprint of the Taylor & Francis Group, an informa business

British Library Cataloguing-in-Publication Data
A catalogue record for this book is available from the British Library

Library of Congress Cataloging-in-Publication Data
Names: Crisp, Beth R., editor. | Taket, A. R. (Ann R.), editor.
Title: Sustaining social inclusion / edited by Beth R. Crisp and Ann Taket.
Description: Abingdon, Oxon ; New York, NY : Routledge, 2020. |
    Includes bibliographical references and index.
Identifiers: LCCN 2019057565 (print) | LCCN 2019057566 (ebook) |
    ISBN 9780367027643 (hbk) | ISBN 9780429397936 (ebk)
Subjects: LCSH: Social integration. | Marginality, Social. | Ecovillages.
Classification: LCC HM683 .S87 2020 (print) | LCC HM683 (ebook) |
    DDC 302.3—dc23
LC record available at https://lccn.loc.gov/2019057565
LC ebook record available at https://lccn.loc.gov/2019057566

ISBN 13: 978-1-03-223631-5 (pbk)
ISBN 13: 978-0-367-02764-3 (hbk)

DOI: 10.4324/9780429397936

Typeset in Times New Roman
by Apex CoVantage, LLC

To all those working for the creation of sustainable communities and societies at levels local, national, regional, and global that encapsulate the idea of 'a fair go for all'

Contents

List of illustrations   xi
List of contributors   xii
List of acronyms   xvi

PART 1
Introduction   1

1   **Approaches to sustaining social inclusion**   3
    BETH R. CRISP AND ANN TAKET

PART 2
Sustainable policies for promoting social inclusion   35

2   **The transformative journey to sustainability for Australia's
    compensation systems: how peer support and restorative
    justice interventions are creating a new inclusive narrative**   37
    JOHN BOTTOMLEY, BETTE PHILLIPS-CAMPBELL
    AND GORDON TRAILL

3   **Sustaining social inclusion: lessons from research,
    intervention, and policymaking**   51
    TAMAR KABAKIAN-KHASHOLIAN, RANA SALEH, JIHAD MAKHOUL
    AND FADI EL-JARDALI

4   **Social policy to support women's reproductive decision-
    making and access to economic participation and resources:
    an Australian case study**   65
    MELISSA GRAHAM, HAYLEY MCKENZIE AND
    GREER LAMARO HAINTZ

5   Not impossible: working with the Deafblind community to
    develop a more inclusive world   77
    ALANA ROY, BETH R. CRISP AND KEITH MCVILLY

PART 3
Sustaining programmes which support social inclusion   91

6   Opening doors: creating and sustaining community
    leadership for promoting social inclusion   93
    ANN TAKET, ALEX MILLS, SALLY-ANN NADJ AND RONDA HELD

7   Responding to hunger in Australia: the role of traditional
    and emerging food distribution measures in addressing food
    insecurity   108
    FIONA H. MCKAY

8   Developing inclusion in a small-town food service   119
    ROHENA DUNCOMBE, JOE FAY, GWEN GOULD, CHARLIE FAY,
    MALCOLM FAY, JULIA HARRINGTON, KUATARINA MOUNT,
    BRIAN NEALE AND SUZANNE ARNOLD

PART 4
Sustaining organisations which promote social inclusion   133

9   How to imagine and make good universities   135
    RAEWYN CONNELL

10 Four decades plus of promoting inclusion to
    higher education   147
    BETH R. CRISP

11 Socially inclusive service development: a new expression of
    democracy for nongovernment organisations delivering
    social care   157
    SARAH POLLOCK

12 The space to think critically: how supervision can support
    sustainable practice in social service organisations   171
    MATT RANKINE AND LIZ BEDDOE

PART 5
Sustainable social inclusion outcomes 187

13 **Embedding change: designing short-term projects for
   sustainable effects** 189
   ELENA JENKIN, ERIN WILSON, ROBERT CAMPAIN, KEVIN MURFITT
   AND MATTHEW CLARKE

14 **Philosophy and ethics: sustaining social inclusion in the
   disability sector** 203
   EMMA RUSH, MONICA SHORT, GISELLE BURNINGHAM AND
   JOAN CARTLEDGE

15 **Spirituality and religion: sustaining individuals and
   communities or replicating colonisation?** 218
   BETH R. CRISP

16 **A 'good news' story of social inclusion: refugee resettlement
   in Australia** 231
   KIM ROBINSON

PART 6
Sustainable social development 245

17 **Strengthening everyday peace formation via community
   development in Myanmar's Rohingya–Rakhine conflict** 247
   VICKI-ANN WARE AND ANTHONY WARE

18 **Sustaining inclusion through work: livelihoods experience of
   rural Indonesian villagers with disability** 262
   EKAWATI LIU, YUHDA WAHYU PRADANA, IRFAN KORTSCHAK, HEZTI
   INSRIANI AND ERIN WILSON

19 **The potential of Information and Communication
   Technology (ICT) to create sustainable caring communities** 277
   ZSOLT BUGARSZKI

20 **Building an accessible and inclusive city** 291
   RICHARD TUCKER, PATSIE FRAWLEY, DAVID KELLY, LOUISE
   JOHNSON, FIONA ANDREWS AND KEVIN MURFITT

**21 Theatre-based programmes: promoting empathy
     and engagement**   304
     ANN TAKET

PART 7
Conclusions   319

22 Strategies for sustaining social inclusion   321
     BETH R. CRISP AND ANN TAKET

Index   333

Illustrations

Figure

21.1   Stages in development of *Being Frank*   310

Tables

1.1   The Sustainable Development Goals and actions required to
       achieve these   5
3.1   The contextualised methodology of citizen engagement in
       comparison with the international literature   55
3.2   Participants' evaluation of the impacts of participatory processes   59
6.1   Community initiatives, their outcomes, and impacts   100
13.1   Change audience, products, and change focus   192
14.1   Examples of ethical frameworks from Codes of Ethics for
       professionals who work in social inclusion contexts   205
17.1   2014 Census data contrasting the situation of the Rakhine with
       all persons in Myanmar   248
19.1   Percentage of requests and offers for help on the Helpific platform   284
20.1   Obstacles to accessibility and inclusion in the built
       environment identified by participants in the STICKE workshop   297
21.1   Sources of feedback from previews and first season   313

Contributors

Fiona Andrews is Senior Lecturer in the School of Health and Social Development, Deakin University, Australia.

Suzanne Arnold is an ESL teacher, working in aged and disability sectors and Homeless and Community Breakfast volunteer, Byron Bay, Australia.

Liz Beddoe is Professor of Social Work in the School of Counselling, Human Services, and Social Work at University of Auckland, New Zealand.

John Bottomley is a member of the Centre for Religion and Social Policy at the University of Divinity, Melbourne, Australia, and Director of Transforming Work.

Zsolt Bugarszki is Lecturer of Social Policy in the School of Governance, Law and Society, Tallinn University, Estonia.

Giselle Burningham is a retired social worker, a former employee of the Department of Human Services, and a self-funded participant of NDIA in Australia.

Robert Campain is Research Fellow in the School of Health & Social Development, Deakin University, Australia.

Joan Cartledge is a community development practitioner and training consultant in Virginia, USA.

Matthew Clarke is Head of School and Alfred Deakin Professor, School of Humanities and Social Sciences, Deakin University, Australia.

Raewyn Connell is Professor Emerita, University of Sydney, and a Life Member of the National Tertiary Education Union in Australia.

Beth R. Crisp is Professor and Discipline Lead in Social Work at the School of Health and Social Development, Deakin University, Australia.

Rohena Duncombe is Lecturer in Social Work and Human Services in the School of Humanities and Social Sciences at Charles Sturt University, Australia.

Fadi El-Jardali is Professor of Health Policy and Systems, Department of Health Management and Policy, and Director of the Knowledge to Policy (K2P) Center at the American University of Beirut, Lebanon.

Charlie Fay is from the Minjungbal tribe of the Bundjalung and Yugambeh nations. He is an Aboriginal and Torres Strait Islander Health Worker with NSW Health, Australia.

Joe Fay is an international humanitarian aid worker—public health, Oxfam and Homeless and Community Breakfast volunteer, Australia.

Malcolm Fay is a Minjungbal man of the Bundjalung and Yugambeh nations. He is active in the Bulgalwena Men's Group, NAIDOC, Kinship Festival, and the Homeless and Community Breakfast, Australia.

Patsie Frawley is Associate Professor in Disability and Inclusion, in the School of Health and Social Development, Deakin University, Australia.

Gwen Gould initiated the Homeless and Community Breakfast. She is a peace activist, community activist, and serial volunteer in Australia.

Melissa Graham is Associate Professor in Public Health in the Department of Public Health, La Trobe University, Australia.

Julia Harrington is a volunteer at the Byron Community Centre, Australia.

Ronda Held is Chief Executive Officer of Council on the Ageing (COTA) in Victoria, Australia.

Hezti Insriani holds a master's degree in anthropology, Gadjah Mada University, Yogyakarta, Indonesia.

Elena Jenkin is an honorary fellow in the School of Humanities and Social Sciences, Faculty of Arts and Education, Deakin University, Australia.

Louise Johnson is Professor of Australian Studies, Deakin University, Australia.

Tamar Kabakian-Khasholian is Associate Professor, Department of Health Promotion and Community Health, American University of Beirut, Lebanon.

David Kelly is a research fellow in the HOME Research Hub, Deakin University, Australia.

Irfan Kortschak is a long-term resident of Jakarta, Indonesia, where he works as a development sector consultant. He has a Master's of International and Community Development from Deakin University, Australia.

Greer Lamaro Haintz is Lecturer in the School of Health and Social Development, Deakin University, Australia.

Ekawati Liu is a doctoral candidate in the School of Health and Social Development, Deakin University, Australia.

Fiona H. McKay is Senior Lecturer in the School of Health and Social Development, Deakin University, Australia.

Hayley McKenzie is Lecturer in the School of Health and Social Development, Deakin University, Australia.

Keith McVilly is Professor of Disability and Inclusion in the School of Social and Political Sciences at the University of Melbourne, Australia.

Jihad Makhoul is Professor in the Department of Health Promotion and Community Health at the American University of Beirut, Lebanon.

Alex Mills is Opening Doors Coordinator at Link Health and Community, Victoria, Australia.

Kuatarina Mount is an artist and costumier. She works with Kupu Kupu Disabled Foundation in Bali. She is an ESL teacher and Homeless and Community Breakfast volunteer in Byron Bay, Australia.

Kevin Murfitt is Senior Lecturer in Disability and Inclusion in the School of Health and Social Development, Deakin University, Australia.

Sally-Ann Nadj was General Manager—Community Wellbeing and Communications in Link Health and Community, Victoria, Australia.

Brian Neale is a retired business manager. He volunteers with many local charities, including the Homeless and Community Breakfast, Byron Bay, Australia.

Bette Phillips-Campbell is Manager of GriefWork for Uniting, Victoria and Tasmania.

Sarah Pollock is Executive Director Research and Advocacy for Mind Australia Limited.

Matt Rankine is Lecturer in Social Work in the School of Counselling, Human Services and Social Work, University of Auckland, New Zealand.

Kim Robinson is Senior Lecturer in Social Work in the School of Health and Social Development at Deakin University, Australia.

Alana Roy is a practising psychologist, mental health social worker, and doctoral candidate in the School of Social and Political Sciences, University of Melbourne, Australia.

Emma Rush is Lecturer in Philosophy and Ethics in the School of Humanities and Social Sciences at Charles Sturt University, Australia.

Rana Saleh is the Advocacy and Evidence Lead Specialist at the Knowledge to Policy (K2P) Centre at the American University of Beirut, Lebanon.

Monica Short is Lecturer in Social Work and Human Services in the School of Humanities and Social Sciences at Charles Sturt University, Australia.

Ann Taket held the Chair in Health and Social Exclusion at the School of Health and Social Development, and was Director of CHASE, Deakin University, Australia until her retirement at the end of 2019.

Richard Tucker is Associate Professor in the School of Architecture and the Built Environment, Deakin University, Australia.

Gordon Traill is Veteran Peer Support for Uniting Victoria and Tasmania.

Yuhda Wahyu Pradana is a co-researcher in the 'Collaborative Research of Livelihoods Voices and Choices of Villagers with Disability in Yogyakarta' project, SIGAB and Deakin University, Australia.

Anthony Ware is Senior Lecturer in International and Community Development, School of Humanities and Social Sciences, Deakin University, Australia.

Vicki-Ann Ware is Lecturer in International and Community Development, School of Humanities and Social Sciences, Deakin University, Australia.

Erin Wilson is the Uniting Kildonan Chair in Community Services Innovation, Centre for Social Impact, Swinburne University of Technology, Australia.

Acronyms

ABC	Australian Broadcasting Corporation
ABCD	asset-based community development
ABS	Australian Bureau of Statistics
ACOSS	Australian Council of Social Services
ADF	Australian Defence Force
AMES	Adult Multicultural Education Services
ASD	Autism Spectrum Disorder
ASRC	Asylum Seeker Resource Centre
AVCC	Australian Vice-Chancellors' Committee
CBOs	community-based organisations
CBR	Community-Based Rehabilitation
CD	community development
CDE	Community Development Education
CEO	chief executive officer
CLS	Communities Living Sustainably
CMN	Creative Ministries Network
CMY	Centre for Multicultural Youth
CRPD	Convention on the Rights of Persons with Disabilities
CSO	civil society organisation
DEET	Department of Employment, Education, and Training
DET	Department of Education and Training
DFAT	Department of Foreign Affairs and Trade
DFID	Department for International Development
DPA	Vanuatu Disability Promotion and Advocacy Association
DPO	Disabled Persons Organisation
DVA	Department of Veterans' Affairs
ECCL	European Coalition for Community Living
EENET	Enabling Education Network
EU	European Union
FAO	Food and Agriculture Organization
FJT	Food Justice Truck
GMB	Group Model Building
GW	GriefWork Support

GWM	GraceWorks Myanmar
HSP	Humanitarian Settlement Programme
ICESCR	International Covenant on Economic Social and Cultural Rights
ICT	information and communication technology
IDP	internally displaced person
IEPCP	Inner East Primary Care Partnership
IESII	Inner East Social Inclusion Initiative
ILO	International Labour Organization
ISP	individual support package
K2P	Knowledge to Policy
KPI	key performance indicator
KT	Knowledge Translation
LBD	Learning by Developing
LGBTIQ	lesbian, gay, bisexual, transgender, intersex, queer
LMICs	low- and medium-income countries
MS	multiple sclerosis
NDIA	National Disability Insurance Agency
NDIS	National Disability Insurance Scheme
NGO	nongovernment organisation
NHS	National Health Service
NPM	New Public Management
NSW	New South Wales
OECD	Organisation for Economic Co-operation and Development
OT	occupational therapist
PHCCs	primary health care centres
PhD	Doctor of Philosophy
PNG	Papua New Guinea
PNG ADP	Papua New Guinea Assembly of Disabled Persons
PNPM	Programme Nasional Pemberdayaan Masyarakat
PR	public relations
PSWs	peer support workers
PTSD	post-traumatic stress disorder
RDSP	Registered Disability Savings Plan
RINDI	Inclusive Village Model (Rintisan Desa Inklusi)
RK	Resilient Kids
SDGs	sustainable development goals
SIGAB	local organisation advocating for the rights of people with disability based in the district of Sleman, Indonesia
SIS	specialised and intensive services
SNAP	Supplemental Nutrition Assistance Program
STEMM	science, technology, engineering, medicine, and mathematics
STICKE	Systems Thinking in Community Knowledge Exchange
SWAN	Scientific Women's Academic Network
TAFE	technical and further education
TCF	The Compassionate Friends

U3A	University of the Third Age
UN	United Nations
UNDP	United Nations Development Programme
UNESCO	United Nations Educational, Scientific and Cultural Organization
UNHCR	United Nations High Commissioner for Refugees
UNICEF	United Nations International Children's Emergency Fund
UNSW	University of New South Wales
VH	Veterans Health
UK	United Kingdom
USA	United States of America
WACHS	Wesley Aged Care Housing Services
WHO	World Health Organization
WRC	Women's Refugee Commission

Part 1

Introduction

1   Approaches to sustaining social inclusion

Beth R. Crisp and Ann Taket

Introduction

This volume is the third in our series of books about social inclusion and exclusion written over the last decade. While we have documented many initiatives which have addressed social exclusion and the impacts of being excluded (see Taket et al. 2009a, 2014), new manifestations of social exclusion continue to emerge. For example, it has been claimed that 'the use of social media and the emergence of fake news has intensified . . . divisiveness and hostility to the so-called Other' (de Souza and Halahoff 2018: 1). In this context, the challenge to create socially inclusive communities in which all members feel they belong and are respected is as necessary as ever.

However, rather than social inclusion, the twenty-first century is increasingly witnessing what has been labelled as 'social seclusion' (Klaufus et al. 2017: 12). Gated communities which provide exclusive enclaves for the wealthy are increasingly prominent in many countries, including in low- and middle-income countries in Africa and Latin America. In South Africa some of these communities are particularly targeting potential residents from a specific religious or cultural group. One gated community in Argentina already has 25,000 residents with the expectation that this will eventually rise to 40,000. Such communities tend to have a high degree of self-containment, providing not only housing but opportunities for employment and socialising, such that residents may have few reasons to leave their enclave (Klaufus et al. 2017).

In our first book, *Theorising Social Exclusion* (Taket et al. 2009a), we explored a wide range of social and cultural factors which have been found to contribute to experiences of inclusion and exclusion by individuals, groups, and communities. Originating in the latter decades of the twentieth century, social exclusion initially referred to entrenched poverty and economic marginalisation and an inability to access the social and cultural resources such as education and employment to move out of poverty. Over time, understandings of social exclusion have developed, such that in our first book we proposed that

> The concept of social exclusion attempts to help us make sense out of the lived experience arising from multiple deprivations and inequities experienced by

people and localities, across the social fabric, and the mutually reinforcing effects of reduced participation, consumption, mobility, access, integration, influence and recognition. The language of social exclusion recognises marginalising, silencing, rejecting, isolating, segregating and disenfranchising as the machinery of exclusion, its processes of operation.

(Taket et al. 2009a: 3)

Understanding social exclusion in this way refers to a diverse range of factors and mechanisms, including but not limited to poverty, which limit acceptance, opportunities equity, justice, and citizenship for individuals, groups, and communities in the broader society. Furthermore, there were others who were also acknowledging the multiplicity of factors and processes which can lead to exclusion. For example, in Tanzania, the *Persons with Disabilities Act* (2010) is concerned with persons 'with a physical, intellectual, sensory or mental impairment and whose functional capacity is limited by encountering attitudinal, environmental and institutional barriers' (Parliament of the United Republic of Tanzania 2010: 9).

Identifying how and why social exclusion occurs has been critical in developing approaches which address exclusion. Thus our second book, *Practising Social Inclusion* (Taket et al. 2014), sought to explore what works and why. In contrast to approaches which have confined understandings of promoting social inclusion to ensuring access to services (e.g. Farrington and Farrington 2005), we were concerned with the fulfilment of civil, political, economic, social, and cultural rights to participation in society as set out in the *Universal Declaration of Human Rights* (United Nations 1948). This involves addressing a range of mechanisms which can promote or deny social inclusion, including policy, service design, service delivery, community life and research (Taket et al. 2014).

At the conclusion of our previous volume, we wrote,

Achieving social inclusion is a continuing challenge which will involve ongoing political will and support from all levels of the community. Undoubtedly, some initiatives to promote social inclusion will be more effective in achieving this goal than others, and there will be ongoing need to reflect and identify factors influencing both success and failure.

(Taket et al. 2014: 256)

Whereas our previous work has been concerned with efforts to promote social inclusion within the fields of health, social care, and education, efforts to address social exclusion are often affected by access to 'the provision of clean water, nutrition, employment, education, shelter, essential medicines, and an unpolluted environment to access to social networks' as well as 'the promotion of freedom from discrimination on the grounds of gender, religion, or race' (Murphy 2012: 20). These are goals which struggle to be met by short-term policy and programme initiatives for which funding is terminated before ongoing change is achieved.

Frameworks for sustaining social inclusion

In previous books (Taket et al. 2009a, 2014), the value of a human rights framework for promoting and protecting social inclusion has been noted. As Sachs (2012) notes, the *Millennium Development Goals* represented a historic method of global mobilisation to achieve important social priorities worldwide. Progress was, however, mixed, both between and within countries. This new book moves the debate further to explore what sustainability means in respect of social inclusion. In recent times there has been much interest and support for the United Nations (2015) *Sustainable Development Goals* (SDGs) which seeks to end extreme poverty, tackle inequality, and take action on climate change by 2030.

United Nations (UN) Secretary-General Ban Ki-Moon's high-level global sustainability panel, appointed in the lead-up to the Rio+20 summit in June 2012, issued a report recommending that the world adopt a set of *Sustainable Development Goals* (SDGs). On 1 January 2016, the 17 *Sustainable Development Goals* (SDGs) of the *2030 Agenda for Sustainable Development*—adopted by world leaders in September 2015 at an historic UN Summit—officially came into force. The goals are shown in Table 1.1

Table 1.1 The Sustainable Development Goals and actions required to achieve these

Number	Goal	Action
1	No poverty	End poverty in all its forms everywhere
2	Zero hunger	End hunger, achieve food security and improved nutrition, and promote sustainable agriculture
3	Good health and well-being	Ensure healthy lives and promote well-being for all at all ages
4	Quality education	Ensure inclusive and equitable quality education and promote lifelong learning opportunities for all
5	Gender equality	Achieve gender equality and empower all women and girls
6	Clean water and sanitation	Ensure availability and sustainable management of water and sanitation for all
7	Affordable and clean energy	Ensure access to affordable, reliable, sustainable, and modern energy for all
8	Decent work and economic growth	Promote sustained, inclusive, and sustainable economic growth and full and productive employment and decent work for all
9	Industry, innovation, and infrastructure	Build resilient infrastructure, promote inclusive and sustainable industrialization and foster innovation
10	Reduced inequalities	Reduce inequality within and among countries
11	Sustainable cities and communities	Make cities and human settlements inclusive, safe, resilient, and sustainable

(Continued)

Table 1.1 (Continued)

Number	Goal	Action
12	Responsible consumption and production	Ensure sustainable consumption and production patterns
13	Climate action	Take urgent action to combat climate change and its impacts
14	Life below water	Conserve and sustainably use the oceans, seas, and marine resources for sustainable development
15	Life on land	Protect, restore, and promote sustainable use of terrestrial ecosystems, sustainably manage forests, combat desertification, and halt and reverse land degradation and halt biodiversity loss
16	Peace, justice, and strong institutions	Promote peaceful and inclusive societies for sustainable development, provide access to justice for all, and build effective, accountable, and inclusive institutions at all levels
17	Partnerships for the goals	Strengthen the means of implementation and revitalize the global partnership for sustainable development

Source: United Nations (2015)

As the UN expressed it, the SDGs

> seek to build on the Millennium Development Goals and complete what they did not achieve. They seek to realize the human rights of all and to achieve gender equality and the empowerment of all women and girls. They are integrated and indivisible and balance the three dimensions of sustainable development: the economic, social and environmental.
>
> (United Nations 2015: Preamble)

The *SDGs* and the set of human rights enshrined in the *Universal Declaration of Human Rights* are closely interlinked; they can be regarded as two different lenses through which the same set of issues can be viewed. Of particular interest here are those that explicitly mention inclusion, quality education, decent work and economic growth, inclusive industrialisation, inclusive settlements and cities, and inclusive societies and institutions (goals 4, 8, 9 11 and 16), but the other goals all have implicit links to social inclusion, as is recognised in the overarching principle of 'Leaving no one behind', a key commitment of the *SDGs*.

> As we embark on this great collective journey, we pledge that no one will be left behind. Recognizing that the dignity of the human person is fundamental, we wish to see the Goals and targets met for all nations and peoples and for all segments of society. And we will endeavour to reach the furthest behind first.
>
> (United Nations 2015: Clause 4)

The ambitious aims of the *SDGs* are reflected in the *High 5 Priority Goals* of the African Development Bank which provide a broad understanding of what is required for social inclusion. These goals are to 'Power Africa; Feed Africa; Industrialize Africa; Integrate Africa; and Improve the Quality of Life for the People of Africa' (African Development Bank Group 2019). Importantly while all five goals are priorities, there is no priority order within this group, as each makes a necessary and complementary contribution to improving the lives of the people of Africa.

The challenges of operationalising 'leaving no one behind' in the context of the *SDGs* has received some attention. For maximum effectiveness, governments and other funding agencies need to ensure investment into all of these goals and not just into those which they consider to be most attractive or most easily achieved (Clark 2018). Some groups in society may also be more likely to be left behind. For example, Elias and Holliday (2019) have considered the difficulties inherent in achieving rights for sex workers, drawing on research conducted in the Southeast Asian region and Cambodia in particular.

Whereas the *SDGs* and the *High 5 Priority Goals* are underpinned by a vision of social inclusion for all, austerity measures in countries like the United Kingdom have seen a move away from a social inclusion agenda to an agenda of protection for the most vulnerable and marginalised members of the community (Parker and Ashencaen Crabtree 2018). As we have demonstrated in our earlier volumes, social exclusion is not only a concern for people living in extreme poverty. Groups affected include childless women (Carey et al. 2009; Graham 2014), women and children who have experienced domestic violence (Barter-Godfrey and Taket 2009), and people who do not fit a heteronormative expectation (e.g. Martin and Pallotta-Chiarolli 2009; Taket et al. 2009b).

One of the reasons why many initiatives aimed at overcoming social exclusion do not achieve their aims is that they fail to take into account the longstanding impact of exclusion on individuals, families, and/or communities. It has been suggested that unless individuals, or others on their behalf, make decisions otherwise, 'the badges of inability resulting from the negatively perceived and assessed attributes of individual/family functioning sustain the negative mechanisms of their possessors life courses and force individuals into biographical traps' (Golczyńska-Grondas 2014: 56). Moreover, the effects of exclusion can last generations. For example, the impact of large-scale emigration of Irish Catholics in the 1840s has been linked with poorer health outcomes and greater likelihood of being in a lower social class, more than a century and a half later for Catholics compared to non-Catholics in Glasgow (Abbotts et al. 1997). As with forced migration, rurality has also been proposed as a factor responsible for storing and transmitting inequality over generations (Shucksmith 2012).

It is hardly surprising that the question has been asked, 'Does exclusion never cease?' (Amin 2019: 4). Yet some countries in which there is considerable ethnic and religious diversity have challenged the intractability of social exclusion and suggest that sustained social inclusion is a real possibility for those who desire inclusion (Amin 2019). In the remainder of this chapter, we outline approaches which would appear to contribute to social inclusion which is sustained. These are policies which promote sustained social inclusion; sustaining programmes and/ or organisations which promote social inclusion; initiatives which lead to social inclusion as a sustained outcome; and sustainable social development.

Sustainable policies for promoting social inclusion

The International Labour Organization (ILO) has developed what it has termed a 'social protection floor' as an

> integrated set of social policies designed to guarantee income security and access to essential social services for all, paying particular attention to vulnerable groups and protecting and empowering people across the life cycle.

It includes guarantees of:

- basic income security, in the form of various social transfers (in cash or in kind), such as pensions for the elderly and persons with disabilities, child benefits, income support benefits, and/or employment guarantees and services for the unemployed and working poor;
- universal access to essential affordable social services in the areas of health, water and sanitation, education, food security, housing, and others defined according to national priorities.

> (ILO 2011: xxii)

The ILO approach has not been to prescribe universal standards but for countries to develop integrated policies which respond to national needs, priorities, and resources and which is sustainable:

> Social protection floor components can be maintained on a long-term basis only if sufficient financial resources are made available, in competition with other claims on a government's spending capacity. Accordingly, it is necessary to consider in some detail the question of how to make available sufficient fiscal space for national programmes. In the past decade, the improvement in macroeconomic conditions, most notably in several middle-income countries, has enabled public institutions to begin to address social deficits and social exclusion.

> (ILO 2011: xxvii)

Addressing lack of access to these essential requirements is critical to sustaining social inclusion, as many of the chapters in this volume attest. Yet as many as 80 per cent of the world's population live without adequate health services and social security systems (ILO 2011). Even in countries which are amongst the wealthiest on the planet, social protection floors may be inadequate in promoting and sustaining social inclusion for some residents. For example, food security is not something which can be taken for granted by many in high-income countries such as Australia (see chapters 7 and 8). Moreover, at least 100 countries, including 22 high-income countries, enacted policy changes between 2010 and 2013 which reduced the coverage of social protection floor measures. On the other hand, some of the world's poorest countries, including Bangladesh, Malawi, and Rwanda, have been increasing the proportion of GDP spent on social protection measures (ILO 2014).

The ILO's social protection floors assume levels of policy coherence at the national level which may not exist. Even when there is policy coherence in theory, coherence does not necessarily result when funding allocations are made. At the end of the twentieth century, Malaysia was undergoing rapid industrialisation from a traditionally agrarian society to one of the fastest-growing economies in Asia. It was recognised that specific endeavours were required to address the poverty of those communities which had traditionally lived off the land. In particular, Malaysia sought to develop a ' "Caring Society" by developing a caring attitude amongst its citizens towards the "less fortunate" ' (Chong 1999: 173). However, 'Though expounded by politicians, this theme has been more political rhetoric than substance' (Chong 1999: 173) in that while policy makers identified critical issues, budget allocations to provide the infrastructure to effect ongoing change was minimal.

Policy coherence may be even more difficult to achieve, let alone sustain, if policy and funding are the responsibility of different authorities. For example, it was government policy in the UK that a specified percentage of rural households had access within a ten-minute walk to buses on an hourly basis. However, the funding for public transport was devolved to local authorities who were not funded to provide that level of service (Farrington and Farrington 2005).

While many of the initiatives described in this volume have received funding as a result of policies which have been enacted, arguably just as importantly, the creation or adoption of policies have symbolic value in making determinations as to who or what is important in a society. Chapter 2 describes the evolution of compensation schemes for injured workers and their families and argues that when 'accidents could be seen as an inevitable business risk', remaining financially profitable may be a higher priority for employers than the needs of injured workers and their dependents. Hence, compensation schemes have often sought to make it difficult for workers and their families to claim compensation and, in doing so, have added to the layers of exclusion being experienced by many. Furthermore, while it is acknowledged that changes have resulted in policies which are less exclusionary, providing support as individuals and families negotiate compensation systems is critical to sustaining their sense of inclusion.

A number of chapters in this book refer to declarations of the United Nations, including the *Universal Declaration on Human Rights* (United Nations 1948), the *Declaration on the Rights of Disabled Persons* (United Nations 2006), and the *Declaration on the Rights of Indigenous Peoples* (United Nations 2007). In becoming a signatory, countries signal their commitment to develop or enact policies which are consistent with declarations, thus contributing to sustainable policy making which promotes social inclusion. However, there are no formal sanctions or penalties for noncompliance for signatories to many declarations. Policy changes which provide sanctions for noncompliance or rewards for compliance can be an effective way of implementing sustained change. For example, the European Union has provided financial incentives for European universities to implement policies to tackle gender discrimination (Carvalho and de Lourde Machado-Taylor 2017). Conversely, in the United Arab Emirates, a lack of obligation to implement affirmative action plans or reporting requirements about groups often marginalised in employment results in no incentive for organisations to tackle issues of marginalisation (Kemp et al. 2017).

In many countries, improving employment opportunities is considered fundamental to social inclusion policy agendas. Policy approaches which tackle structural problems in the labour market are likely to result in more sustainable outcomes in respect of social inclusion, but many countries adopt approaches which are premised on the basis that social inclusion is achieved by redressing the deficits of unemployed individuals. The latter approach has limited impact in the longer term, particularly when funding is provided for employers to accept individuals for limited-term job placements. Such schemes typically result in those unemployed persons who are most employable being offered employment for a short period, only to find themselves once more unemployed once the placement has been completed (Perkins 2010). Furthermore, temporary workers are those most likely to lose jobs during downturns. For example, job losses in Spain as a result of labour-market adjustments were disproportionately accounted for by temporary workers (Muñoz de Bustillo and Antón 2015).

Policies which aim to promote social inclusion can have the opposite effect if implementation has not been carefully planned and executed. Chapter 4 discusses policies around motherhood and employment, which are designed to enable women to return to work after having a child. However, it is left to individual women and their employers to make this work in practice. Lack of affordable childcare and other supports which mothers need to enable them to participate in the workforce are often absent, sometimes placing parents in an invidious position of taking up employment or leaving them in unsuitable childcare arrangements. Hence, although society as a whole benefits from children, if individual employers are left with paying the costs of maternity leave, then it is not surprising that some are resistant to employing women whom they may perceive will soon be having children.

Another example of failure to consider issues of implementation can be found in our previous volume. This concerned a funding programme to support people with disability living in the community acquire assistive technologies. In order to enhance independence and facilitate community involvement, the scheme included support for people to purchase vehicles and specialised equipment, as well as modifications to the home. While the aims of the programme seemed to promote social inclusion, the demand for the service was much more than could be delivered. Hence, decisions as to who received assistance exacerbated the experience of exclusion for those who did not receive services they believe they needed and were eligible to receive (Layton and Wilson 2014).

One of the reasons why policies which aim to promote social inclusion strug-gle to do so is lack of consultation with those members of the community whom particular policies are expected to support. Chapter 3 provides one possible solu-tion to this problem through a discussion of citizen consultations in Lebanon. While it is too early to know the long-term effects of these in respect to childhood obesity, the focus of these consultations, getting agreement from diverse sectors of the community is an important starting point. Nevertheless, Lebanon is a coun-try where policymaking rarely involves community consultation, and given the high satisfaction with the process as revealed by many participants indicating their willingness to be involved in further consultations, the process outlined in chapter 3 provides one possible model for the development of sustainable policies which promote social inclusion.

For some groups and communities, standard methods of consultation are unlikely to be appropriate or effective. Chapter 5 notes that research and consulta-tion processes commonly assume participants are part of a hearing and sighted world. Consequently, people who are Deafblind are rarely included in community consultations. This need not be the case, but new methods of consultation need to be developed as a step toward sustainable policymaking.

Policy processes rarely meet the needs of all members of a society and can often promote social exclusion, either by intention or because the consequences for some members of society were not adequately considered. Sometimes com-promises are made on the basis that getting a piece of policy partially ratified is better than not having it adopted at all. In our previous volume, Barter-Godfrey and Shelley (2014) explored the inclusion of conscience clauses into health policies in some countries. Essentially these allow service providers to refuse a request for a service to which they have a moral objection, such as contraception or abortion. The insertion of such clauses may be promoted as providing for the needs of both service users and service providers. However, as Barter-Godfrey and Shelley noted, the implications of refusal have far more negative impact on those seeking a service than on those refusing to provide, particularly if there is no onus for refusers to refer individuals to a service which can assist them. Con-sequently, policies which sustain social inclusion need to ensure fairness to all and not privilege those who provide over those who require services.

Inclusive practice can also be facilitated by social policy processes which recommend priorities for legislation, funding, service design principles, and the research paradigms used to justify the need for or evaluate social programmes. Policies underpinned by social inclusion principles often have long-lasting effects in respect of promoting social inclusion. In Chapter 9, it is argued that 'we need to think about sustainability in a much longer frame than the policymakers and managers generally do'. Such comments are particularly apt, given that policy ini-tiatives which explicitly sought to tackle social exclusion in Britain and Australia were early casualties of incoming conservative governments (Slay and Penny 2013; Sustainable Governance Indicators 2016; Wilson et al. 2013). Hence, at a policy level, bilateral political support is crucial, so if there is a change of govern-ment, an initiative does not face being defunded (Baum et al. 2010).

Sustaining programmes which promote social inclusion

It is recognised that social exclusion is not always easily overcome and that the effects of exclusion can be multi-generational (Abbotts et al. 1997). Such exclusion will not be overcome with short-term programmes or policies. Nevertheless, at times of financial constraint, funding for programmes which seek to reduce the impact of social exclusion, e.g. programmes in fields such as health, welfare, and education, are most at risk of being discontinued. It was recently observed in the United Kingdom that

> There have been more than 100 government programmes funded over the last thirty years aimed at tackling problems faced by young people. Few have survived for more than three years, whilst disadvantage amongst 10–20% of young people persists.
>
> (Duxbury 2016: 11)

One of the reasons why many programmes fail is that they are developed by experts whose understandings of those they are seeking to assist are simplistic and fail to recognise the complexity and diversity of the lived experiences of those targeted by their programmes. For example, employment programmes are proposed for those living in poverty which fail to take into account that social exclusion is often multidimensional (Chambers 2010).

Organisations are often willing to take on new programmes when they receive funding to do so. Yet it is not uncommon for the funding of such programmes to be ceased on a whim rather than based on any evidence as to whether the programme was achieving its goals. This includes situations in which evaluations have been commissioned but have yet to be completed, even when anticipated date of completion is within agreed timelines. Unless alternate funds can be acquired quickly, programmes which are tackling social exclusion will often be discontinued or replaced by programmes which fit the current funding priorities of governments, corporations, and philanthropists. The acceptability of programmes to a community can vary, and for a programme which is perceived by the community as having been inappropriately terminated, any replacement programme cannot necessarily expect the support received by its predecessor (Hafford-Letchfield et al. 2014).

Funding bodies may seek to leverage sustainability by requiring host organisations to demonstrate a commitment to continuing to provide the programme after the initial additional funding has finished (Keating et al. 2010). However, it is important that this initial funding takes into account that the establishment of programmes which sustain social inclusion can take some years. The recent evaluation of *Communities Living Sustainably* (CLS), a five-year programme to assist 12 local communities in England to tackle issues associated with climate change but where many of the projects also tackled social inclusion, found that even five years of initial funding was not long enough for some of these communities to be able to sustain these projects once funding ceased. The project evaluation noted

Ensuring the changes brought about are sustained and the structures put in place are embedded in the local community is a complex task that can't be rushed.

After five years some of the community assets and organisations developed through CLS are just beginning their journey and their long-term survival beyond the end of grant funding is by no means assured. This needs to be set against the current context of many community organisations surviving from year to year in a very uncertain funding climate.

(Groundwork UK 2017: 26)

Alternately, some programmes rely on voluntary labour which can also be difficult to sustain over a long period (Brault et al. 2018). Nevertheless, some programmes manage to survive long term with limited or precarious funding. This includes the *Homeless and Community Breakfast* in a rural Australian town which is described in chapter 8. This has been running for 15 years with a very limited budget, relying on a range of donations from local businesses, fundraising efforts, and volunteer labour, and demonstrates how long-lasting services have the capacity to adapt to changing resources available and demands (Crossland and Veitch 2005). Not being reliant on a single source of funding has meant that when an individual supporter was no longer able to contribute money, food, or labour, the programme was not held ransom to the changing fortunes or interests of an individual supporter. Furthermore, the magnitude of each contribution was not large so that alternate sources of support could readily be located within the community, but this did require the programme to be continually active in building and maintaining networks of support within the wider community.

Supporting programmes which are effective in addressing social inclusion is not always a priority of local businesses. This was the experience of the *Opening Doors* programme, described in chapter 6. Despite developing community leaders who have developed more than 100 initiatives involving 15,000 members in their local communities, attempts to secure corporate sponsorship of the programme have been unsuccessful. Although funded by a mix of resources and grants from community agencies and local government, the programme has been hosted by a local community health agency which considers the aims of *Opening Doors* to be within the agency's remit of addressing social inclusion. The role of the host organisation entails underwriting the cost of the programme coordinator and administrative costs and hence ensuring that appropriately qualified staff can be recruited and retained whether or not various funding applications are successful. Many of the initiatives which have been established by graduates of *Opening Doors* such as support networks for carers, people living with disabilities, or providing opportunities for people from culturally and linguistic communities to meet, are in fact the types of programmes which other organisations with a similar remit provide resources, including staff, to run. However, while it takes courage for an organisation to decide to run a programme, such as *Opening Doors*, in which it does not have control over initiatives its graduates ultimately develop, the overall reach into the community is far greater than the more traditional approach of community health agency staff running programmes for selected groups in the community which they have the skills and resources to support.

An alternate model of funding has been adopted for the *Food Justice Truck* which is described in chapter 7. Operating on a business rather than charity model, this has been established as a social enterprise, which provides heavily discounted food to asylum seekers while others pay full price. Because the enterprise relies on patronage from community members, the service provides opportunities for asylum seekers to mix with the broader community as they engage in the common task of buying nutritious food for their households.

Sustaining social inclusion includes ensuring that individuals and communities will feel they can access services which are provided on their behalf. A further factor contributing to the sustainability of the *Opening Doors*, the *Homeless and Community Breakfast*, and the *Food Justice Truck* is their attractiveness to participants. A recent survey of social workers in the US found that more than two-thirds (69 per cent) reported that inadequate food was an issue for their clients (Nesmith and Smyth 2015). Yet as noted in chapter 8, many programmes established to provide food aid dehumanise potential participants, many of whom will opt out rather than accept charity. The authors note the importance of ' "solidarity with" rather than "charity for" '.

Similarly, *Opening Doors* (chapter 6), seeks to build on the existing skills, networks, and enthusiasm of participants to enable them to achieve their aims in the community. While both programmes have professionals from the health and community services sectors providing support, they seek to minimise status differentials between the various participants. For example, the *Homeless and Community Breakfast* sought to have all participants involved in all aspects of the programme, including food preparation and serving. These aims were challenged when another group who used the building wanted to redesign the space, which, had their plans been realised, would have resulted in volunteers being physically separated from the intended programme recipients. Hence, sustaining a programme which is socially inclusive may require an ongoing commitment to a model of service provision alternate to that provided for by more traditional paradigms (Crossland and Veitch 2005). This, however, does not mean that programmes remain static and unchanging, but rather as the examples in this volume demonstrate, there is a commitment to ongoing reflection and evaluation and adapting the programme to maintain relevance (Scheirer 2005).

Not all programmes need to be sustained indefinitely, as the need can disappear. For example, during the first half of the twentieth century, the local community health service in one inner Melbourne suburb provided bathing facilities for the many households in the area which did not have their own bathrooms. After a major programme of slum redevelopment, with the replacement housing all being equipped with bathrooms, this programme was no longer needed (Lindsay 1994). Other programmes may be discontinued when evidence emerges which contradicts claims about programme effectiveness or the programme is no longer aligned with community values and beliefs (Muir-Gray 1999).

One programme we might hope is not required in future generations is *Athena SWAN*. This grew out of a UK-funded project involving the Scientific Women's Academic Network (SWAN) and arising out of concerns as to the status and career opportunities for women academics in science, technology, engineering, medicine, and mathematics (STEMM) disciplines. From this emerged the *Athena SWAN Charter* in 2005 in which universities and research institutes seeking to join the *Charter* must agree:

- To address gender inequalities requires commitment and action from everyone, at all levels of the organisation
- To tackle the unequal representation of women in science requires changing cultures and attitudes across the organisation
- The absence of diversity at management and policymaking levels has broad implications which the organisation will examine
- The high loss rate of women in science is an urgent concern which the organisation will address
- The system of short-term contracts has particularly negative consequences for the retention and progression of women in science, which the organisation recognises
- There are both personal and structural obstacles to women making the transition from PhD into a sustainable academic career in science, which requires the active consideration of the organisation.

(Equality Challenge Unit 2018a)

Over time, the scope for *Athena SWAN* has broadened to include other academic disciplines and become concerned with the broader workforce within higher education and research institutes, including professional, technical, and support staff as well as academics. The *Charter* has also found an administrative base in the Equality Challenge Unit which receives public funding to monitor equity, diversity, and inclusion issues in higher education in the United Kingdom (Advance HE 2018). Institutions, or departments thereof, wishing to sign up to the *Athena SWAN Charter* must submit a portfolio of evidence including data about gender equity within their organisation and an action plan outlining further work to be done. Applications are expected not just to meet legislative requirements but to provide examples of 'good practice' which goes beyond these. Applicants can apply for recognition at the Bronze (lowest), Silver, or Gold (highest) levels (Barnard 2017).

In the first few years, there was little incentive for organisations which were struggling with gender equity to apply to join the *Charter*. However, a 2011 announcement from British Medical Research Council in which future applicants for the National Institute of Health Research funding would be expected to have attained at least silver status in *Athena SWAN* saw a massive increase in applications to join the charter. *Athena SWAN* programmes have also been established in other countries, including Australia and Ireland (Barnard 2017).

For organisations submitting an application to *Athena SWAN*, the monetary cost is negligible at UK£500 per application in 2018. However, to successfully maintain their status, members of the Charter must reapply every four years (Equality Challenge Unit 2018b). With only a few departments and no whole institution yet attaining gold status, there have been suggestions that even those departments with gold status could still improve opportunities for women, particularly those employed at senior levels (Barnard 2017). With an ongoing need, a structure which is predominantly self-funding, and incentives for organisations to participate in *Athena SWAN*, this is a programme that should be able to be sustained in the long term or as long as gender equity is still an issue in higher education and research institutes. Furthermore, versions of the programme having been adopted in other countries suggests *Athena SWAN* provides a model of a sustainable programme which can traverse national borders.

Some programmes are developed and implemented through a collaboration of a number of organisations, which may be located in different sectors, and have different mandates and resources they can contribute. Sustaining programmes run by collaborations requires ongoing commitment from each of the partners, or the capacity and willingness of remaining partners to offer the programme should one or more partners withdraw. At least one collaborating partner needs to have the capacity to provide any infrastructure support that might be required, including administrative support and access to finance and other resources as required. Such a partner may add a perception of legitimacy or credibility to a collaboration (Chalk and Pilkinton 2018).

Sustaining organisations which promote social inclusion

It is often assumed that sustaining a programme requires it to be embedded in an organisation which hosts or provides a range of initiatives (Groundwork UK 2017). This logic is based on the presumption that although funding of individual programmes can come and go, organisations tend to survive, particularly if their income is derived from a range of sources (Crossland and Veitch 2005). Furthermore, co-locating individual staff from a range of programmes in a single setting enables staff to feel less isolated and more able to engage in collaborations and makes recruitment and retention easier (Taylor et al. 2001). Nevertheless, many organisations have a limited life span, lasting only as long what they can offer is still regarded as required by the communities they serve. This includes organisations which seek to promote social exclusion (Ozanne and Rose 2013).

South Australia's Social Inclusion Board was funded by the South Australian Government but purposely established as a separate organisation and not as a government entity. An evaluation of the first five years found the effectiveness of the board in tackling social exclusion was attributed by informants to having a high profile and strong champion whose mandate was to advocate for South Australia's Social Inclusion Initiative:

> The mandate given by the Premier to the SI Board is to act in a much stronger capacity than just an advisory board role, so that it has the power and authority

from the Head of Government to intervene to address social exclusion, to obtain information and confront issues which might otherwise be seen as too difficult or too hard, to strongly advise on joined up government at various levels and to work with government agencies and service providers to achieve change.

(in Baum et al. 2010: 478)

However, there was concern that the board's capacity to remain an effective player in addressing social inclusion would 'depend upon continued quality leadership, should there be a change of Chair' (Baum et al. 2010: 479). The importance of leadership which regards social inclusion as important in practice and not just in rhetoric is also discussed in chapter 11 of this volume. However, effective leadership is not enough if the organisation does not pay sufficient attention to its management, including ensuring staff had access to appropriate staff development to enable them to carry out their work (Baum et al. 2010).

Ironically, organisations which were developed with a specific mission of promoting social inclusion are not necessarily good at promoting an internal culture which is inclusive. While priding itself on its provision of free healthcare to Britons for 70 years (Simpson et al. 2015), within Britain's National Health Service (NHS), individual staff, and patients often report being marginalised, disempowered, and/or silenced (Pope 2019; Simpson and Esmail 2011). Hence, chapter 11 describes an organisational framework developed by a nongovernment organisation, which identifies several elements which make a crucial difference in enabling service users to feel included, i.e. that they are part of the organisation and not just a client receiving a service.

The NHS, like health services in several of the wealthiest countries on this planet including US, Canada, Australia, New Zealand, and Canada, is highly reliant on international recruitment of professional staff (Simpson et al. 2010; Simpson and Esmail 2011), often to the detriment of employers and service users in the country of origin of those employees, particularly in developing countries which cannot afford the high salaries on offer in the developed world (Ahmad 2005; Kirk 2002). While it is understandable why individuals move internationally to take up employment possibilities, overreliance by health systems on foreign-trained workers is not an ethical method for sustaining healthcare provision if it is based on recruiting staff from poorer countries where there are already shortages (Ahmad 2005). Nor does it encourage organisations to fix problems which lead to local staff leaving their professions (Kirk 2002).

A study of after-hours medical services in Queensland, Australia, identified five key factors as being common amongst services which were long-lasting. These were appropriate management structures which supported the work of clinicians, collaborative relationships with other service providers, and the presence of unambiguous protocols or practice guidelines which identified how different aspects of the service would operate, and effective staff recruitment and retention strategies which included ensuring workers were receiving an appropriate levels of remuneration (Crossland and Veitch 2005). In short, these were good working environments which were attractive to both existing and prospective staff.

Similarly, the need for good working environments which value staff is noted in chapter 9. It is proposed that organisations which are socially inclusive and democratic are far more attractive places to work than organisations where high status results in privilege and arrogance being accepted norms. In particular, 'working conditions and workplace relations matter' and all staff—not just an elite subset—need to be respected and valued:

> Universities can get by without the millionaire managers and the gleaming tower blocks; we cannot get by with a demoralised or disintegrating workforce. . . . There is an occupational culture here that embeds the passion for knowledge, and makes workers of all kinds proud to be working specifically for a university.
>
> (Connell 2015: 95)

Although Connell is writing about universities, her arguments apply more broadly. For example, nursing graduates who found it difficult to implement what they believed to be good nursing practice were more likely to become disillusioned and leave the profession or keep swapping jobs with the hope of finding a role they were happy in. Those who retained their ideals for holistic care tended to work in fully staffed units, where there was a supportive environment on the ward, and to engage in ongoing professional education (Maben et al. 2007).

Organisations which achieve longevity also tend to be those which also nurture the passion and ideals of staff, which may complement practices of individual staff members to sustain their hope and commitment to promoting social inclusion (Wallin et al. 2003). Increasing technical and organisational capacity typically means investing in staff and not expecting staff to bear all the cost in terms of fees and time required to complete continuing professional education or upgrade qualifications (Keating et al. 2010).

One very effective means of sustaining the passions and ideals of health and social care practitioners as they work to promote social inclusion is the provision of professional supervision as observed in chapter 12. Not only can professional supervision enable practitioners to continue doing very difficult work in fields such as child protection, but also good supervision can be critical for encouraging more inclusive approaches to be adopted. Although in times of fiscal constraint, organisations may consider it as unnecessary to provide ongoing professional supervision to qualified staff, it is argued this is short-term thinking which challenges organisational sustainability. The long-running efforts of unions (Connell 2015) and professional associations (Harris et al. 2009; St Pierre Schneider et al. 2009) in supporting workers to obtain working conditions so they can continue in roles in which they are actively engaged in promoting and sustaining social inclusion has also been critical.

In order to continue to operate effectively, evidence would suggest long-lasting services must have the capacity to adapt to changing resources available and changing needs, in order to keep challenging social exclusion (Crossland and Veitch 2005). Organisational change is difficult to achieve, with more than two-thirds of organisational change initiatives failing to achieve their goals. This is particularly so when initiatives are reactive and introduced without proper consideration as to what is required to successfully implement change (By 2005). Fostering a learning culture is one mechanism to help an organisation to become more inclusive. This includes an ability to plan and implement new ways of working and review and modify as required. Unintended consequences and constraints are recognised and addressed by the organisation as a whole and not by punishing individual staff for poor performance (Rowe and Boyle 2005).

As the discussion of *Athena SWAN* earlier in this chapter demonstrated, reforms in the broader policy context may require organisations to adapt or modify if they are to remain in existence (Giffords and Dina 2003). An Irish university, which regards itself as inclusive, increased the proportion of female professors from 0 to 34 per cent from 1997 to 2012. However, the policies and culture of the university did not change substantially over this time. By 2015, committees which had a mandate to oversee equal opportunities mechanisms within the university were disbanded, and the proportion of female professors had started to drop. With a lack of policies and processes which enable women to be appointed to senior positions within the institution and the lack of sanctions from the Higher Education Authority for the institution not meeting statutory requirements for at least 40 per cent representation by both genders on the university's governing body, a 'leaving it to chance' modus operandi is not an adequate approach to sustaining high levels of female employment at the highest levels (O'Connor 2017).

Maintaining an ethos in which social inclusion is central to the organisation's mission is much easier than trying to encourage an organisation to become more inclusive. Chapter 10 examines Deakin University in Australia, which has for more than 40 years regarded social inclusion as central to its mission. As such, it is a very different feel of an organisation from the universities which Connell (2015) describe in which prestige is intricately associated with privilege. A long commitment is however no guarantee that social inclusion will continue to be central, particularly when organisations are merged to form new entities. Mergers are often premised on the basis that a larger organisation is more sustainable. However, key elements of a vision, including a vision in which social inclusion is a central pivot, can readily be lost in a merged organisation unless identified as critical to retain (Giffords and Dina 2003).

While it is arguably easier for organisations which have always had the promotion of social inclusion as integral to their mission to continue to do so, it is possible for others to radically change to place social inclusion as pivotal. Stellenbosch University played a critical role in the establishment and maintenance of the ideologies which enabled apartheid to become a dominant political ideology in South Africa for much of the twentieth century. Established as an Afrikaans-language university, the university attracted students and staff who were attracted to the promotion of an agenda in which opportunity was based on race and not capability. However, once governments supporting apartheid were overturned in the 1990s, Stellenbosch had to change or risk redundancy. A new vice chancellor not only developed a vision statement in which the university committed itself to contributing to the good of all South Africans, but had to ensure that staff and students, most of whom had benefitted from apartheid, were enabled to see a new future for the institution. One of the most important acts was for the university to host the African National Congress in 2002. Held every four years, the Congress attracts thousands of delegates, few of whom were white. This was a pivotal moment in proclaiming that Stellenbosch University welcomed people of all races and not just white Afrikaaners (Brink 2018).

The type and location of buildings out of which organisations operate can also facilitate and sustain social inclusion. In recent decades, the closure of large institutions for people living with severe mental illness and/or other disabilities has occurred in many countries in the Western world. Often built on the outskirts of towns and cities, there was little expectation of residents interacting with the wider community. As such, it has been noted that 'under this model, large institutions emerged as facilitators of social exclusion, not medical innovation' (Rowe and Boyle 2005: 110). Former institutions have often been demolished, and services have been moved to new purpose-built facilities which are integrated into local communities. While new buildings can facilitate more inclusive ways of working, there nevertheless must also be both a willingness and capacity to change to more inclusive ways of working, particularly if exclusionary ways of working are long entrenched (Rowe and Boyle 2005). As the findings of the recent Royal Commission into the mental health system in Victoria, Australia, indicate (Armytage et al. 2019), it is hard to ensure that the new facilities are appropriately provided.

Sustainable social inclusion outcomes

Sigmund Freud wrote of the need to work for enduring change more than a century ago (Clack 2013). Yet for much of the twentieth century, health and welfare professionals justified their existence on the basis of how many people they provided services to rather than the effectiveness of their efforts (Crisp 2000) and only later considering the magnitude of effect of their efforts (Hawe et al. 1997). Recognising that many initiatives which seek to address social exclusion are only funded for limited time periods, sustainable outcomes, in terms of ongoing social inclusion, has much more recently become an expectation (Swerissen and Crisp 2004).

International aid and development agencies typically provide funds for a limited time frame with the expectation that outcomes will be continued once funding has ceased. As poor health frequently places limits on people's ability to participate fully in society, it is unsurprising that ensuring health services are available for all is a priority both within many countries and for providers of foreign aid. However when the funding is provided by private corporations, their priorities may be to sponsor initiatives which provide the greatest opportunities for brand recognition rather than for outcomes associated with social inclusion (Adams 2016) or to support the status quo rather than to risk financial uncertainty by being associated with the recognition of rights for women and other marginalised sections of society (Durano and Bidegain Ponte 2016). Short-term funding from charitable organisations can also result in pragmatic decisions which may conflict with a social inclusion agenda. This was the impression that Gorik Ooms, who worked in Mozambique leading a Médecins Sans Frontières team, developed in respect of the decision-making of Ministry of Health (MoH) officials:

> if you are an MoH staff member of a low-income country and you receive a grant of US$ 50,000, you could buy an ambulance or you could hire 50 nurses for a year. If you know the grant will be continued year after year, you will do better to hire 50 nurses, as they will save a lot more lives than an ambulance. But if you think the grant will not be repeated, you had better buy the ambulance, as it will not protest if it is "fired" next year.
>
> (Ooms 2012: 35)

Pressure to spend funds quickly can result in flawed decisions, which might have been avoided had time been spent consulting with the communities who were supposed to benefit from initiatives. For example, international aid agencies may feel pleased with their efforts in building a school, but if the buildings are inaccessible to children with a disability, they reinforce exclusion for those who are already marginalised (Shakespeare 2018). Developing meaningful ways of consulting with the recipients of funding is taken up in chapter 13. Working with children who have a disability in Papua New Guinea and Vanuatu, the authors demonstrate the many benefits from giving members of the community whose voices tend not to be heard, the chance to speak and be listened to by those making decisions concerning them.

The importance of listening to those who have long experienced exclusion is also discussed in chapter 15 as essential when working with Indigenous peoples. A recent study using official data from 187 countries found that differences in religion and ethnicity were among the leading contributors to exclusion (Amin 2019). However, as argued in chapter 15, while respecting the spirituality of Indigenous peoples is a step toward inclusion, there are also benefits for settler societies who are open to learning from their Indigenous peoples who were denigrated by centuries of colonisation.

Lack of consultation also occurs in local initiatives when wrong assumptions guide decision-making. For example, community gardens often provide a place for people to meet and develop relationships with others in their community, as well as enabling the possibility of culturally appropriate and nutritional food at a low cost for participants (Gichunge and Kidwaro 2014). However, there will be families in the community who lack the capacity or interest in such projects for whom other sustainable solutions will be required. Of 371 low-income families in Toronto, only 12 had participated in community gardens in the 12 months prior to interview. Some families were open to the idea; however for one quarter (24.2 per cent) of the families, there was no community garden in their area, while others were unaware of how to become involved in such programmes (28.4 per cent) or did not know what a community garden is (11.7 per cent). While these issues can potentially be addressed, there were more than one third (38.7 per cent) of the families who perceived the community garden as not being a viable long-term option in addressing their need for an affordable and nutritious food, with lack of time (23.4 per cent) or lack of interest (11.7 per cent) being cited as the main reasons (Loopstra and Tarasuk 2013). Such lack of consultation with the community as to how best meet their needs, prior to implementing programmes, can prove to lead to an expensive waste of resources (Osmani 2008).

Flawed decision-making processes can also lead to service provision being deemed not necessary. Settlement support programs for recently arrived migrants and refugees often provide support for a set period of time on the assumption that over time people will become integrated with their local communities. In particular, it is assumed that they will find support from others who have come from the same place who arrived earlier and have established themselves in their new country. However, failure to properly assess the level of social capital in a community can results in programmes being less effective than anticipated (Cuthill 2010). Factors such as ethnicity or religion which can create division and exclusion within societies do not necessarily disappear in a new context. For example, when a group of Christian Syrian refugees were settled in a northern suburb of Melbourne, there was no support available from Muslim Syrians living in the area (Colic-Peisker and Dekker 2017). As religion has frequently been used to create social divisions and is often implicated in arguably the most extreme form of social exclusion involving exile from one's homeland, lack of support from Syrians of other religions is not surprising. Nevertheless, as argued in chapter 15, there are times when religion and spirituality can be powerful tools in creating and sustaining social inclusion.

Effective refugee settlement can lead to sustained social inclusion for new arrivals as argued in chapter 16. However, this requires a range of services to be made available to meet the various needs of communities, as well as organisations having a clear understanding of the philosophical underpinning of the models of practice by which they operate. As discussed in chapter 13 with examples from their lived experiences, *how* a service is provided makes a critical contribution to whether participants feel included or excluded.

In chapter 16, it is observed that service providers cannot agree as to whether refugees are consider to be 'victims' or 'survivors' and whether they are 'vulnerable' or 'resilient'. The capacity for language to promote and sustain, or conversely hinder, social inclusion should not be underestimated (Garrett 2018). As we wrote in our first volume, 'we make sense of the world, our understandings of it, and our place in it, through language; our use of language creates, contests and recreates power, authority and legitimation' (Taket et al. 2009a: 5). Language can communicate to individuals or groups that they matter (Crisp and Fox 2014) or marginalise them as those who are 'othered' (Barter-Godfrey and Taket 2009). Hence, persons enrolled in a university feel as if they are valued members of the organisation when known as 'students' but reduced to a commodity when labelled as 'customers' or 'clients' (Connell 2014). In chapter 8, the authors recall a conversation between some of them as to what to call participants in a community breakfast programme. Although they struggled to agree on what language should be used, they recognised that they did 'not like terms such as "client" that inherently imply hierarchy between programme providers and the recipients of a service'.

Language is also important when it comes to how services are described. In our previous volume, the parents of children participating in a programme run by a large welfare agency had a clear preference for the language of 'help' rather than 'support':

> "Help" was important to service users because it stressed the personal relationship between the parents and the staff who assisted them, and brought to the fore elements of working together and caring, whereas "support" was redolent of a professional discourse with more distant relationships and overtones of neediness and dependency.
>
> (Pollock and Taket 2014: 86–7)

In the case of people who in the twenty-first century are often considered to have 'learning difficulties', this is far more neutral language than labels used by previous generations, such as 'cretin' or 'sub-normal' which made pejorative statements about individuals *per se* and which excused their exclusion from the broader society (Hastings and Remington 1993). It has been argued that 'the adoption of labels with the most positive, or least negative, connotations may be the first step in encouraging more positive attitudes towards, and interaction with, people with mental handicap' (Hastings and Remington 1993: 240). Yet the adoption of popular labels can be problematic when it comes to programme outcomes. It has been proposed that for social programmes which have 'resilience' as an explicit objective, social inclusion may be relegated to being a byproduct at best or, at worst, lost as an objective (Béné et al. 2012; Garrett 2018).

Inclusive processes are not the same as inclusive outcomes, and it is misleading to assume that the former necessarily results in the latter (Barton 2015). Policies which have been developed to maximise social inclusion do not necessarily achieve the desired outcome when implemented. Chapter 14 explores the lived experience of cash-for-care policies, which have been developed with the intention of promoting agency for people living with disability. However, the promise of agency often fails to materialise, and the authors discuss the potential of different ethical frameworks to assist in the implementation of socially inclusive policy.

At times, social inclusion outcomes can occur despite lack of community involvement. For example, bureaucratic decision-making with limited community consultation can produce cityscapes in which people are encouraged to walk, which leads to the potential for social interactions and increased connectedness that does not occur in cities designed to be traversed by individual drivers in cars (Corburn 2015). Alternately, social inclusion outcomes which are more readily achievable may be overlooked. In countries such as the UK and US, people living with mental illness are often disenfranchised from voting in elections, even though the act of voting can reinforce one's sense of inclusion in society. Nash (2002) has commented that societal views are often that people residing in psychiatric care lack the capacity to make judgements at the ballot box, and yet studies have found no difference in the distribution of votes of people with mental illness compared to total votes cast in the jurisdictions they are voting in. As such he has argued that

> Ensuring voting is accessed by the mentally ill may be a foundation that social inclusion is based on, or the goal to which it aspires. Voting may be a real measure of how well people have integrated into society. Not only is it a fundamental right, it may also be easier for mental health staff to accomplish in comparison with finding employment opportunities or wrestling with housing issues.
>
> (Nash 2002: 702)

Sustainable social development

Finally, we are interested in sustainability in respect of social development. The *SDGs* propose that

> Sustainable development recognizes that eradicating poverty in all its forms and dimensions, combating inequality within and among countries, preserving the planet, creating sustained, inclusive and sustainable economic growth and fostering social inclusion are linked to each other and are interdependent.
>
> (United Nations 2015: Clause 13)

Social development is a concept which is still evolving but recognises that social factors including social cohesion, equity, and the ability to fully participate in civic society underpin sustainable development (Murphy 2012). While outcomes which sustain social inclusion are important, they should not come at the expense of marginalising the voices of those who are expected to benefit from initiatives.

> The freedom to participate is related to the process aspect of freedom, and as such it is very much a constituent of development, not just a means of achieving it. As a constituent it may be valued just as much as the final outcomes. For instance, while people value freedom from hunger, they are not indifferent to the process through which this outcome is achieved. In particular, they have reason to value a process in which they have the freedom to participate actively in the choice of pathways leading to freedom from hunger as compared to a process in which this outcome is gifted to them by a benevolent dictator.
>
> (Osmani 2008: 3)

This can lead to different decisions being made in different contexts. When two Indian states developed mechanisms to ensure women's voices were part of decisions about how funds for local communities were spent, the desire of many women to increase access to drinking water was reflected in the funding allocations of jurisdictions where women were appointed to decision-making bodies (Chattopadhyay and Duflo 2004). Similarly, several chapters in this volume provide examples of how involving different people in decision-making processes is crucial in making a society more inclusive. This includes the community development approach described in chapter 17, which is seeking to build peace between the Rohingya and Rakhine communities, which have long been in conflict in Myanmar. As Helen Clark, former prime minister of New Zealand and former administrator of the United Nations Development Programme has advocated:

> We need big picture thinking here—the peace needed for sustainable development will not be the product of early warning systems to spot tensions, nor of the dispatch of mediators or peacekeepers. Rather, enduring peace will be the outcome of long term developmental processes, including governance capacities.
>
> (Clark 2018: 7)

Leaving no one behind will often require new ways of working to ensure the voices of those most affected are not relegated to being less important than those of distant bureaucracies. Situations such as local officials in Haiti reporting feeling like strangers in their hometown three months after an earthquake should not arise. However, given that humanitarian aid is often determined by the donors with little consultation with recipients, the sidelining of locals is not surprising. Yet it is not just in emergency situations in which the intended recipients of goods or services are excluded from making decisions which affect them (Sanderson 2018). Rather it is the exception in which affected communities are involved in decision-making at more than tokenistic level. Yet as some of the examples in this volume testify, there are huge benefits from including individuals and communities in decision-making rather than being the beneficiaries of decisions made on their behalf. These include involving people living with disability in the management of employment programmes as part of anti-poverty initiatives in Indonesia (chapter 18) and in urban planning in a regional city in Australia (chapter 20). Both of these examples demonstrate the rich possibilities which emerge from 'new ways of inspiring and supporting . . . people to become active citizens and community leaders and new models to make that engagement self-sustaining' (Duxbury 2016: 9). Nevertheless, the extent of capacity building required for such engagement to be meaningful tends to be underestimated and limits the sustainability of many initiatives (Cosijn et al. 2018).

In recent years, concerns about climate change have stimulated interest in sustainable social development, often in response to events which have had serious consequences for those most likely to be excluded including children, the elderly, those with health issues, and the poor (Frumkin et al. 2008). For example, a developer in Kenya on deciding to build new apartments on a river flood plain also built a flood wall to keep the apartments safe. As a consequence, floodwaters were diverted into an already impoverished existing neighbourhood which had sanitation systems not designed to deal with this flooding, and human excrement and disease were spread throughout the community (Willett 2015). Hence, social inclusion in the form of 'environmental justice' (Nesmith and Smyth 2015: 485) has been proposed. This requires that '1) the burden of environmental hazards or degradation is shared equally across all demographic groups or communities, and 2) there is equal decision-making processes that result in environmentally related policies and actions' (Nesmith and Smyth 2015: 485). Hence, banning agricultural practices which are harmful to the environment but not enabling farmers to take up alternate processes which are less harmful fails to acknowledge the survival mechanisms of workers whose livelihood is threatened (Shajahan and Sharma 2018). As such, sustainable social development involves the creation of conditions which enable individuals, groups, and communities to experience an inclusive society without compromising the capacity of future generations to have their needs met (Anåker and Elf 2014). This involves the utilisation of universal design principles to enable places and products to be able to be used by as many people as possible without the need for adaptation or special measures for some individuals or groups (Vavik and Keitsch 2010).

Freiburg in Germany, which was extensively rebuilt in the second half of the twentieth century following bombing of much of the city during World War II, is an example of a city in which the principles of environmental sustainability and a good quality of life for all residents were paramount. Although social inclusion per se was not the primary objective, it has been argued that adoption of social inclusion principles has been one of the critical factors in Freiburg's success in sustaining its vision of being an environmentally sustainable and inclusive city over several decades of growth (Grant and Barton 2015).

On a smaller scale, in the United Kingdom, a private company developed a plan for the development of a new community including 400 homes as well as basic services including a local shop and medical centre. What made the plan unusual was the design which 'created a series of safe and attractive open spaces, varying in size, function and character, including a community orchard and allotments for local food production, wildlife habitats and walking and cycling corridors' (de Havilland and Burgess 2015: 336). However, it was recognised that for these shared spaces to achieve their objectives on an ongoing basis, the development of a community infrastructure to take responsibility for the ongoing running of these community facilities would be required. As there was no existing community, the developer recognised that they would need to facilitate this process and not just leave it to chance.

> The house builder involved with this proposal understands the difficulties of ensuring the longevity of responsibility and governance required to sustain the community places and spaces. In response to this, the house builder is establishing a community trust to ensure that the community spaces are managed in an inclusive manner with the full involvement of stakeholders, new residents and occupiers. A community trust is a neighbourhood government vehicle that allows the developer to provide seed funding to establish the long-term management of community assets. The ownership of the assets is

transferred to the trust along with an ongoing management charge paid by the new community, providing a future income for the trust. This provides a mechanism to ensure that the provision of important elements within the design are realised and funded.

(de Havilland and Burgess 2015: 336–7)

Nevertheless, while physical infrastructure such as an appropriate mix of housing and space for leisure are important, ensuring critical services can be readily accessed is also crucial. It has been argued that if we are serious about tackling social exclusion, primary and secondary prevention services such as postnatal services, parenting programs, paediatric assessments, and adolescent mental health need to be present in the most disadvantaged communities (Vinson 2007).

Building a new inclusive community on an empty site is arguably much easier than retrofitting existing infrastructure (Marco and Burgess 2015). Sustainable social development may require new ways of working to ensure social inclusion (Goodman 2011). Emerging technologies are providing opportunities for finding 'new modes of local citizenship, which in turn have the potential to drive stronger democratic engagement' (Duxbury 2016: 9). One such example is *Helpific* which is a digital platform that enables people with disabilities or mental health problems to post requests for help and others in their neighbourhood to respond to requests. Operating in Estonia, Ukraine, Hungary, and Croatia, one of the unanticipated outcomes was that many of those requesting help were also providing assistance to others, thus breaking down traditional distinctions between helper and helpee. Further information about *Helpific* is presented in chapter 19.

Another key aspect of sustainable social development which is highlighted in some of the chapters in this book is challenging exclusionary attitudes at a societal level. Chapter 21 presents a number of examples of theatre-based programmes which not only promote empathy for and understanding of groups of people who are often excluded but build the capacity of audience members to take action against words and actions they witness which seek to entrench exclusion. Theatre was also used as a medium for reporting back research findings in the anti-poverty initiatives to research participants living with disability in Indonesia (chapter 18) and the arts as part of peace-making initiatives in Myanmar (chapter 17).

Conclusion

This chapter has introduced five different broad approaches by which social inclusion can be sustained. In some instances, the retention of programmes or organisations which promote social inclusion will be critical, but in some circumstances, sustained social inclusion does not require ongoing external support. Legislation and decision-making processes which value social inclusion and changes in community attitudes resulting in less acceptance and tolerance of exclusionary practices also contribute to sustaining social inclusion.

Sustaining social inclusion is difficult, and this chapter has identified many ways in which attempts to promote and sustain social inclusion may be thwarted, often unintentionally. This includes initiatives that while promoting social inclusion, at the same time are contributing to experiences of exclusion. Nevertheless, as the remainder of this book demonstrates, there are many opportunities for promoting and sustaining social inclusion, and the need for ongoing research and practice development to increase our understanding of how to ensure that that societal development truly leaves no one behind.

References

Abbotts, J., Williams, R., Ford, G., Hunt, K. and West, P. (1997) 'Morbidity and Irish Catholic descent in Britain: an ethnic and religious minority 150 years on', *Social Science and Medicine*, 45: 3–14.

Adams, B. (2016) 'United Nations and business community: out-sourcing or crowding in?' *Development*, 59: 21–8.

Advance HE (2018) 'About advance HE's Athena SWAN charter'. Online. Available at www.ecu.ac.uk/equality-charters/athena-swan/about-athena-swan/ (accessed 4 November 2019).

African Development Bank Group (2019) 'The high 5 for transforming Africa'. Online. Available at www.afdb.org/en/high5s (accessed 4 November 2019).

Ahmad, O.B. (2005) 'Managing medical migration from poor countries', *British Medical Journal*, 331: 43–5.

Amin, S. (2019) 'Diversity enforces social exclusion: does exclusion never cease?' *Journal of Social Inclusion*, 10(1): 4–22.

Anåker, A, and Elf, M. (2014) 'Sustainability in nursing: a concept analysis', *Scandinavian Journal Caring Sciences*, 28: 381–9.

Armytage, P., Fels, A., Cockram, A. and McSherry, B. (2019) *Royal Commission into Victoria's Mental Health System: Interim Report*. Online. Available at www.parliament.vic. gov.au/file_uploads/6183-RCVMHS-InterimReport__Web_Ready__R2_GKyv8v04. pdf (accessed 8 December 2019).

Barnard, S. (2017) 'The Athena SWAN Charter: promoting commitment to gender equality in higher education institutions in the UK', in K. White and P. O'Connor (eds) *Gendered Success in Higher Education: Global Perspectives*, London: Palgrave Macmillan.

Barter-Godfrey, S. and Shelley, J. (2014) 'Your rights to a conscience ends at my right to safe, legal and effective health care', in A. Taket, B.R. Crisp, S. Goldingay, M. Graham, L. Hanna and L. Wilson (eds) *Practising Social Inclusion*, London: Routledge.

Barter-Godfrey, S. and Taket, A. (2009) 'Othering, marginalisation and pathways to exclusion in health', in A. Taket, B.R. Crisp, A. Nevill, G. Lamaro, M. Graham and S. Barter-Godfrey (eds) *Theorising Social Exclusion*, London: Routledge.

Barton, H. (2015) 'Planning for health and well-being: the time for action', in H. Barton, S. Thompson, S. Burgess and M. Grant (eds) *The Routledge Handbook of Planning for Health and Well-being*, London: Routledge.

Baum, F. Newman, L. Biedrzycki, K. and Patterson, J. (2010) 'Can a regional government's social inclusion initiative contribute to the quest for health equity?' *Health Promotion International*, 25: 474–82.

Béné, C., Godfrey-Wood, R., Newsham, A. and Davies, M. (2012) *Resilience: New Utopia or New Tyranny? Reflection About the Potentials and Limits of the Concept of Resilience in Relation to Vulnerability Reduction*, Brighton: Institute of Development

Studies, Working Paper 405. Online. Available at https://onlinelibrary.wiley.com/doi/abs/10.1111/j.2040-0209.2012.00405.x (accessed 29 July 2019).

Brault, M.A., Brewster, A.L., Bradley, E.H., Keene, D., Tan, A.X. and Curry, L.A. (2018) 'Links between social environment and health care utilization and costs', *Journal of Gerontological Social Work*, 61: 203–20.

Brink, C. (2018) *The Soul of a University: Why Excellence Is Not Enough*, Bristol: Bristol University Press.

By, R.T. (2005) 'Organisational change management: a critical review', *Journal of Change Management*, 5: 369–80.

Carey, G.E., Graham, M., Shelley, J. and Taket, A. (2009) 'Discourse, power and exclusion: the experiences of childless women', in A. Taket, B.R. Crisp, A. Nevill, G. Lamaro, M. Graham and S. Barter-Godfrey (eds) *Theorising Social Exclusion*, London: Routledge.

Carvalho, T. and de Lourde Machado-Taylor, M. (2017) 'The exceptionalism of women rectors: a case study from Portugal', in K. White and P. O'Connor (eds) *Gendered Success in Higher Education: Global Perspectives*, London: Palgrave Macmillan.

Chalk, K. and Pilkinton, J. (2018) 'How does networked civil society change?' *Development Bulletin*, 79: 93–7.

Chambers, R. (2010) *Paradigms, Poverty and Adaptive Pluralism*, Brighton: Institute of Development Studies, Working Paper 344. Online. Available at https://onlinelibrary.wiley.com/doi/abs/10.1111/j.2040-0209.2010.00344_2.x (accessed 29 July 2019).

Chattopadhyay, R. and Duflo, E. (2004) 'Women as policy makers: evidence from a randomized policy experiment in India', *Econometrica*, 72: 1409–43.

Chong, G. (1999) 'Information technology and social work education in Malaysia', *Computers in Human Services*, 15: 171–84.

Clack, B. (2013) *Freud on the Couch: A Critical Introduction to the Father of Psychoanalysis*, London: One World Publications.

Clark, H. (2018) 'Partnering for impact on sustainable development', *Development Bulletin*, 79: 5–8.

Colic-Peisker, V. and Dekker, K. (2017) *Religious Visibility, Disadvantage and Bridging Social Capital: A Comparative Investigation of Multicultural Localities in Melbourne's North: Final Report*, Melbourne: Centre for Global Research, RMIT. Online. Available at www.cgr.org.au/research-reports/ (accessed 26 July 2019).

Connell, R. (2014) 'Love, fear and learning in the market university', *Australian Universities' Review*, 56(2): 56–63.

Connell, R. (2015) 'The knowledge economy and university workers', *Australian Universities' Review*, 57(2): 91–5.

Corburn, J. (2015) 'Urban inequalities, population health and spatial planning', in H. Barton, S. Thompson, S. Burgess and M. Grant (eds) *The Routledge Handbook of Planning for Health and Well-being*, London: Routledge.

Cosijn, M., Williams, L. and Hall, A. (2018) 'Partnering for developmental impact: innovation in Indonesian agricultural systems', *Development Bulletin*, 79: 73–7.

Crisp, B.R. (2000) 'A history of Australian social work practice research', *Research on Social Work Practice*, 10: 179–94.

Crisp, B.R. and Fox, J. (2014) 'Enabling new students to feel that they matter: promoting social inclusion within the university community', in A. Taket, B.R. Crisp, S. Goldingay, M. Graham, L. Hanna and L. Wilson (eds) *Practising Social Inclusion*, London: Routledge.

Crossland, L. and Veitch, C. (2005) 'After-hours service models in Queensland Australia: a framework for sustainability', *Australian Journal of Primary Health*, 11(2): 9–15.

Cuthill, M. (2010) 'Strengthening the social in sustainable development: developing a conceptual framework for social sustainability in a rapid urban growth region in Australia', *Sustainable Development*, 18: 362–73.

de Havilland, J. and Burges, S. (2015) 'Delivering healthy spaces: the role of the private sector', in H. Barton, S. Thompson, S. Burgess and M. Grant (eds) *The Routledge Handbook of Planning for Health and Well-being*, London: Routledge.

de Souza, M. and Halahoff, A. (2018) 'Introduction', in M. de Souza and A. Halahoff (eds) *Re-enchanting Education and Spiritual Well-being: Fostering Belonging and Meaning-Making for Global Citizens*, London: Routledge.

Durano, M. and Bidegain Ponte, N. (2016) 'A feminist perspective on the follow-up process for financing for development', *Development*, 59: 32–9.

Duxbury, G. (2016) 'Young green leaders: promoting social action to sustain green spaces'. Online. Available at www.groundwork.org.uk/ygl-promoting-social-action-uk (accessed 2 October 2018).

Elias, J. and Holliday, J. (2019) 'Who gets "Left behind"? Promises and pitfalls in making the global development agenda work for sex workers: reflections from Southeast Asia', *Journal of Ethnic and Migration Studies*, 45: 2566–82.

Equality Challenge Unit (2018a) 'History of Athena SWAN (pre May 2015)'. Online. Available at www.ecu.ac.uk/equality-charters/athena-swan/about-athena-swan/history-of-athena-swan/ (accessed 3 October 2018).

Equality Challenge Unit (2018b) 'Athena SWAN FAQs'. Online. Available at www.ecu.ac.uk/equality-charters/athena-swan/athena-swan-faqs/ (accessed 3 October 2018).

Farrington, J. and Farrington, C. (2005) 'Rural accessibility, social inclusion and social justice: towards conceptualisation', *Journal of Transport Geography*, 13: 1–12.

Frumkin, H., Hess, J., Luber, G., Malilay, J. and McGreehin, M. (2008) 'Climate change: the public health response', *American Journal of Public Health*, 98: 435–45.

Garrett, P.M. (2018) *Welfare Words*, London: Sage.

Gichunge, C. and Kidwaro, F. (2014) 'Utamu wa Afrika (the sweet taste of Africa): the vegetable garden as part of resettled African refugees' food environment', *Nutrition and Dietetics*, 71: 270–5.

Giffords, E.D. and Dina, R.P. (2003) 'Changing organizational cultures: the challenge in forging successful mergers', *Administration in Social Work*, 27: 69–81.

Golczyńska-Grondas, A. (2014) 'Badges of social valuing and the biography. Natalia's interview in the perspective of the sociologist of poverty and social exclusion', *Qualitative Sociology Review*, 10: 38–58.

Goodman, B. (2011) 'The need for a "sustainability curriculum" in nurse education', *Nurse Education Today*, 31: 733–7.

Graham, M. (2014) 'The invisibility of childlessness in research: a more inclusive approach', in A. Taket, B.R. Crisp, S. Goldingay, M. Graham, L. Hanna and L. Wilson (eds) *Practising Social Inclusion*, London: Routledge.

Grant, M. and Barton, H. (2015) 'Freiburg: green capital of Europe', in H. Barton, S. Thompson, S. Burgess and M. Grant (eds) *The Routledge Handbook of Planning for Health and Well-being*, London: Routledge.

Groundwork UK (2017) *Our Place, Our Planet: Helping Communities Become Champions of Climate Change,* Birmingham: Groundwork UK. Online. Available at www.groundwork.org.uk/wp-content/uploads/2019/08/Our-Place-Our-Planet.pdf (accessed 4 November 2019).

Hafford-Letchfield, T., Lambley, S., Spolander, G. and Cocker, C. (2014) *Inclusive Leadership in Social Work and Social Care*, Bristol: Policy Press.

Harris, N., Pisa, L., Talioaga, S. and Vezeau, T. (2009) 'Hospitals going green: a holistic view of the issue and the critical role of the nurse leader', *Holistic Nursing Practice*, 23: 101–11.

Hastings, R.P. and Remington, B. (1993) 'Connotations of labels for mental handicap and challenging behaviour: a review and research evaluation', *Mental Handicap Research*, 6: 237–49.

Hawe, P., Noort, M., King, L. and Jordens, C. (1997) 'Multiplying health gains: the critical role of capacity-building within health promotion programs', *Health Policy*, 39: 29–42.

International Labour Office (ILO) (2011) *Social Protection Floors for Social Justice and a Fair Globalization*, Geneva: ILO. Online. Available at www.ilo.org/wcmsp5/groups/public/@ed_norm/@relconf/documents/meetingdocument/wcms_160210.pdf (accessed 26 July 2019).

International Labour Organization (ILO) (2014) *World Social Protection Report: Building Economic Recovery for Inclusive Development and Social Justice 2014/5*, Geneva: ILO. Online. Available at www.ilo.org/global/research/global-reports/world-social-security-report/2014/lang--en/index.htm (accessed 26 July 2019).

Keating, S.F.J., Thompson, J.P. and Lee, G.A. (2010) 'Perceived barriers to the sustainability and progression of nurse practitioners', *International Emergency Nursing*, 18: 147–53.

Kemp, L.J., Gitaski, C. and Zoghbor, W. (2017) 'Negotiating space for women's academic leadership within the Arab Gulf States', in K. White and P. O'Connor (eds) *Gendered Success in Higher Education: Global Perspectives*, London: Palgrave Macmillan.

Kirk, M. (2002) 'The impact of globalisation and environmental change on health: challenge for nurse education', *Nurse Education Today*, 22: 60–71.

Klaufus, C., van Lindert, P., van Noorloos, F. and Steel, G. (2017) 'All-inclusiveness versus exclusion: urban project development in Latin American and Africa', *Sustainability*, 9(2038): 1–15.

Layton, N. and Wilson, E. (2014) 'Practising inclusion in policy design for people with disabilities', in A. Taket, B.R. Crisp, S. Goldingay, M. Graham, L. Hanna and L. Wilson (eds) *Practising Social Inclusion*, London: Routledge.

Lindsay, A. (1994) *Dancing in the Kitchen: Portraits of Collingwood's Older Women*, Collingwood, Victoria: Carlton Collingwood Fitzroy Health Service.

Loopstra, R. and Tarasuk, V. (2013) 'Perspectives on community gardens, community kitchens and the good food box program in a community-based sample of low-income families', *Canadian Journal of Public Health*, 104: e55–9.

Marco, E. and Burgess, S. (2015) 'Healthy housing', in H. Barton, S. Thompson, S. Burgess and M. Grant (eds) *The Routledge Handbook of Planning for Health and Well-being*, London: Routledge.

Martin, E. and Pallotta-Chiarolli, M. (2009) '"Exclusion by inclusion": bisexual young people, marginalisation and mental health in relation to substance abuse', in A. Taket, B.R. Crisp, A. Nevill, G. Lamaro, M. Graham and S. Barter-Godfrey (eds) *Theorising Social Exclusion*, London: Routledge.

Maben, J., Latter, S. and Macleod Clark, J. (2007) 'The sustainability of ideals, values and the nursing mandate: evidence from a longitudinal qualitative study', *Nursing Inquiry*, 14: 99–113.

Muir-Gray, J.A. (1999) 'Postmodern medicine', *The Lancet*, 354: 1550–3.

Muñoz de Bustillo, R. and Antón, J-I. (2015) 'Turning back before arriving? The weakening of the Spanish welfare state', in D. Vaughan-Whitehead (ed) *The European Social Model in Crisis: Is Europe Losing Its Soul?* Geneva: International Labour Organization.

Murphy, K. (2012) 'The social pillar of sustainable development: a literature review and framework for policy analysis', *Sustainability: Science, Practice and Policy*, 8: 15–29.

Nash, N. (2002) 'Voting as a means of social inclusion for people with a mental illness', *Journal of Psychiatric and Mental Health Nursing*, 9: 697–703.

Nesmith, A. and Smyth, N. (2015) 'Environmental justice and social work education: social workers' professional perspectives', *Social Work Education*, 34: 484–501.

O'Connor, P. (2017) 'Changing the gender profile of the professoriate: an Irish case study', in K. White and P. O'Connor (eds) *Gendered Success in Higher Education: Global Perspectives*, London: Palgrave Macmillan.

Ooms, G. (2012) 'Three and a half arguments for global social protection for health (a personal story)', in J. Holst (ed) *Global Social Protection Scheme: Moving from Charity to Solidarity*, Frankfurt: Medico International and Merelbeke, Belgium: Hélène de Beir Foundation.

Osmani, S.R. (2008) 'Participatory governance: an overview of issues and evidence', in *Participatory Governance and the Millennium Development Goals (MDGs)*, New York: United Nations. Online. Available at http://unpan1.un.org/intradoc/groups/public/docu ments/un/unpan028359.pdf (accessed 29 July 2019).

Ozanne, E. and Rose, D. (2013) *The Organisational Context of Human Service Practice*, South Yarra, Victoria: Palgrave Macmillan.

Parker, J. and Ashencaen Crabtree, S. (2018) *Social Work with Disadvantaged and Marginalised People*, London: Sage.

Parliament of the United Republic of Tanzania (2010) *The Persons with Disabilities Act 2010*. Online. Available at http://parliament.go.tz/polis/uploads/bills/acts/1452071737-ActNo-9-2010.pdf (accessed 16 September 2019).

Perkins, D. (2010) 'Activation and social inclusion: challenges and possibilities', *Australian Journal of Social Issues*, 45: 267–87.

Pollock, S. and Taket, A. (2014) 'Inclusive service development: exploring a whole-of-organisation approach in the community service sector', in A. Taket, B.R. Crisp, S. Goldingay, M. Graham, L. Hanna and L. Wilson (eds) *Practising Social Inclusion*, London: Routledge.

Pope, R. (2019) 'Organizational silence in the NHS: "hear no, see no, speak no" ', *Journal of Change Management*, 19: 45–66.

Rowe, P.A. and Boyle, M.V. (2005) 'Constraints to organizational learning during major change at a mental health services facility', *Journal of Change Management*, 5: 109–17.

Sachs, J.D. (2012) 'From millennium development goals to sustainable development goals', *The Lancet*, 379: 2206–11.

Sanderson, D. (2018) 'Shifting from supply to demand: opportunities for improving humanitarian response in urban disaster settings', *Development Bulletin*, 79: 63–7.

Scheirer, M.A. (2005) 'Is sustainability possible? A review and commentary on empirical studies of program sustainability', *American Journal of Evaluation*, 26: 320–47.

Shajahan, P.K. and Sharma, P. (2018) 'Environmental justice: a call for action for social workers', *International Social Work*, 61: 476–80.

Shakespeare, T. (2018) 'Foreword', in S. Mitra (ed) *Disability, Health and Human Development*, New York: Palgrave Macmillan.

Shucksmith, M. (2012) 'Class, power and inequality in rural areas: beyond social exclusion?' *Sociologica Ruralis*, 52: 377–97.

Simpson, J.M., Checkland, K., Snow, S., Voorhees, J., Rothwell, K. and Esmail, A. (2015) 'Access to general practice in England: time for a policy rethink', *British Journal of General Practice*, 65: 606–7.

Simpson, J.M. and Esmail, A. (2011) 'The UK's dysfunctional relationship with medical migrants: the Daniel Ubani case and reform of out-of-hours services', *British Journal of General Practice*, 61: 208–11.

Simpson, J.M., Esmail, A., Kalra, V.S. and Snow, S. (2010) 'Writing migrants back into NHS history: addressing a "collective amnesia" and it policy implications', *Journal of the Royal Society of Medicine*, 103: 392–6.

Slay, J. and Penny, J. (2013) *Surviving Austerity: Local Voices and Local Action in England's Poorest Neighbourhoods*, London: New Economics Foundation. Online. Available at https://neweconomics.org/uploads/files/630d61e59ee7ff259a_jbm6bujah.pdf (accessed 4 November 2019).

St. Pierre Schneider, B., Menzel, N., Clark, M., York, N., Candela, L. and Xu, Y. (2009) 'Nursing's leadership in positioning human health at the core of urban sustainability', *Nursing Outlook*, 57: 281–8.

Sustainable Governance Indicators (2016) 'United States'. Online. Available at www.sgi-network.org/2016/United_States/Social_Policies (accessed 4 November 2019).

Swerissen, H. and Crisp, B.R. (2004) 'The sustainability of health promotion interventions for different levels of organization', *Health Promotion International*, 19: 123–30.

Taket, A., Crisp, B.R., Goldingay, S., Graham, M., Hanna, L. and Wilson, L. (eds) (2014) *Practising Social Inclusion*, London: Routledge.

Taket, A., Crisp, B.R., Nevill, A., Lamaro, G., Graham, M. and Barter-Godfrey, S. (eds) (2009a) *Theorising Social Exclusion*, London: Routledge.

Taket, A., Foster, N. and Cook, K. (2009b) 'Understanding processes of social exclusion: silence, silencing and shame', in A. Taket, B.R. Crisp, A. Nevill, G. Lamaro, M. Graham and S. Barter-Godfrey (eds) *Theorising Social Exclusion*, London: Routledge.

Taylor, J., Blue, I. and Misan, G. (2001) 'Approach to sustainable health care service delivery for rural and remote South Australia', *Australian Journal of Rural Health*, 9: 304–10.

United Nations (1948) 'Universal declaration of human rights'. Online. Available at www.refworld.org/docid/3ae6b3712c.html (accessed 4 November 2019).

United Nations (2006) 'Convention on the rights of persons with disabilities'. Online. Available at www.un.org/development/desa/disabilities/convention-on-the-rights-of-persons-with-disabilities/convention-on-the-rights-of-persons-with-disabilities-2.html (accessed 4 November 2019).

United Nations (2007) 'Declaration on the rights of indigenous peoples'. Online. Available at www.un.org/esa/socdev/unpfii/documents/DRIPS_en.pdf (accessed 4 November 2019).

United Nations (2015) 'Transforming our world: the 2030 agenda for sustainable development'. Online. Available at https://sustainabledevelopment.un.org/post2015/transformingourworld/publication (accessed 4 November 2019).

Vavik, T. and Keitsch, M.M. (2010) 'Exploring relationships between universal design and social sustainable development: some methodological aspects to the debate on the sciences of sustainability', *Sustainable Development*, 18: 295–305.

Vinson, T. (2007) *Dropping off the Edge: The Distribution of Disadvantage in Australia*, Richmond, Victoria: Jesuit Social Services.

Wallin, L., Boström, A.M., Wikblad, K. and Ewald, U. (2003) 'Sustainability in changing clinical practice promotes evidence-based nursing care', *Journal of Advanced Nursing*, 41: 509–18.

Willett, J.L. (2015) 'Exploring the intersection of environmental degradation and poverty: environmental injustice in Nairobi, Kenya', *Social Work Education*, 34: 558–72.

Wilson, T., Morgan, G., Rahman, A. and Vaid, L. (2013) *The Local Impacts of Welfare Reform: An Assessment of Cumulative Impacts and Mitigations*, London: Local Government Association. Online. Available at www.learningandwork.org.uk.gridhosted.co.uk/wp-content/uploads/2017/01/The-local-impacts-of-welfare-reform-version-7.pdf (accessed 4 November 2019).

Part 2

Sustainable policies for promoting social inclusion

2 The transformative journey to sustainability for Australia's compensation systems

How peer support and restorative justice interventions are creating a new inclusive narrative

John Bottomley, Bette Phillips-Campbell and Gordon Traill

Introduction

Organisational and personal transformations are two critical factors that sustain social inclusion outcomes for peer support and restorative justice interventions in veterans' and workers' compensations systems. Integrating these two transformations cultivates the solidarity which may sustain an alternative narrative to challenge the historic justification of these medico-legal systems. In this chapter, we will examine the experience of two Australian social development intervention programmes provided by the Melbourne-based Creative Ministries Network (CMN).

CMN began in 1984 as an initiative of Methodist ministers in Victoria who had moved from parish ministry into paid employment to minister with people in their working lives. There they discovered unanticipated levels of work-related harm through injury, illness, and death. As well as researching occupational health and safety, CMN established a self-help support programme for injured workers (1985) and later a self-help programme for families bereaved by an industrial death (1996). CMN provided GriefWork Support (GW) from 1999, a peer support programme for families bereaved by work-related deaths, and Veterans Health (VH) from 2003, a peer support programme for Australian Defence Force (ADF) veterans.

The two peer support programmes have in common their clients' experiences of trauma from either the death of a loved one due to work or the death of workmates or personal injury while on active war or peacekeeping service. The chapter describes the historical background to the first workers compensation schemes and identifies the critical assumptions that are embedded almost universally in compensation systems today. From listening to the pain and grief of those traumatised by work-related deaths, the CMN Board then embraced their own individual experiences of grief and vulnerability, which challenged their personal and corporate assumptions about the processes of healing and justice. We next trace the unfolding stages of two staff, Bette Philips-Campbell and Gordon Traill, as we recount their journey from trauma exposure to volunteering as peer support workers (PSWs) with bereaved families on a state-based workers compensation scheme and with federal Department of Veterans' Affairs (DVA) compensation for veterans, respectively.

Historical context for workers and war service compensation

The rapid industrialisation of the nineteenth century broke down traditional village and family structures and wrought devastation on workers and families injured or killed at work. For families affected by a worker's injury or death, poverty was almost always an inevitable consequence. Perhaps it is no surprise that this state of affairs helped to fuel the establishment of trade union and socialist organisations intent on radical programmes of social and economic redress. So one intent of the first state insurance workers' compensation schemes in Germany (1884) was to mitigate trade union demands while marginalising the political agendas of a range of socialist/revolutionary groups (Gurtler 1989; Kleeberg 2003; van Meerhaeghe 2006). The British Workers' Compensation Act (1897) embedded the removal of political/legal considerations of righting an individual wrong with its focus on providing financial/medical benefits for the victims of work-related harm (Gurtler 1989).

Workers compensation began 'as an instrument of government, serving the political and economic objectives of minimising a cause for industrial conflict and maximising capital accumulation, while simultaneously managing the conduct of the injured worker' (Duncan 2003: 454). This led to similar legislation being almost universally implemented as the first social insurance programme for 106 out of 136 countries (Schiller 2006). From 1902 to 1914, Australian states in turn readily adopted the UK compensation scheme (Duncan 2003), thus implementing the strategic change that shifted the historic obligations between injured workers and employers. With workers' compensation, the employer now accepted responsibility for a worker who may be injured at work 'as a normal and predictable risk of business' (Duncan 2003: 453). Work accidents could be seen as an inevitable business risk.

The medico-legal basis of the compensation system focussed attention on the definitions of 'injured worker' and 'dependent'. Both were removed from their social and political contexts so that traumatised people became isolated victims to be managed by expert means 'that are sanctioned by law and controlled by the agents of insurance institutions' (Duncan 2003: 455). As victims of work-related harm, injured workers and dependents were deprived of their agency by the compensation system, rendering them powerless in relation to their trauma. Feeling powerless is a truthful reading of their experience of trauma. But in the rational medico-legal world of objective cause-effect explanation, the compensation system denied victims of work trauma any public agency for emotions such as powerlessness (Bottomley 2015). Their suffering is legally defined and confined to an economic loss. Brueggemann (2014: 47) described this process as the politics of death, by which social power is organised to seem completely 'rational', but is 'unrestrained by any sense of the possibility of human solidarity'. The social isolation of injured workers and dependents was evident by the 1970s, as few trade unions provided social support to their injured members, and there was even less support for families bereaved by work-related deaths (Bottomley 1988). The emerging self-help movement of the 1970s and 1980s provided a conceptual framework for groups of people to organise around their shared experiences, and this seemed as true for Vietnam Veterans associations from about 1980, as it was for injured workers groups in Victoria from the mid-1980s (Bottomley 1988), and our experience with work-related bereavement advocacy groups in the mid-1990s.

Governance: creating the possibility of human solidarity

We submit that a matter of first importance was that the CMN board, management, and staff had a shared vision with clients for their social inclusion and a commitment to sustaining this vision when both the veterans and workers compensation systems shared historic assumptions that militated against social inclusion. The shared vision emerged from CMN's painful experience of establishing a self-help work-related bereavement and advocacy programme.

One of our authors was the CEO of CMN at the time. Because the grieving founders of the programme felt unable to lead the grief support group sessions, the CEO facilitated them. Then over time, tensions developed over control of the programme, its funding, and his role as a participant in the group, until a group of participants split from the agency and formed their own self-help organisation. Reflecting on this later, the CEO wrote,

> I had been captive to my masculine identity that too often separated feelings from thinking. Cut off from my own feelings, I often found myself allowing the group members' feelings fill the void of my own emotional landscape. I had ignored my feelings as unimportant and justified my decisions on the flawed view that feelings of victims of injustice spoke of a larger truth than my own feelings.

The self-help community development model hid the CEO's own pain from him through his belief he functioned as a value-free facilitator. But

> to hear voices of suffering without massive distortion it is necessary also to hear the grief and rage within ourselves. Without knowledge of our own wounds, the abyss in the lives of others will terrify us and make compassion impossible.
>
> (O'Connor 2002: 95)

This fundamental insight underpinned CMN's commitment to transform its programme for families bereaved by a work-related death to a peer support programme. So the agency board and staff devoted regular times at meetings to attend to their own experiences of grief, injustice, suffering, and vulnerability. The agency's journey toward sustainable social inclusion for traumatised people began with the board's governance commitment to a self-reflective practice embracing the vulnerability of their personal woundedness. Peer support was the social intervention that gave expression to the agency's commitment to our clients, but the context for this commitment was the board's solidarity through their shared lived experience of grief, injustice, suffering, and vulnerability.

Peer support

As with self-help programmes, peer support is 'a system of giving and receiving help founded on key principles of respect, shared responsibility and mutual agreement of what is helpful' (Mead et al. 2001: 135) amongst people with similar experiences. Peer support has emerged most strongly in the mental health arena with a challenge to the way the cultural mainstream defines behaviour, forcing people to understand their situation in ways that disconnect them from the social and political factors that contribute to their experience of injustice and suffering. Peer support operates at a face-to-face level, but its potential to become a sustainable social development depends on peer programmes giving voice not only to the suffering experienced by victims of a traumatic event, but also giving voice to the injustices and suffering caused to trauma victims by institutions of care that have failed to meet their needs.

What does it take to become a peer support worker?

Time for healing

Bette was bereaved by her son's death at his workplace and was the first staff person at CMN for the new peer support programme for families bereaved by a work-related death. She began as a volunteer to develop a role as a PSW. But what does it take to become a PSW? It took Bette seven years from the day her son died at work to the day she contacted CMN to offer herself as a volunteer. Reflecting on this length of time ten years after her son's death, Bette wrote,

> I began a journey that I felt would never end. I remember even months later walking to the letterbox and believing this is a dream. I will wake up! Yet I just wanted to stay in bed. I did not want to face the world. Yet I wanted to tell everyone who might listen that I had lost my only son. I wanted to act like it never happened, for then it would not have. I sat in the shower each morning shedding my tears; it was the only place that I felt it was safe to do so. I could not lose control, I might never regain it. This is the chaos that is everyday grief and it seems like it will never end.

The traumatic death of her son touched a far deeper reality than just her emotional chaos at the physical loss of her loved one from her life, as Bette next recounted.

My everyday issues were about loss of identity and self-confidence. I could not find the energy to go back to work, even though I loved to do the kind of work that I do. I wanted to be a mother. I wanted to be a grandmother. All my dreams for the future were shattered. . . . I wanted my life back as it was, with my son still in it.

CMN's peer support worker in the veterans' programme, Gordon, also took seven years between his exposure to the trauma of death and destruction on active service with the ADF in Iraq and to the time when he felt like living again. He said,

My head was like Swiss cheese. I was afraid of going out. I had five years of excruciating pain from my neck and back until surgery fixed it. I was hospitalised for PTSD while in the army after breaking down while speaking at a programme for wives to prepare them for their husband's return from Iraq. I was discharged after 12 months, and began seeing a psychiatrist every two months. It took me time to accept that I needed medical help.

This experience is congruent with the observation that 'where peers are employed to provide support in services, the peer employed in the support role is generally considered to be further along their road to recovery' (Repper and Carter 2011: 395). But what is it that unfolds over this extended period that equips a survivor of trauma to develop the role of a PSW as a sustainable social development?

From pain as pathology to shared pain as indicator of injustice

Perhaps the first important transformation is that the trauma survivor understands their personal pain. Mead (n.d.) has emphasised how Western culture has individualised and pathologised pain as if it were a byproduct of a wound or symptom of an illness. This is how the army and the DVA responded to Gordon's pain from his exposure to the trauma and destruction of war. He was treated as if he were ill, with a series of hospitalisations and clinics. During treatment, Gordon was supported by his wife, a doctor, a psychiatrist, and a chaplain, who together helped him to see how much damage to himself he had endured, to accept his vulnerability and need for help, and to understand his pain was a result of military service rather than his personal pathology. A turning point for Gordon was a phone call he received from another veteran after a story in the local paper featured Gordon's story. Gordon felt an immediate connection with the caller, who followed up by calling Gordon a number of times and then meeting him for coffee. Because Gordon sensed this veteran had walked in his shoes, their shared pain became a point of connection and mutual support: a new and healing experience for Gordon.

Bette recalled how the workers' compensation system gave no acknowledgement of her pain as a bereaved family member. In part, this was because she did not fit the criteria of dependent to be a beneficiary of the system and in part due to the dehumanising processes of the legal and investigative aspects of the system. As the mother of a deceased worker, she was not a dependent and therefore had no legal claim under workers' compensation legislation. The 1897 British legislation defined a dependent as a member of a worker's family 'as were wholly or in part *dependent upon the earnings* of the workman at the time of his death' (Clegg 1898: 97) (our italics). This legal understanding of pecuniary compensation payable for a work-related death is reaffirmed in the *Victorian Accident Compensation Act* (Victorian Parliament 1985), which states that a dependent is a person who 'at the time of the death of a worker was *wholly, mainly or partly dependent on the earnings* of the worker' (Victorian Parliament 1985: 10) (our italics).

The nineteenth-century beliefs about family life that assumed women were economically incorporated into their husband's identity is the basis of today's policy that dependent spouses (mostly wives) and children will be the only beneficiaries of workers' compensation. The definition of eligibility not only excludes family members who are not dependents but excludes all non-economic bases of work-related harm, including pain and suffering. While her pain was dismissed from the purview of the workers' compensation system, over seven years Bette was able to begin the process of understanding that her pain need not be confined to the sphere of her private grief.

Being connected through mutual support and life energy

Bette's transformative process from victim of trauma to volunteer was also enabled by her gradual awareness that her marriage was blocking her capacity to deal with the pain of her traumatic experience. A family law solicitor provided valuable support in disentangling her post-traumatic pain from the pain of a failing marriage. On the tenth anniversary of her son's death, she said,

> I was not encouraged to talk about my feelings with my husband. He did not want to know that I was not coping with the stress. Some issues had become a problem for my husband and I, so now I needed to deal with my grief and a failing marriage. So a relationship already fragile disintegrated. We parted some 4 years ago.

After her son's death, Bette bought a horse and, through her daily riding, found her horse helped her to reconnect with her humanity. A further support for Bette came from her decision to join The Compassionate Friends (TCF), a self-help organisation for parents of a child who had died. Like Gordon, Bette experienced the fruits of mutual support with others (as bereaved parents) who shared her experience of trauma.

Sharing stories evokes the gift of healing

Bette quickly became a volunteer with TCF and found that the opportunity to help other bereaved parents gave her renewed self-confidence and a new sense of identity with her volunteer role. It was similar with Gordon. The veteran who reached out to Gordon was a member of the CMN board, so that in time Gordon responded to tell his story as a guest speaker at an annual church service to remember the wounds of war and later was guest speaker at the agency's annual remembrance eve dinner. Both Bette and Gordon learned from these volunteer roles that they were ready with something to offer from their trauma that could support others with whom they shared a common experience.

Trauma transformed: discovering a spiritual connection

Finally both Gordon and Bette had a spiritual experience in the seven years before they became PSWs, which appears vital to the sustainability of their future roles. In theological terms, both Bette and Gordon experienced a deep inner conviction that they were being called to a new vocation. Bette attributed this to the deepening of her long-held belief that people came into her life for a reason and that her son's life and death had set her on a new path, which she continues to be on nearly twenty years after joining CMN as a volunteer. Looking back, Bette feels her son's influence on her life is stronger today than ever before, and she trusts that the spiritual connection she has with him is ongoing and purposeful. The result of this inner strength is that Bette can embrace the challenges of her work and life's journey with deep gratitude for her son's leading in her life. Gordon's sense of vocation in a PSW role emerged from his personal response to a calling to become a Christian, following other members of his family's interest in Christian faith. At a time when he felt unhappy, Gordon recounts attending his adult son's baptism and being touched by the feeling he needed to explore this further. He then realised he wanted to become a Christian, and with his wife, they did so. For Gordon, a burden was lifted from his heart, and he experienced the inner peace of being at ease with his life. Like Bette, there is an inner strength Gordon brings to his commitment to become a PSW.

The importance of the spiritual experience both Bette and Gordon received during the seven years from trauma exposure to volunteering as a PSW is an unexpected contribution to the sustainability requirements for a PSW. The CMN agency described this as 'companioning peer support'. For both Bette and Gordon, their personal spiritual companion (her son and Jesus Christ, respectively) had suffered trauma uniquely in their own deaths, and both Bette and Gordon experienced their connection with their spiritual companions in forgiveness, peace, and their calling to the new vocation of PSW.

Peer support as a model for social inclusion: recovering a holistic vision for human life

Three critical issues for sustaining a transformed interior life for trauma victims

Mead's (n.d.) description of peer support captures the endpoint reality of Gordon and Bette's seven-year journeys from trauma exposure to taking up their new vocations. There were three critical issues that needed to be resolved in that extended period of time for them to be equipped to be PSWs.

1   Finding a new source of meaning in their lives, despite the harm living in the world causes.

Peer supports can offer a fundamentally different framework for making meaning about our experiences and perceptions of our past, present, and futures. It can provide us with opportunities to find new ways of understanding our world and our experiences and of finding new ways to respond to it. In peer support, we can learn to form relationships outside of the definition or context of 'illness' that pathologises pain and to talk about the effects of trauma and abuse in our lives.

2   Accepting compassionately their own internal chaos equips PSWs to listen compassionately to the objectively recounted distress of others.

We can share our stories with each other, and we can begin to question how and why other people have learned to tell their stories in the ways that they do. We can begin to listen to each other in new ways, hearing the story rather than evaluating and assessing the problem.

3   Refusing to pathologise pain and so respecting pain as messages about the world of harm.

We can be witnesses to each other's pain. And most importantly, we can validate the reality of each other's' feelings, perceptions, and experiences. (Mead n.d.)

Integrating the separation between public and private realities

A fourth issue emerges from their work of being a PSW. It comes from being engaged with the harm others have experienced but arises from providing support to others from the harm inflicted by the compensation system (Pollock et al. 2014). The 'no-fault' liability for employers established by the German and UK compensation legislation separated the state's public liability for economic compensation from the sufferers' personal emotional, physical, spiritual, and social experience of work-related harm. The liability is minimised to an economic 'fact', and every other dimension of liability is relegated to the privatised world of the trauma victim.

The nineteenth-century laws limited compensation to economic considerations, while determining whether the cause of injury or death was work-related was given to medical science. But Bette and Gordon's experiences highlight how the traumas they each experienced created more than merely economic needs. In their roles as PSWs, both workers have also encountered numerous clients where they have advocated for peers who have been denied access to compensation because medical science was unable to provide conclusive evidence that the client's suffering was related to the trauma they experienced. In particular, research by CMN into work factors in suicide (Bottomley 2015) and injured workers suicidality (Pollock et al. 2014), accompanied by Bette's growing caseload of clients bereaved by their loved one's work-related suicide, has contributed to some clients successfully receiving a compensation payment. Such advocacy is a vital contribution to strengthening the social inclusion of the peer support programmes.

The recovery of a holistic vision for human life brings a further important insight into the role of PSWs. While Bette and Gordon both found the practice of peer support vital to establishing their foundations in a new sphere of work after their trauma experience, their development of new skills as they creatively responded to the needs of clients, has changed their self-understanding of their current work. We propose that peer support is better understood as a way of being in their work rather than a set of skills. The vitality of peer support is in the capacity for being alongside another victim of trauma rather than the 'doing' of a role. Bette and Gordon bring different skills to their support for clients, honed and developed over many years. But what they share is a heart and soul forged from the bitter pain of trauma and a hard-won wisdom that has enabled them to develop a professional skill set that takes their work beyond an ascribed role. This insight circles back to the initial commitment of the CMN board for all its members to share their own stories and journey as board members as the foundation for the exercise of their governance. So it is vital to the social inclusion project that board, management, and staff share a commitment to both the interior and objective realities of formation for peer support rather than limiting PSW to a staff role that then mirrors the isolation of victims in compensation systems.

Restoring justice to what it means to be human

The compensation system imagines the trauma felt by victims as an individual and private matter for each person and so treats the consequences of the work-related harm they experience as an individual and private matter. For example, the removal of the employer's legal liability for 'fault' from the system removed the possibility for a widow to seek justice for the death of her husband, herself, and her family. Their husbands' deaths were minimised as matters of public responsibility or accountability, and widows themselves were left in an 'uncertain, socially unsupported and vulnerable' position (Mellor and Shilling 1993: 417). Then the compensation system imposed upon the widow a burden of moral and economic regulation to ensure she was worthy of the entitlement and compliant with the regulatory requirements. Bette encountered this experience as a bereaved mother and so developed the resources to deal with it while working for CMN. Bette had shared her yearning to meet with her son's employer with her CEO, and together they discussed how to approach him so that she might find answers to some matters that still affected her. Reflecting on the tenth anniversary of her son's death, Bette recalled her meeting with her son's boss.

> This was the first time we had met since the inquest. I cannot tell you how important that this was for me. While it was not easy for either one of us, I now have some of my answers. . . . How sad and unjust it is that our adversarial

legal and compensation system could build a wall between us, and keep our grief apart for so long . . . how difficult it is for those work-mates that are left to deal with the aftermath. The effect ripples on. Those first months in particular are the most difficult—doing the same work as you were at the time. The support for the worker is severely lacking. This seems to be the case in almost all of the companies where a death has occurred. The expectation is that the worker will eventually get over it.

Bette's experience of being cut off from the employer was often repeated in the stories of her clients, but particularly when a prosecution was being mounted by the health and safety authority, where it was almost impossible for clients to meet with an employer. Yet the experience of healing and reconciliation that Bette experienced from meeting with her son's employer encouraged CMN to explore the possibility of developing a restorative justice service.

Restorative justice

With funding from a government agency, CMN carried out research into the feasibility of establishing a restorative justice service for parties affected by a work-related death. While the findings from the research and an all-parties round-table recommendation supporting a preferred model (Brookes 2009) were not sufficient to secure funding in 2009, the need for a restorative justice service as part of the government's response to work-related harm is again under public policy consideration in 2018. Such an initiative would strengthen the social inclusiveness of the PSW model pioneered by CMN by strengthening the healing process for bereaved family members and providing a 'safe place within the justice system for people to interact in a more human way to achieve a range of benefits not so readily available under the criminal justice system' (Brookes 2009: 106).

However, to achieve this outcome will require the transformation of one of the historic assumptions of the workers' compensation system. It will require the sacrosanct status of employer's 'no-fault' liability in the criminal justice system to be twinned with a restorative justice process where employers accept personal responsibility for work-related harm in their business. The proposed benefits for both bereaved families and employers are greatly improved healing and reconciliation outcomes at a personal and inter-personal level. But perhaps the potential benefits for the company and similar industries are equally compelling in overcoming the stultifying dualism that exists between work-related harm prevention and harm compensation. Brookes argues that when companies interact in a more human way, it may help them to better understand the consequences of work-related death and to embed their commitment to occupational health and safety at the personal level in the corporate culture. Further, the restorative justice service's capacity to record data and conduct evaluations of its casework may help to identify 'hidden' factors that contribute to prevention of work-related deaths (Brookes 2009).

Social inclusion establishes social justice as a new horizon for social change

All compensation insurance rests on a devastating paradox: the lives it compensates for injury and death caused by the industrial system or war service are objectified as an economic cost of the system's 'success' and 'progress', or society's 'peace'. 'Workers were increasingly viewed as extensions of, or accessories to, machinery—the breakdown of which . . . could be expected to happen every so often' (Duncan 2003: 465). Workers' compensation insurance changed the nature of the employer-employee relationship to an essentially utilitarian affair where the employer's responsibility to work-injured employees is viewed in impersonal, almost amoral, terms. The injured or deceased worker is no longer viewed as an individual-in-relationship but as a normal and predictable risk to the business. This view also predominates in federal compensation legislation for military service, where injury and death on active service are regarded as a risk of war service in the cause of 'peace'.

The removal of employer fault through the introduction of workers' compensation legislation was accompanied by the assignment of moral hazard to the injured or deceased worker. The insurance concept of 'moral hazard', which refers to the supposedly innate character of the insured person to be prone to exploit an insurance contract for gain through deliberate 'accidents' or false claims, (Duncan 2003) justified the introduction of a cap on benefits for injury and death. The economic priority of employers' financial concerns cannot be underestimated as a key driver of the first workers' compensation scheme, and this priority is still in evidence today in both workers' and veterans' compensation schemes.

Both CMN programmes counter this dehumanising spirit with public ceremonies, events, rituals, and services of remembrance that honour the humanity and dignity of those who have died on war service or from work-related causes. The two PSWs provide a range of art therapy interventions to support clients establishing their own peer relationships of mutual support. The physicality of working with clay or planning a photograph, the stimulation of writing a book, or a time of reflective contemplation are just some of the techniques that ensure the inclusiveness of their peer support activities. Mead reinforces the importance of how these public and inter-personal shared experiences may contribute to a more fundamental transformation of compensation systems historically designed to treat those recovering from work-related and war service trauma as autonomous individuals.

> As we unite in shared experiences and begin to expose the very structures that have kept us silenced, we find that "doing" social action becomes inextricably linked to healing—personally, relationally and culturally. People who have seen themselves as powerless suddenly find that they are not alone in their perceptions.
>
> (Mead n.d.)

The Enlightenment thinkers who nurtured the belief structure of the Industrial Revolution viewed work—and we suggest, war—as objective public realities, while grief was viewed as a subjective private reality to be managed by each bereaved individual or family (Bottomley 2015). Compensation systems were designed to redress the publicly objective economic harm suffered by individual widows after the death of their bread-winning husband. By assuming grief was merely emotion and therefore 'private', unjust death and grief were removed from the public sphere of justice. Compensation's medical-legal structure thus dismissed from public scrutiny public liability for state-sponsored killing and employer negligence. But peer-supported public rituals, ceremonies, and events break the system-imposed silence by integrating trauma victims' public lament with their personal pain (Bottomley 2015). Doing social action is inextricably linked to healing: the personal is political, and work-related and war-related deaths are reinstated in the public domain by the personal healing processes of trauma victims. The sustainability of social inclusion outcomes for peer support programmes rests upon the transformation of trauma victims from 'powerless' victims silenced by the state's beneficence to active agents of their personal and shared futures. When public rituals of remembrance embody a holistic vision of the human person, the pain of unjust and violent death is embraced, and the grief of the bereaved is, in a sense, made holy. Such reverencing of pain due to the traumatic violence and injustice of corporations and nations generates a cry for justice and establishes a new horizon for truth-speaking (Brueggemann 2010).

The experience at CMN suggests its vision for peer support did not set its horizon on simply fitting in with existing compensation systems that have held victims of trauma in an isolated and isolating space. Social inclusion for trauma victims of war and work-related deaths will require a broader horizon of health and community service systems as well as compensation systems to also be transformed by the inclusion of peer support and restorative justice practices. To further this transformative challenge to state-run services and private enterprise insurers, the Uniting Church's 2016 decision to amalgamate CMN into Synod's (Victoria/Tasmania) new community services entity, 'Uniting', provides an exciting possibility for strengthening the sustainability of CMN's social development innovations. Uniting has an opportunity to pioneer a solidarity compact across its mental health, veterans, and work-related harm programmes. Uniting may ensure the sustainability of the former CMN programmes by pursuing an inclusive vision integrating peer support and restorative justice programmes from its diverse client experiences of injustice and trauma, while nurturing a holistic commitment to healing and justice—personally, relationally, and organisationally.

Conclusion

From the nineteenth-century beginnings of state-run compensation schemes, the welfare of individual workers, dependents, and veterans has been couched within a political and legal narrative designed to protect powerful industrial, commercial, and political interests. For more than 100 years, Victorians and Australians have died from the prevailing ideological assumptions that social progress and peace are only achieved at the price of lives sacrificed to these ends. This reality dictates that the challenges to state-based compensation systems of sustainable peer support and restorative justice social development interventions is at profound risk.

If the gains of these social development interventions continue to challenge the ultimate status of such work-related and war deaths, sacrifices which have been incorporated into the narrative assumptions of compensation systems, it is an open question whether these interventions will continue to be funded by the state. So the challenge for the future sustainability of the former CMN's programmes rests with their incorporation into the new structure of Uniting and whether the agency is able to enter into its own cultural transformation through its broad-based solidarity with its clients' reality of pain and grief as victims of trauma. We submit both peer support and restorative justice better strengthen social inclusion outcomes of healing and justice when holistically integrated in the auspice organisation's self-understanding.

References

Bottomley, J. (1988) *We're All in the Same Boat: A Literature Review on the Role of Support Groups for Injured Workers as a Preventative Measure in Community Mental Health*, Melbourne: Urban Ministry Network.

Bottomley, J. (2015) *Hard Work Never Killed Anybody: How the Idolisation of Work Sustains This Deadly Lie*, Northcote: Morning Star Publishing.

Brookes, D. (2009) *Restorative Justice and Work—Related Death: Consultation Report*, Melbourne: Creative Ministries Network.

Brueggemann, W. (2010) *Journey to the Common Good*, Louisville: Westminster John Knox Press.

Brueggemann, W. (2014) *The Practice of Homefulness*, Eugene, OR: Cascade Books.

Clegg, A. (1898) *Commentary on the Workmen's Compensation Act, 1897*, Edinburgh: William Green & Sons.

Duncan, G. (2003) 'Workers' compensation and the governance of pain', *Economy and Society*, 32: 449–77.

Gurtler, P.R. (1989) 'The workers' compensation principle: a historical abstract of the nature of workers' compensation', *Hamline Journal of Public Law and Policy*, 9: 285–96.

Kleeberg, J. (2003) 'From strict liability to workers' compensation: the Prussian Railroad Law, the German Liability Act, and the introduction of Bismarck's Accident Insurance in Germany, 1838–1884', *International Law and Politics*, 36: 53–132.

Mead, S. (n.d.) *Trauma Informed Peer Support*. Online. Available at http://citeseerx.ist.psu.edu/viewdoc/download?doi=10.1.1.516.2074&rep=rep1&type=pdf (accessed 16 October 2018).

Mead, S., Hilton, D. and Curtis, L. (2001) 'Peer support: a theoretical perspective', *Psychiatric Rehabilitation Journal*, 25: 134–41.

Mellor, P. and Shilling, C. (1993) 'Modernity, self-identity and the sequestration of death', *Sociology*, 27: 411–31.

O'Connor, K. (2002) *Lamentations and the Tears of the World*, Maryknoll, NY: Orbis Books.

Pollock, S., Bottomley, J. and Taket, A. (2014) *Workers' Compensation and Mental Health: Examining the Mental Health Impacts of Involvement in the Victorian WorkCover*

System from the Perspective of Long-term Injured Workers, Melbourne: Creative Ministries Network.

Repper, J. and Carter, T. (2011) 'A review of the literature on peer support in mental health services', *Journal of Mental Health.* 20: 392–411.

Schiller, R. (2006) *Behavioral Economics and Institutional Innovation*, Cowles Foundation Discussion Paper No.1499, Cowles Foundation for Research in Economics, Yale University. Online. Available at www.econ.yale.edu/~shiller/pubs/p1150.pdf (accessed 16 October 2018).

van Meerhaeghe, M. (2006) 'Bismarck and the social question', *Journal of Economic Studies*, 33: 284–301.

Victorian Parliament (1985) Accident Compensation Act 1985 No. 10191 of 1985.

3 Sustaining social inclusion

Lessons from research, intervention, and policymaking

*Tamar Kabakian-Khasholian, Rana Saleh,
Jihad Makhoul and Fadi El-Jardali*

Introduction

Participatory approaches around the world have witnessed a surge in the recent decades. Social movements and advocacy have challenged unfair policies resulting in a rise of socially inclusive practices in service design and delivery, community participatory research, and public participation in policymaking (Taket et al. 2014). Public participation in policymaking is considered a key component in the process of development of socially inclusive policies. The right of individuals/citizens to be involved in the decision-making process that will affect their lives is recognised as a human right (World Health Organization 1978) and operationalised by the Organisation for Economic Co-operation and Development (OECD) guiding principles for policymaking. The *Sustainable Development Goals* (SDGs) agenda also calls for ensuring responsiveness, inclusiveness, and participatory approaches in the decision-making processes at all levels in the health system to promote peaceful and inclusive societies (United Nations 2015). Engaging the public in policies allows the development of policies that are sensitive to their needs, priorities, and expectations (Bruni et al. 2008; Oxman et al. 2009). It also leads to improvements in public education, policy implementation, and compliance, better quality services, and thus improved health outcomes. Public participation also encourages public accountability, transparency, and advocacy (Oxman et al. 2009; Williamson 2014). Empowering citizens to take part in the decisions affecting their health also increases their trust and confidence in the healthcare system (Bruni et al. 2008).

Several countries of the Global North, such as Canada, Australia, and members of the European Union (EU), have moved forward with national agendas and policy reform toward social inclusion. National policies developed by EU countries in the early twenty-first century, for example, served as models for countries to develop their own policies based on common EU objectives for social inclusion (Commission of the European Communities 2005). In 2009, the OECD updated its 10 guiding principles for open and inclusive policymaking for countries to develop their policies and services (OECD 2009). In 2007, the Australian government joined this trend of introducing social policy with its Social Inclusion Agenda whose aim is to increase social and economic participation, described as having the potential to make a substantive contribution to the social determinants of health of the Australian population (Carey et al. 2012).

These advances in the Global North toward socially inclusive policies were not witnessed in Arab countries, which have lagged behind in the attention to social inclusion and particularly socially inclusive policymaking. There is a great need in the Arab world for policies that improve social inclusion to improve economic performance in the region (Devarajan et al. 2016). The region is characterised by its long history of armed conflicts and struggles against colonialism, constant forced migration, inequitable social development, and poor social and health policies (Makhoul and El-Barbir 2006). An estimated two thirds of the Arab world population is young, with a mean age below 25 years old (United Nations Development Programme [UNDP] 2016). Very few of the 22 countries have developed cross-sectoral and integrated national youth policies. Out of 22 countries in the region, only nine have either developed youth policies or are in the process of formulating them (United Nations 2010). The demographic pressure of a large youth cohort has made it difficult for their countries to absorb all of the youth labour market needs (Silver 2007). In addition to youth, other population groups have been found to experience injustices and marginalisation based on gender, economic, political, religious, or ethnic differences (Monshipouri and Whooley 2011; UNDP 2016). This widespread social exclusion has ignited resistance to social and political domination and exclusion in the form of national struggles, Palestinian *intifadas*, and Arab uprisings, in many instances, resulting in violence, armed conflict, unjust welfare systems, and further social exclusion (Barron et al. 2006).

Despite the recognition and commitment to socially inclusive policies in the Global North, the actual implementation of a process that ensures development of policies equitable to all groups of the population is seen challenging and not always successfully implemented (Taket et al. 2014). Further, since most of the social inclusion frameworks have been developed in the Global North (Mitton et al. 2009), little is known about how these frameworks fit in the context of low- and medium-income countries (LMICs).

Lebanon, for example, does not have systems in place that facilitate the inclusion of its citizens' voices and values in the policy development process. There are also no platforms for citizen engagement in health policy and decision-making and no requirement from a governmental perspective that such an engagement is necessary. Health policies in Lebanon are mainly initiated by the executive or legislative branch of the government (World Intellectual Property Organization 1995) following a top-down approach, influenced by sectarianism and favouritism, based on the political agendas and priorities of the ruling political parties (El-Jardali et al. 2014), and adopting policies which have been implemented elsewhere in the globe instead of developing policies which take into account the context in Lebanon.

A few success stories of civil society movements of initiating social/health policies have been documented in Lebanon (domestic violence, tobacco control). Multiple efforts from national and international organisations have started programmes to engage youth in political and democratic decision-making (United Nations

Educational, Scientific and Cultural Organization [UNESCO] 2011; World Bank 2014; Youth Forum for Youth Policy 2012), but not specifically in public health policies.

The Knowledge to Policy (K2P) Centre, the only centre in the Arab region specialised in evidence-informed health policies, initiated a public participation programme in an attempt to shift the focus toward inclusive health policies in Lebanon. The programme includes trying out different modalities for the engagement of all relevant stakeholders related to a public health problem, such as researchers, policymakers, decision-makers, media, and citizens, with a focus on including citizens in policy development through identifying priorities and developing contextualised bottom-up policies that are responsive to their needs, priorities, and expectations. This programme is in line with the Knowledge Translation (KT) scientific methodology (El-Jardali and Fadlallah 2015) that K2P Centre employs. KT is a 'dynamic and iterative process that includes the synthesis, dissemination, exchange and ethically sound application of knowledge to improve health, provide more effective health services and products, and strengthen the healthcare system' (Straus et al. 2009: 165). Given the limited capacity and the novelty of the concept of public participation in Lebanon, K2P Centre has not engaged the public in health policy in the past. Nonetheless, the Centre moved forward with public participation processes for the issue of childhood obesity. The exemplar shown later describes the iterative process that K2P Centre employed to engage citizens for the first time in health policy in Lebanon through citizen consultations, its process and outcome evaluation, barriers, and the lessons learned about social inclusion in policymaking in this context.

Citizen engagement in policies for childhood obesity prevention in Lebanon

Childhood obesity is an emerging priority public health issue in Lebanon given the evident increase in its prevalence and associated consequences (Nasreddine et al. 2012, 2014) that requires the development and implementation of national policies and legislations. Accordingly, K2P Centre addressed this priority public health concern through KT. This KT methodology starts by prioritising a specific public health problem in a participatory process with multiple stakeholders (policymakers, decision-makers, researchers, local and international organisations, and civil society) via focused discussions and priority setting (El-Jardali et al. 2010). High-quality evidence on the known policy solutions for this problem, along with implementation barriers and facilitators, are gathered and synthesised into a policy brief. Then all relevant stakeholders are engaged again in the process of drafting the policy brief by providing their feedback on the feasibility, applicability, and soundness of the emerging policy options within the local context. This policy brief then informs a national policy dialogue with all the involved stakeholders to discuss the policy options and identify the best way forward toward the policy implementation in the local context. This extensively engaging process ensures policymakers' buy-in, and as such, the policy dialogues often result in a road map for the stakeholders on the implementation of the evidence-informed policy options. Further strategies are also suggested for implementation and to ensure policy uptake such as advocacy, media, and further stakeholder engagement (El-Jardali and Fadlallah 2015).

Developing the policy brief

Using the previously mentioned methodology, K2P Centre developed a policy brief on school policies for the prevention of childhood obesity summarising the available global, regional, and international evidence about policy options at schools (Saleh et al. 2019). The aim of the policy brief was to inform deliberations with policy and decision-makers in a national policy dialogue based on evidence-informed school policies for childhood obesity prevention. This policy brief was developed while engaging an impact team of content experts, an advocacy and policy advisor, a lawyer, and a communication specialist, all serving as a steering committee. The final phase of development involved the K2P Centre holding 16 in-depth individual interviews with researchers, policymakers, and other stakeholders to further refine the brief and ensure it was appropriately contextualised. A supplementary policy brief was developed specifically for citizens that is short, easy to read, colourful, and supported by supplementary infographics and animated videos.

Developing a consultation process

Throughout the development of the policy brief, the problem of childhood obesity prevention policies within Lebanese schools appeared to be within the implementation of existing policies and decisions. With these challenges not being found in the international literature, local experiences needed to be documented by engaging stakeholders involved in school health. It also became apparent to the researchers that the issue of childhood obesity in Lebanon is politically and interest-charged. Multiple transnational corporations and local industries interfere with local researchers and the government to market their products in school premises. Hence, the inclusion of the public's opinion was considered to influence the local authorities on the adoption of policies pertaining to the school food environment.

Published methods of public participation in health policy and decision-making were identified and reviewed. A process of public participation was developed and piloted based on a methodology that would be appropriate and acceptable in the context. Table 3.1 shows the identified methods for public participation in the literature and how these methods were contextualised for the Lebanese context in order to elicit citizen values, expectations, and experiences around a high-priority public health problem and its policy elements. This process aims to support a full discussion of the contextual considerations of the research evidence about the policy elements in order to inform the action of key stakeholders based on not only research evidence but also citizen values and expectations.

Table 3.1 The contextualised methodology of citizen engagement in comparison with the international literature

	Public participation methodology from the international literature	*Public participation methodology chosen in Lebanon*	*Rationale for the methodology adaptations*
Aim of public participation	Broad system design and system planning functions Goal-setting level in specific decisions about sites or programmes; Less common in monitoring or evaluation	Broad system design and system planning functions	Inform deliberations about policies
Level of engagement	Communication Consultation Participation	Consultation	Time and resources of the Centre No previous citizen engagement activities in health policy to learn from
Inclusion/ exclusion criteria	The informed public as citizens (with previous experience or trained) Civil society Consumers of health policy Interest group representatives Disadvantaged populations	The public as citizens Civil society Consumers of health policy Interest group representatives Disadvantaged populations	It was not possible to know beforehand if the citizens were informed
Sampling	Purposive recruitment Random Self-selection	Purposive Per governorate, chosen by gatekeeper	No sampling frame Last census 1930s No previous engagement activities in health policy in Lebanon
Channels of recruitment	Targeted, personal invitations Wide advertising Use of mass media Contact by telephone, mail, or email	Targeted, personal invitations/telephone by community gatekeeper letters Different channels per region (between personal invitations, phone calls, and emails)	Websites, online platforms not popular among all age groups and urban vs. rural Urban settings could be reached with emails

(Continued)

Table 3.1 (Continued)

	Public participation methodology from the international literature	*Public participation methodology chosen in Lebanon*	*Rationale for the methodology adaptations*
Data collection methods	Briefs, surveys, and evaluations pre, during, and after engagement events Engagement exercises are rarely formally evaluated	Citizen brief sent before citizen engagement Evaluation only conducted after the citizen engagement	Culture of data collection not common People engage with minimum requirement from their side Citizens didn't receive and/or didn't read the Citizen brief sent before 77 per cent response rate to the evaluation
Method of public participation	Written consultation Public hearing Hotline Opinion poll or survey Standing citizens' advisory panel Interviews Citizens' jury Electronic consultation Town meeting with voting Focus groups Consultation document with select persons or groups Consumer panels Committee membership	Consultation document with select persons or groups	Online does not reach everyone Low rate of response to surveys Time and resources of the Centre No culture of engagement in Lebanon No previous examples of engagement activities in Lebanon and the region to learn from
Design of engagement activity	Activities, scenarios, group work, and group discussion Face-to-face/online Ongoing/one-time/ one-time multiple days	Face-to-face One-time Group work, group discussion	Experience of gatekeepers with citizen activities Experience of researchers with previous community participatory activities Reflexive design adapting each context and learning from each citizen consultation

	Public participation methodology from the international literature	*Public participation methodology chosen in Lebanon*	*Rationale for the methodology adaptations*
Follow-up strategies with the participants	There is a lack of practical guidance for integrating public input with other forms of evidence Email Phone calls Further panels	Social media: WhatsApp and Facebook Email Phone calls Through gatekeepers Results were sent to participants and integrated into the Policy Brief	The choice of follow-up method was individualised based on the preference of each participant and after their request of follow-up with us

Sources: Abelson et al. 2010, 2013; Mitton et al. 2009; Oxman et al. 2009

Four citizen consultations were then conducted across different Lebanese governorates (administrative regions) to inform citizens about the evident problem of childhood obesity, present the evidence-informed policy options, and identify contextual barriers and facilitators for the implementation of the suggested policies. Key features of the citizen consultations include addressing a current issue in Lebanon with a focus on different underlying factors; exploring two policy elements of a comprehensive approach; being informed by a pre-circulated K2P Citizen Brief; discussing the full range of factors that can inform ways to approach the problem with policy elements for addressing it; bringing together citizens from different backgrounds who would be involved in or are affected by future decisions related to the issue; engaging a facilitator to assist with the deliberations; and encouraging frank discussions following the Chatham House rule which allows the use of participants' de-identified input and does not require consensus.

K2P citizen consultations

With the help of several local community councils across the country (municipalities) and primary healthcare centres (PHCCs), we accessed citizens for the consultation process. Seventy-one participants attended four citizen consultations. There was socioeconomic, demographic, religious, and gender diversity, as well representation from rural and urban communities. Most participants had university degrees or an equivalent higher education (73 per cent), around 19 per cent had secondary education or its equivalent, and the rest were school students. The participants included those who are directly and indirectly involved in school nutrition and physical activity programmes, such as public and private school directors, teachers, school canteen owners, nurses/health workers, municipality/community/PHCCs representatives, physicians, dietitians, social workers, parents, children, and youth. Three quarters (76 per cent) were 30 years of age or over, and 72 per cent indicated not having previously been part of a participatory dialogue or a group discussion (Table 3.1).

All participants received a copy of the policy brief prior to the consultation. During the four citizen consultations, information about childhood obesity in Lebanon, its consequences, and underlying factors were displayed using innovative data visualisation tools, including animated videos and PowerPoint presentations, followed by a discussion. The evidence-informed policies were then presented together with the implementation barriers and facilitators. Participants were then provided with the opportunity to discuss various policy options in facilitated groups.

In the first two citizen consultations, the facilitated discussions were within the larger group. However, participants reported unsatisfactory experiences in terms of the level of engagement in the general discussion. In the final two consultations, participants broke into small groups for facilitated discussions, with some groups composed of members with the same occupation. All the groups convened later for a general discussion.

The citizens identified the policies that they perceived could be implemented in their communities. They identified the different approaches that could be implemented in rural or urban settings and in public or private schools of varying governance structures and policies. They also pointed to the gaps in the current system and suggested corrective strategies, ways to overcome conflict of interest and pragmatic details for effective implementation unrecognised by the international literature. It was evident throughout all the consultations that citizens believed the government is the primary body responsible for policy implementation. With a strong-voiced mistrust in the system, they called for transparent policy implementation and monitoring.

The data obtained from citizen consultation discussion notes, citizen written feedback about policy options and implementation considerations, and evaluation forms were subject to thematic analysis, and the findings were summarised in another brief. Together with the initial policy brief document, it will inform the discussions in the national policy dialogue. Interested citizens who received a summary of the consultation findings were engaged in further advocacy efforts on the initiative (Saleh 2019).

Evaluation

Fifty-five participants completed evaluation forms for the consultation process. The majority of participants reported that the dialogue achieved its overall goal, and they agreed that the content especially the policy options and their implementation considerations was presented in a comprehensive manner. Participants also gave positive feedback on the process of the citizen consultations, finding the facilitated group discussions helpful, particularly those that involved members of the same occupation. They preferred to be engaged with multiple stakeholders during these discussions, something that was reported to enrich the discussion with tacit knowledge that each stakeholder brings to the table, and increase the chances of generating contextualised solutions. They recommended making the citizen brief available prior to the animation videos and the PowerPoint presentations in future consultations.

Table 3.2 Participants' evaluation of the impacts of participatory processes

Consultation ability	Very helpful	Moderately helpful	Slightly helpful	Neutral	Slightly unhelpful	Moderately unhelpful	Very unhelpful	Total
	%	%	%	%	%	%	%	N
To affect decision-maker	18.2	32.7	10.9	25.5	7.3	5.5	0.0	55
To allow joint decision-making with citizens	21.8	36.5	7.3	18.2	10.9	1.8	3.6	57
To allow citizen advocacy	40.7	33.3	7.4	3.7	5.6	9.3	0.0	54

Table 3.2 shows that participants were positive as to the usefulness of the citizen consultations in decision-making. This is reflected in the majority of responses that indicate that the dialogue can be helpful in affecting decision-makers (62 per cent), stating that it will allow joint decision-making (65 per cent) and will enable citizen advocacy for this cause (81 per cent).

All of the 47 participants who filled the follow-up request forms asked for updates on the process, agreed to take part in the Centre's future activities, and wanted to move forward and advocate for the issue. They further expressed their willingness to be part of an advocacy workshop that the Centre might conduct at a later stage (80 per cent). Citizens showed interest in continuing their efforts through raising awareness among parents/families and school directors, moving forward with implementing the solutions in their work (schools) using participatory approaches, increasing activities and awareness efforts in schools, starting their own advocacy efforts, and conducting municipality level activities to prevent childhood obesity.

Discussion

The citizen consultation around childhood obesity was a first attempt to follow a process of public participation in policy development in Lebanon. A positive view of the participants on the content of the citizen consultation is in line with the recommendations that deliberations in health policy should discuss the problem parameters and the policy implementation-related issues (Lavis et al. 2009). The use of multiple means to present data and issues to the participants was welcomed. The findings of the evaluation highlight citizens' willingness to engage in the process of decision-making and advocacy, especially in politically and interest-charged topics. In turn, this participation will lead to improvements in public education, public accountability, transparency, and advocacy (Oxman et al. 2009; Williamson 2014). Our findings also indicate citizens' positive perception of the usefulness of their engagement in the policy development process highlighting the necessity of the application of this participatory approach in health policy to enhance social inclusion and ensure positive outcomes of the policies.

In addition to the evaluation findings, as one of the first applications of public participation in health policy in Lebanon, there are major lessons learned in the process of conducting citizen consultations. The public participation frameworks, developed by countries of the Global North, are not always applicable in varied and more challenging contexts. These have to be adapted to the local contexts of the countries adopting them, both nationally and subnationally (e.g. rural vs. urban settings) using various methods of engagement.

In countries such as Lebanon, which lack national databases facilitating citizen recruitment, other contextually relevant approaches can be adopted. The use of community gatekeepers for access is one such approach that proved to be useful in our case. Our approach also allowed for flexibility in the implementation in order to overcome the challenges as were encountered. One important challenge is the almost nonexistent practice of public engagement in decision-making and health policy in systems, and this reflects the little attention to citizens' rights. The participants in our citizen consultations were engaged for the first time in such an initiative. As such, they did not have clear expectations about the process and the commitment to this matter. In fact, during the first two consultations, the citizens were focusing on complaints about the system rather than providing a clear description of the problem and its solutions. To overcome this challenge, the Centre ensured that for the last two consultations, citizens were engaged in smaller homogenous constructive group discussions guided by a facilitator. This led to filtering the feedback to the most relevant and specific policy options. Further awareness and capacity building of citizens on the engagement processes might be warranted.

Another important barrier to the public participation in health policy in Lebanon is the Lebanese people's lack of trust in the system. This affected their motivation to participate in the consultations and to provide constructive feedback and their trust in the ability of these consultations to affect decision-making process. Nonetheless, transparent citizen engagement activities have been shown to enhance citizens' trust in the system (Mitton et al. 2009). Consequently the public's trust in the system facilitates inclusive policymaking.

Investing more time and effort in building a transparent process for public participation is much needed. This process would include a rights-based perspective in building the awareness of citizens about the importance of their engagement, setting clear communication and follow-up methods and maintaining the engagement with citizens after the consultation.

Different priority health topics might require including participants of particular characteristics, multiple methods of engagement, and variations of the recruitment and follow-up processes. Based on these lessons learned, the K2P Centre has initiated a more detailed study to develop a contextualised model for citizen engagement in health policy tailored to the context of Lebanon. This study involving key informant interviews with selected stakeholders as well as data from focus group discussions with citizens aimed at identifying the different methods required for different topics within the Lebanese context. The process and lessons learnt can be tested and applied to other contexts around the world and documented to inform the development of socially inclusive policymaking.

A number of implications follow from this exemplar of inclusive consultation for policymaking. To sustain social inclusion in the policymaking process, challenging ground preparation work for citizen consultation needs to take place, at the level of both citizens and policymakers themselves. Such socially inclusive initiatives may take place in contexts of the Global South where citizens do not have trust in or may be apprehensive of the sociopolitical system they live in and believe that any involvement of theirs will not result in social improvements for them or their societies. Dialogue with community gatekeepers and groups will help in improving the prospects of a successful sustainable process and reduce the risk of abrupt discontinuity of citizen participation. In such contexts, policymakers will also have been using nonparticipatory approaches to develop and implement policies and therefore may see very little value of an inclusive and evidence-informed process. Policymakers need to be convinced of the benefit of this innovative approach and aware of the added value of citizen participation to enable them to listen to people and take their perceptions seriously.

Researchers or moderators need to be transparent, inclusive, and dynamic, and they need to network to continue to involve groups of citizens from different backgrounds, especially the marginalised among them, and in all aspects of the policymaking process. They need to continue to involve citizens in evaluating the implementation of policies to sustain the people's ownership and social inclusion. Policymakers will benefit from integrating time for reflection, dialogue, and collective discussion with communities to build capacities, partnerships, and opportunities for learning for everyone involved. Sharing experiences gained in this process with others who might be involved in research or policymaking is very important. This can be done through workshops and dialogues and continually documenting the process to make it publicly accessible.

Equitable participation is important to consider to avoid citizen burnout and placing burdens on some groups of people in the participatory process over others. Participation in citizen dialogue or citizen involvement needs to be voluntary to avoid exploitation or coercion. Involuntary participation or participation for expected incentives is more probable in resource-poor societies where there is an imbalance of power between general citizens, researchers, and policymakers and participation in the policy development process may be out of perceived access to services. Benefits/incentives for citizens need to be tangible for participants and also carefully considered to ensure continued interest in citizen involvement in the process.

References

Abelson, J., Bombard, Y., Gauvin, F-P., Simeonov, D. and Boesveld, S. (2013) 'Assessing the impacts of citizen deliberations on the health technology process', *International Journal of Technology Assessment in Health Care*, 29: 282–9.

Abelson, J., Montesanti, S., Li, K., Gauvin, F-P. and Martin, E. (2010) *Effective Strategies for Interactive Public Engagement in the Development of Healthcare Policies and Programs*, New Brunswick: Canadian Health Services Research Foundation.

Barron, M., Graham, B. and Hartwell, M. (2006) *Social Exclusion and Conflict: Analysis and Policy Implications*, Oxford: Center for Research on Inequality, Human Security and Ethnicity (CRISE).

Bruni, R.A., Laupacis, A., Martin, D.K. and for the University of Toronto Priority Setting in Health Care Research Group (2008) 'Public engagement in setting priorities in health care', *Canadian Medical Association Journal*, 179: 15–18.

Carey, G., Riley, T. and Crammond, B. (2012) 'The Australian government's "social inclusion agenda": the intersection between public health and social policy', *Critical Public Health*, 22: 47–59.

Commission of the European Communities (2005) *Working Together, Working Better: A New Framework for the Open Coordination of Social Protection and Inclusion Policies in the European Union*, Brussels: Communication from the Commission to the Council, the European Parliament, The European Economic and Social Committee and the Committee of the regions.

Devarajan, S., Mottaghi, L., Do, Q.T., Brockmeyer, A., Joubert, C., Bhatia, K. and Abdel-Jelil, M. (2016) *Middle East and North Africa Economic Monitor, October 2016: Economic and Social Inclusion to Prevent Violent Extremism*, Washington, DC: World Bank. Online. Available at https://openknowledge.worldbank.org/handle/10986/25087 (accessed 20 March 2019).

El-Jardali, F., Bou-Karroum, L., Ataya, N., El-Ghali, H.A. and Hammoud, R. (2014) 'A retrospective health policy analysis of the development and implementation of the voluntary health insurance system in Lebanon: learning from failure', *Social Science and Medicine*, 123: 45–54.

El-Jardali, F. and Fadlallah, R. (2015) 'A call for a backward design to knowledge translation', *International Journal of Health Policy and Management*, 4: 105.

El-Jardali, F., Makhoul, J., Jamal, D., Ranson, M.K., Kronfol, N.M. and Tchaghchagian, V. (2010) 'Eliciting policymakers' and stakeholders' opinions to help shape health system research priorities in the Middle East and North Africa region', *Health Policy and Planning*, 25: 15–27.

Lavis, J.N., Permanand, G., Oxman, A.D., Lewin, S. and Fretheim, A. (2009) 'SUPPORT tools for evidence-informed health Policymaking (STP) 13: preparing and using policy briefs to support evidence-informed policymaking', *Health Research Policy and Systems*, 7(1): S13.

Makhoul, J. and El-Barbir, F. (2006) 'Obstacles to health in the Arab world', *BMJ*, 333: 859.

Mitton, C., Smith, N., Peacock, S., Evoy, B. and Abelson, J. (2009) 'Public participation in health care priority setting: a scoping review', *Health Policy*, 91: 219–28.

Monshipouri, M. and Whooley, J. (2011) 'Minorities and marginalized communities in the middle east: the case for inclusion', in M. Monshipouri (ed) *Human Rights in the Middle East*. New York: Palgrave Macmillan.

Nasreddine, L., Naja, F., Akl, C., Chamieh, M.C., Karam, S., Sibai, A.M. and Hwalla, N. (2014) 'Dietary, lifestyle and socio-economic correlates of overweight, obesity and central adiposity in Lebanese children and adolescents', *Nutrients*, 6: 1038–62.

Nasreddine, L., Naja, F., Chamieh, M.C, Adra, N., Sibai, A.M. and Hwalla, N. (2012) 'Trends in overweight and obesity in Lebanon: evidence from two national cross-sectional surveys (1997 and 2009)', *BMC Public Health*, 12: 798–808.

Organisation for Economic Co-operation and Development [OECD] (2009) *Focus on Citizens: Public Engagement for Better Policy and Services*, Paris: OECD.

Oxman, A.D., Lewin, S., Lavis, J.N. and Fretheim, A. (2009) 'SUPPORT Tools for evidence-informed health Policymaking (STP) 15: engaging the public in evidence-informed policymaking', *Health Research Policy and Systems*, 7(1): S15.

Saleh, R. (2019) *K2P Citizen Consultations: School Policies for Childhood Obesity and Overweight Prevention in Lebanon*, Beirut: Knowledge to Policy (K2P) Center. Online. Available at www.aub.edu.lb/k2p/Documents/K2P%20Citizen%20Consultation%20 on%20School%20Policies%20for%20Childhood%20Obesity%20Prevention-%20 March%202019.pdf (accessed 5 November 2019).

Saleh, R., Nakkash, R. and El-Jardali, F. (2019) *K2P Policy Brief: Promoting Effective School Policies for Childhood Overweight and Obesity Prevention in Lebanon*, Beirut, Lebanon: Knowledge to Policy (K2P) Center. Online. Available at www.aub.edu.lb/ k2p/Documents/K2P%20Policy%20Brief-%20School%20Policies%20for%20Child hood%20Obesity%20Prevention%20in%20Lebanon-March%202019.pdf (accessed 5 November 2019).

Silver, H. (2007) 'Social exclusion: comparative analysis of Europe and middle east youth', Middle East Youth Initiative Working Paper No. 1. Online. Available at https://papers. ssrn.com/sol3/papers.cfm?abstract_id=1087432 (accessed 15 October 2018).

Straus, S.E., Tetroe, J. and Graham, I. (2009) 'Defining knowledge translation', *Canadian Medical Association Journal*, 181: 165–8.

Taket, A., Crisp, B.R., Graham, M., Hanna, L. and Goldingay, S. (2014) 'Scoping social inclusion practice', in A. Taket, B.R. Crisp, M. Graham, L. Hanna, S. Goldingay and L. Wilson (eds) *Practising Social Inclusion*, London: Routledge.

United Nations (2010) 'Regional overview: youth in the Arab region'. Online. Available at https://social.un.org/youthyear/docs/Regional%20Overview%20Youth%20in%20the %20Arab%20Region-Western%20Asia.pdf (accessed 20 March 2019).

United Nations (2015) 'Transforming our world: the 2030 agenda for sustainable development'. Online. Available at https://sustainabledevelopment.un.org/post2015/transform ingourworld/publication (accessed 4 November 2019).

United Nations Development Programme [UNDP] (2016) *Arab Human Development Report 2016: Youth and the Prospects for Human Development in Changing Reality*, New York: UNDP. Online. Available www.arab-hdr.org/reports/2016/english/Execu tiveENG.pdf (accessed 15 October 2018).

United Nations Educational, Scientific and Cultural Organization [UNESCO] (2011) *Arab Youth: Civic Engagement and Economic Participation*, Beirut: UNESCO Regional Bureau. Online. Available at www.unesco.org/new/fileadmin/MULTIMEDIA/FIELD/ Beirut/pdf/YCE%20_EN.pdf (accessed 20 March 2019).

Williamson, L. (2014) 'Patient and citizen participation in health: the need for improved ethical support', *The American Journal of Bioethics*, 14(6): 4–16.

World Bank (2014) 'Strategic framework for mainstreaming citizen engagement in world bank group operations: engaging with citizens for improved results'. Online. Available at http://documents.worldbank.org/curated/en/266371468124780089/Strategic-frame work-for-mainstreaming-citizen-engagement-in-World-Bank-Group-operations-engag ing-with-citizens-for-improved-results (accessed 23 February 2017).

World Health Organization (1978) *Declaration of Alma Ata: Report of the International Conference on Primary Health Care*, Geneva: World Health Organization.

World Intellectual Property Organization (1995) *The Lebanese Constitution.* Online. Available at www.wipo.int/edocs/lexdocs/laws/en/lb/lb018en.pdf (accessed 15 October 2018).

Youth Forum for Youth Policy (2012) 'The document of youth policy in Lebanon'. Online. Available at www.youthforum-lb.org/en/index.php?option=com_content&view=article&id=87%3Ayouth-policy-in-lebanon-document&catid=47%3Arelevent-information&Itemid=155 (accessed 23 February 2017).

4 Social policy to support women's reproductive decision-making and access to economic participation and resources

An Australian case study

*Melissa Graham, Hayley McKenzie
and Greer Lamaro Haintz*

Introduction

Reproductive decision-making is complex, dictated by interconnected political, religious, social, and cultural beliefs and traditional gender roles. Tensions exist between women's reproductive rights and the highly regulated and politicised context in which reproductive decisions are made and carried out (Graham et al. 2016).

The social policy context for reproductive decision-making is based on international conventions to which Australia is a signatory and has adopted (United Nations 1948), ratified (United Nations 1979), or acceded to (United Nations 1999). Governments 'are obliged under international law to promote, protect, and fulfil people's fundamental rights. Nevertheless, through laws criminalising and regulating women's reproductive behaviors, governments indirectly and directly violate women's human rights' (Uberoi and de Bruyn 2013: 166). This is evident in the Australian context as the way in which these conventions have been enacted within the policy landscape has created a disconnect between women's reproductive rights and their ability to fully act on these rights (Graham et al. 2016). This is exacerbated by policy relating to reproduction being both a state and territory government responsibility; however, the broader social policy context is the responsibility of the federal government. Furthermore, there is inconsistency in reproductive policy across Australian states and territories. While policy can be used to promote and sustain inclusion, it can also be punitive (Uberoi and de Bruyn 2013).

This chapter explores how to create a social policy context which supports women and sustains their inclusion in economic participation and access to resources regardless of their reproductive intentions, desires, and choices. Rather than a possibility, it should be an expectation that social policies ensure women's reproductive rights and their full access to economic participation and resources.

This chapter draws on data from in-depth interviews with women, which explored the Australian social policy context in relation to women's reproductive decision-making. In particular, this research explored the role of policy on and support for reproductive decision. While this chapter has a specific focus on economic participation and access to resources, sustainable inclusive social policy could be explored focusing on other policy areas, recognising that social inclusion is broader than economic participation.

For the purpose of this chapter, economic participation and access to resources refers to women's participation in the labour force and associated resources to support labour force participation, for example, leave entitlements and flexible workplace arrangements. Illustrative quotes are used and are denoted by the participant's pseudonym and age. The next section explores challenges to women's economic participation and their access to resources to support it before the chapter moves on to consider four elements that can move social policy in a more helpful direction.

Challenges to women's access to economic participation and resources

Reproductive policies are generally considered to be those that relate specifically to fertility, family planning, abortion, and maternal mortality. The influence of social policy on reproductive policy must be considered when exploring how to ensure policies to support women's reproductive decision-making and their access to economic participation and resources. Social policy influences women's reproductive decision-making, and women's reproductive decision-making and choices are regulated through social policies (Graham et al. 2016).

Pronatalism underpins Australia's social policy landscape (Dever 2005; Jackson and Casey 2009). This ideological positioning of women's purpose as procreators conflicts with the increasing demand for and by women for access to other life choices and pathways through education, employment, economic independence from men and the state, equality, and freedom to make their own reproductive choices, including if, when, and how many children to have along with access to affordable reliable contraception and termination of pregnancy. Furthermore, positioning women solely as mothers conflicts with competing policies which situate women as economic contributors to society. As such, the social policy landscape has created a context whereby women are dual citizens with competing demands: women as mothers and women as workers. This conflict is described by Lily as a burden, and she questions how social policies designed to support women as mothers and workers are equitably supporting all women and their reproductive choices, highlighting the gendering of caring responsibilities.

> I suppose I say burden because that's how I feel it's portrayed that women are a burden on society if they're receiving payments or they're out of the workforce and you know their partner's there to pay for them or support the family. I suppose I see it as or the way things influence me is that I think I need to be a productive member of society and that's how we've been raised to be productive members of society and I feel that unfortunately the way society views that is to be working. . . . That being a financial contributor to

the country is really your duty and if you're taking time out to have a family, you're expected that you will go back to work, hopefully as soon as six months but no more than 12 months really. . . . How do you manage your finite sick leave, carer's leave, annual leave that doesn't actually match up with the same impacts of school holidays and illness and everything else? I suppose, I don't know that is equally shared between both the male and the female when making those decisions in a heterosexual relationship.

(Lily, aged 30)

Amelia highlights the conflict in social policy designed to return women to the workforce once their child reaches a certain age and the lack of support in social policy to actually achieve this.

I don't know how women cope now, given that that pension's [Parenting Payment] not available and I guess once their child turns eight, expecting them to just magically find a job is quite bizarre, especially women coming from generational poverty and things like that. They might not have the capacity to learn new skills and knowledge in terms of to go and get employment, and the majority of employers want someone with experience so if the government isn't providing those women with formal training to get a qualification, so not only have they not got the qualification, but they haven't got the experience, so they're not going to be able to get a job, so to put them on Newstart [unemployment benefit] puts them and their children at a disadvantage.

(Amelia, aged 42)

Social policies, including parental leave, childcare subsidies, flexible work arrangements, leave entitlements, and gender equality, presumably have been designed to support equity for women by making motherhood more compatible with labour force participation and therefore access to economic participation and resources. However, these types of social policies also have a degree of pronatalist purpose which does not necessarily support sustaining women's social inclusion in economic participation, thus creating a conflict. While these social policies appear to have dual agendas, it does not necessarily mean they are incompatible; however, it is indicative of disconnect and conflict and creates challenges for women, their reproductive decision-making and economic participation, and access to resources, and thus it challenges their sustained inclusion.

Analysis of 18 federal level social policies which influence reproductive decision-making suggests these policies 'aim to regulate, control and selectively support women's reproduction while silencing, marginalising and reprimanding some groups of women, subsequently failing to allow for alternative discourse or positions to be represented' (Graham et al. 2018: 161). Furthermore, this study found a lack of ideological coherence both within and between the social policies and that they failed to consider the diversity of women and their lives (Graham et al. 2018). The consequence of this incoherence for women's reproductive decision-making is a social policy landscape which fails to sustain women's inclusion in and access to economic participation and resources. The following sections discuss potential solutions to these challenges.

Creating social policy to support women's reproductive decision-making and access to economic participation and resources

The Australian social policy context requires women to navigate a range of complex policy systems at both the federal and state or territory level when deciding if to have a child, timing of a pregnancy, returning to work, breastfeeding in the workplace, discrimination in the workplace, superannuation, financial security, and independence through income. However, it is through the design, delivery, and review of these policies that inclusion is sustained and particularly women's economic participation and access to resources. Inclusive policy has been defined as

> transparent, evidence driven, accessible and responsive to as wide a range of citizens as possible. It strives to include a diverse number of voices and views in the policy-making process, including traditional cultures. To be successful, these elements must be applied at all stages of the design and delivery of public policies and services. While inclusive policy making enhances transparency, accountability and public participation and builds civic capacity, it also offers a way for governments to improve their policy performance by working with citizens, civil society organizations (CSOs), businesses and other stakeholders to deliver concrete improvements in policy outcomes and the quality of public services.
>
> (Organisation for Economic Co-operation and Development [OECD] 2013: 146)

Sevciuc (2014: 111) provides a useful analytical framework for inclusive policy design and demonstrates the need for multiple layers of action, emphasising that 'inclusive policy is concerned with adequate inclusion of all parties in the process of policy design and delivery and, at the same time, with producing the outcome of inclusion'. Markers of inclusive policy should be considered based on contextual factors and the intended outcomes of social policy (Sevciuc 2014) rather than addressing all layers of action for all policy, noting that no single policy can create sustainable social inclusion; it is the combination and coherence of social policy that has the potential to sustain inclusion. Yet as demonstrated, Australia's social policy context for women's reproductive decision-making and full access to economic participation and resources is not coherent. To address the shortcomings, sustainable inclusive social policy to support women's reproductive decision-making and their full access to economic participation and resources requires women's participation in the design, delivery, and review of policy and that all social policy is examined for gender impact. The following sections outline four different elements of a potential solution: assessing social policy for gender impacts; shifting gender norms in policy; including the voices of women; and implementing policy.

Assessing social policy for gender impacts

In Australia, gender impact assessment of social policy is not routinely undertaken (OECD 2013). This has consequences for women as social policy is not gender neutral and can affect women's economic participation and access to resources. Social policies such as the *Paid Parental Leave Act* (Office of Parliamentary Counsel 2013) and the *Workplace Gender Equality Act 2012* (Office of Parliamentary Counsel 2012) affect men and women differently and have a greater impact on women as mothers, the presumed primary carer of children. Analysis of Australian federal level social policy revealed the discourses and regulatory mechanisms implicit in policies that positioned women primarily as mothers and carers and secondly as workers. For instance, the *Paid Parental Leave Act* positioned women as the primary carer of children, requiring them to manage their mothering responsibilities and their return to paid employment. In contrast, men are not required to manage these two competing responsibilities despite the scheme's aim to promote equality between genders and a balance between work and family life (Graham et al. 2018). Similarly, the *Workplace Gender Equality Act 2012* was found to unconsciously promote traditional gender roles of women as carers, placing caring burden on women rather than men (Graham et al. 2018). Both these social policies, while arguably designed to support women manage their dual roles as mothers and workers, perpetuate pronatalist ideology reinforcing women's role as mother and men's roles as breadwinners. This is further discussed in the following section on *Shifting gender norms in policy*.

Gender impact assessment has the potential to redress the gender inequity in social policy which has consequences for women and their full access to economic participation and resources. Redressing inequity in gender-blind social policy through gender impact assessment can make women visible in social policy and enable the differential impacts on women and men to be addressed. However, it must also be acknowledged that social policies do not affect all women in the same way, and as such, gender impact assessment needs to take an intersectional approach since women are not a homogenous group. An intersectional approach would consider the diversity of women's socio-demographic characteristics and position, the intersections between these characteristics, and the intersections with institutional processes of power and oppression (Hankivsky 2012; Hankivsky et al. 2009).

Applying an intersectional gender impact assessment lens would support the operationalisation of multiple international rights conventions, including the *Universal Declaration of Human Rights* (United Nations 1948), the *Declaration on the Rights of Disabled Persons* (United Nations 2006), and the *Convention on the Elimination of All Forms of Discrimination Against Women* (United Nations 1979). As previously highlighted, social policy does not work in a silo, and rather a multitude of factors representing and recognising diversity need to be taken into consideration to ensure a comprehensive and inclusive social policy landscape. Furthermore, ensuring that social policy is underpinned by and consistent with a human rights approach and more specifically, in this instance, reproductive rights can work toward creating sustained inclusion for women in social policy. Creating a social policy context which takes account of gender and intersectional differences has the potential to positively impact women's daily lived experiences of reproductive decision-making and their full access to economic participation and resources.

Shifting gender norms in policy

> This is what we were meant to be able to do, to balance our lives and choose what we wanted to do with our lives.
>
> (Ruby, aged 44)

The preservation of socially ascribed gender roles for women is apparent in much Australian social policy. The gender mainstreaming efforts that have taken place (Hankivsky 2008) have not necessarily addressed traditional gender roles and norms which are still perpetuated in social policy positions, for example, the Paid Parental Leave scheme. Beyond and in addition to strengthening gender mainstreaming, additional approaches are required.

Social and cultural norms influence social policy design, delivery, and review and, as such, can remove women's agency and prevent advances in gender equity (Domingo et al. 2015). As discussed under *Assessing policy for gender impacts*, traditional gender roles continue to pervade social policy and, as such, affect women's full economic participation and access to resources. Within this policy discourse, women's financial dependence on the state is viewed as problematic while women's financial dependence on men is not (Graham et al. 2018). To create sustainable, inclusive social policy, women's dependence on men should also be viewed as problematic, and social policy should advocate for, promote, and facilitate women's financial independence. This requires a shift in policy discourse which can be achieved through removing assumptions about women's roles and positions in society and applying a gender lens to the design, delivery, and review of social policy: a process known as gender-transformative policy and practice.

A shift from the neoliberal discourse of men as breadwinners and women as mothers and carers is required along with challenging the pervasive representation of the traditional family archetype: mum, dad, and children. From this perspective, not only is a gender-impact lens required along with gender mainstreaming, but so too is a reconsideration of how 'family' is defined and how the traditional construct of 'family' pervades social policy, which is not inclusive of all women or family types. If social policies shift from an assumption of traditional family structures and ascribed gender norms to account for the changing roles of women and men in society, the impact of social policies on women's reproductive decision-making and their constrained access to economic participation and resources would be reduced. Ideally in the future, women's economic participation and access to resources would not be influenced by reproductive decision-making, and women's reproductive decision-making would not influence economic participation and access to resources in the way it currently generally does not for men. Furthermore, such a shift in social policies could influence social and cultural beliefs about women's role in society and consequently improve equity. However, it must be acknowledged that social change is a slow process, with a long lead time between a change to social policy and social change. Women's experiences of traditional gender roles and constructs of family in relation to economic participation and access to resources is discussed further in the section on policy implementation.

Including the voices of women

Women's voices have historically been and continue to be absent in the design, delivery, and review of social policies. This exclusion removes women's agency and power in relation to their reproductive decision-making process as their 'choices' are restricted by policy and legislation:

> just not treating women as though they have power over their own bodies.
>
> (Mia, aged 45)

Schofield and Goodwin (2005: 17–18) argue in their analysis of gender politics in policymaking that a number of conditions are required to advance gender equality in the policymaking processes, including 'participation by community-based, feminist advocacy groups throughout the process'. The exclusion of women's voices from the social policymaking process can be addressed through meaningful consultation in the design, delivery, and review of policy. The OECD has produced guidelines for inclusive policy making which states that

> all citizens should have equal opportunities and multiple channels to access information, be consulted and participate. Every reasonable effort should be made to engage with as wide a variety of people as possible' and 'public engagement should be undertaken as early in the policy process as possible to allow a greater range of solutions and to raise the chances of successful implementation. Adequate time must be available for consultation and participation to be effective.
>
> (OECD 2009: 17)

Osborne et al. (2010) provide a useful discussion on the types of consultation and how community consultation inclusive of women can be achieved. Some social policies, for example, the *National Women's Health Policy 2010* (Australian Government Department of Health and Ageing 2010), include the voice of women; however not all women are included or represented. Not only are women's voices through co-production essential in social policy design, delivery, and review, but also a diverse representation of women is required. Moving away from policy focusing on traditional families through gender-transformative policy and practice would support the inclusion of a diversity of women's voices. An intersectional lens can ensure that a diversity of women's voices is included. In doing so, social policies will acknowledge the heterogeneity of women's unique needs in relation to economic participation and access to resources.

Implementing policy

There are a range of social policies designed to increase women's inclusion in relation to economic participation and access to resources, particularly in relation to women as mothers and carers and less so in relation to women who are not mothers or women more generally, further highlighting the need for an intersectional lens. However, it is how these policies are designed and enacted that provides the potential to not only improve women's inclusion but also sustain their inclusion across the life course. For example, Ellie described a situation relating to women employees of reproductive age and maternity leave entitlements where her employer expressed their discontent with employing women as they will become pregnant and take leave.

> I had my last boss say to me that he had one of the girls I worked with fell pregnant and it kind of annoyed him that he was the one who had to take care of paying her maternity leave. And he said it's frustrating and it's really hard sometimes as an employer to hire people around my age when they're thinking of having kids, because if they fall pregnant it falls on them. And I think that makes me nervous. . . . I think that's going to affect me getting a job, so I feel like that makes me nervous.
>
> (Ellie, aged 27)

This motherhood penalty, which assumes all women are or will be mothers, penalises all women on the grounds that they may require time out of the workforce to have and care for children and that employers suffer the consequences. Social norms do not apply this same discourse to men. Social policies are designed to protect women from the discrimination expressed by Ellie's employer; however it is how policy is applied within the workplace that can positively impact women and sustain inclusive social policy, enabling women to have full economic participation and access to resources. A positive experience of the application of policy in the workplace is demonstrated by Zoe.

> I guess the policies that women can return to work after having your baby. I know that in my Mum's day, Mum said women couldn't return to work, so it was comforting to know that if you want to return to work once you've had a baby that you are allowed to in our society. And there's breastfeeding policies to allow babies to be fed wherever babies are allowed to be, which

includes the workplace, which assisted in giving me the confidence to be able to continue breastfeeding once I returned to work.

(Zoe, aged 36)

For others, they highlighted the practicalities of putting these policies into practice and the everyday experiences within the policy environment:

I'm not saying the workplace isn't family friendly, but when I think when you break it down to individual managers, especially if it's not being reported through—and that's my other issue as well that I need to speak to HR: where do I gain support from the organisation if I find my manager isn't supporting me to be family friendly? Yeah and for me the added frustration is when you're dealing with women who have got families and it's like 'well you did this' and I think again, that generation gap, they probably just took time off, had their kids and then came back into the workplace either later on or—I'm not sure, I've never had a conversation with them, but I just get this impression that they didn't have—they had policies available to them and they're fine, so why should need that? That's the feeling I get.

(Renee, aged 30)

While social policies may be in place, it is how women experience the delivery or implementation of policies that has the greatest impact on women in terms of their economic participation and access to resources. Policy is not uniformly applied to all women and situations. For example, previous research has identified that women without children have less access to workplace entitlements, including flexible work arrangements, work hours/shifts, and leave compared with mothers. Furthermore, women without children have reported being overlooked for employment and promotion because they did not have children (Graham et al. 2019; Turnbull et al. 2017, 2018). Women should be protected from this type of discrimination through social policies; however, the failure of policies to protect women does not necessarily lie within the policy design but rather how it is applied.

The implementation of social policy at the individual level is dictated by beliefs about women and men's roles and social-cultural norms. This suggests that addressing the implementation of social policy lies within the shifting of gender norms in policy as previously discussed. Social policies more inclusive of women and men's changing social roles would remove assumptions of women as mothers and men as breadwinners enabling equitable implementation of policies, placing the same expectations of women on men and vice versa. In doing so, the discrimination of women by employers, as expressed by Ellie, could be reduced as men would equally be recognised as fathers and therefore have caring responsibilities and women would be acknowledged as also being breadwinners. In this way, both women and men would be dual citizens, more evenly distributing and balancing economic participation and access to resources. There are numerous useful tools to support workplaces to apply gender equity practices (e.g. Nally et al. 2019) which would arguably aid in the redressing of the inequitable implementation of social policy at the individual level. However, it is beyond the scope of this chapter to explore these further as they sit outside of the broader social policy context.

Conclusions

Social policy is a complex web of competing interests, often promoting and encouraging certain pathways, as explored throughout in this chapter. This chapter has discussed the Australian social policy context in relation to women's experiences of their reproductive decision-making specifically in relation to sustaining their inclusion in economic participation and access to resources. It has highlighted that despite numerous policies in place to support women's reproductive decision-making, further work is required to ensure and sustain inclusion in social policy, including that specific to economic participation and access to resources. While this chapter has focused on the Australian policy context, it raises issues and offers considerations which are relevant elsewhere in similar social and cultural contexts.

Reproductive decision-making and reproductive-related policy cannot be considered in isolation from broader social policy. Underpinning this is Engeli's (2012) perspective on the reproductive policy making context as multifaceted and multilayered (involving various levels of stakeholders), emphasising the interactive nature of reproductive policy and social policy. Sevciuc's (2014) analytical framework for inclusive policy design also underscores the need for multiple layers of action in this area.

Furthermore, the broader social policy context is fluid. Social policy is dynamic and shifting with changes in society, such as the changing nature of gender norms, women's roles, and family structures. Thus, social policy must evolve and be responsive to contemporary contexts. As gender and family norms shift, social policy needs to continue to reflect these changes in a timely manner, with particular attention given to the diversity of women's roles and lives, their reproductive decisions and choices, and how these impact on economic participation and access to resources. As discussed, for example, when ensuring workplace flexibility, both women and men need to be considered in order to move beyond the perspective of 'mother as carer and father as breadwinner'. Responsive social policy would also include an intersectional gender impact assessment. This would enable recognition of the diversity of women and ensure this is at the forefront of policy design, delivery, and review.

Also notable for policymakers is the equal importance of both policy design and the implementation of policy. The chapter highlighted that social policy designed and appropriately *applied* to shift gender norms is needed. However, to support this, more conscientious effort is needed in areas of advocacy and accountability in the implementation of policy. This also highlights the necessity for continual monitoring of policy development and implementation and the intended and unintended impacts of social policy on reproductive decision-making for women's economic participation, access to resources, and sustained inclusion.

For Australia, the chapter highlights opportunities to explore more inclusive policy design. In particular, four key areas for creating policy which sustains inclusion were identified: assessing social policy for gender impacts; shifting gender norms in policy; including the voices of women; and implementing policy. Various tools have been identified to assist policymakers in this, including gender impact assessment, intersectional policy analysis (Hankivsky 2008, 2012; Hankivsky et al. 2009, 2014), and Sevciuc's (2014) analytical framework for inclusive policy design.

References

Australian Government Department of Health and Ageing (2010) *National Women's Health Policy 2010*, Canberra: Australian Government Department of Health and Ageing. Online. Available at www.health.gov.au/internet/main/publishing.nsf/Content/3BC 776B3C331D5EECA257BF0001A8D46/$File/NWHP.pdf (accessed 13 March 2019).

Dever, M. (2005) 'Baby talk: the Howard Government, families, and the politics of difference', *Hecate*, 31: 45–61.

Domingo, P., Holmes, R., O'Neil, T., Jones, N., Bird, K., Larson, A., Presler-Marshall, E. and Valters, C. (2015) *Women's Voice and Leadership in Decision-making: Assessing the Evidence*, London: Overseas Development Institute. Online. Available at www.odi. org/sites/odi.org.uk/files/odi-assets/publications-opinion-files/9627.pdf (accessed 13 March 2019).

Engeli, I. (2012) 'Policy struggle on reproduction: doctors, women, and Christians', *Political Research Quarterly*, 65: 330–45.

Graham, M., McKenzie, H. and Lamaro, G. (2018) 'Exploring the Australian policy context relating to women's reproductive choices', *Policy Studies*, 39: 145–64.

Graham, M., McKenzie, H., Lamaro, G. and Klein, R. (2016) 'Women's reproductive choices in Australia: mapping federal and state/territory policy instruments governing choice', *Gender Issues*, 33: 335–49.

Graham, M.L., McKenzie, H., Turnbull, B. and Taket, A.R. (2019) ' "Them and us": the experience of social exclusion among women without children in their post-reproductive years', *Journal of Research in Gender Studies*, 9: 71–104.

Hankivsky, O. (2008) 'Gender mainstreaming in Canada and Australia: a comparative analysis', *Policy and Society*, 27: 69–81.

Hankivsky, O. (2012) *An Intersectionality-Based Policy Analysis Framework*, Vancouver, BC: Institute for Intersectionality Research and Policy, Simon Fraser University. Online. Available at https://data2.unhcr.org/en/documents/download/46176 (accessed 13 March 2019).

Hankivsky, O., Cormier, R. and de Merich, D. (2009) *Intersectionality: Moving Women's Health Research and Policy Forward*, Vancouver, BC: Women's Health Research Network. Online. Available at http://bccewh.bc.ca/2014/02/intersectionality-moving-wom ens-health-research-and-policy-forward/ (accessed 13 March 2019).

Hankivsky, O., Grace, D., Hunting, G., Giesbrecht, M., Fridkin, A., Rudrum, S., Ferlatte, O. and Clark, N. (2014) 'An intersectionality-based policy analysis framework: critical reflections on a methodology for advancing equity', *International Journal for Equity in Health*, 13: 119.

Jackson, N. and Casey, A. (2009) 'Procreate and cherish: a note on Australia's abrupt shift to pro-natalism', *New Zealand Population Review*, 35: 129–48.

Nally, T., Taket, A. and Graham, M. (2019) 'Exploring the use of resources to support gender equality in Australian workplaces', *Health Promotion Journal of Australia*, 30: 359–70.

Office of Parliamentary Counsel (2012) *Workplace Gender Equality Act 2012 (Act No. 91 of 1986 as amended)*, Canberra: Commonwealth of Australia Office of Parliamentary Counsel.

Office of Parliamentary Counsel (2013) *Paid Parental Leave Act 2010 (No. 104, 2010 as amended)*, Canberra: Commonwealth Government Office of Parliamentary Counsel.

Organisation for Economic Co-operation and Development [OECD] (2009) *Focus on Citizens: Public Engagement for Better Policy and Service*, Paris: OECD Publishing.

Organisation for Economic Co-operation and Development [OECD] (2013) *Government at a Glance 2013*, Paris: OECD Publishing.

Osborne, K., Bacchi, C. and MacKenzie, D.C. (2010) 'Gender analysis and community participation: the role of women's policy units', in C. Bacchi and J. Eveline (eds) *Mainstreaming Politics: Gendering Practices and Feminist Theory*, Adelaide: University of Adelaide Press.

Schofield, T. and Goodwin, S. (2005) 'Gender politics and public policy making: prospects for advancing gender equality', *Policy and Society*, 24: 25–44.

Sevciuc, I. (2014) 'Analytical framework for inclusive policy design: of what, why and how MOST Working Document', *International Social Science Journal*, 65: 109–32.

Turnbull, B., Graham, M. and Taket, A. (2017) 'Pronatalism and social exclusion in Australian society: experiences of women in their reproductive years with no children', *Gender Issues*, 34: 333–54.

Turnbull, B., Graham, M. and Taket, A. (2018) 'Understanding the employment experiences of women with no children', in N. Sappleton (ed) *Voluntary and Involuntary Childlessness: The Joys of Otherhood?* Bingley: Emerald Publishing Limited.

Uberoi, D. and de Bruyn, M. (2013) 'Human rights versus legal control over women's reproductive self-determination', *Health and Human Rights*, 15: 161–74.

United Nations (1948) 'Universal declaration of human rights'. Online. Available at www.refworld.org/docid/3ae6b3712c.html (accessed 4 November 2019).

United Nations (1979) *Convention on the Elimination of All Forms of Discrimination Against Women*. Online. Available at www.ohchr.org/Documents/ProfessionalInterest/cedaw.pdf (accessed 5 November 2019).

United Nations (1999) *Optional Protocol to the Convention on the Elimination of All Forms of Discrimination Against Women*. Online. Available at www.ohchr.org/Documents/HRBodies/CEDAW/OP_CEDAW_en.pdf (accessed 5 November 2019).

United Nations (2006) 'Convention on the rights of persons with disabilities'. Online. Available at www.un.org/development/desa/disabilities/convention-on-the-rights-of-persons-with-disabilities/convention-on-the-rights-of-persons-with-disabilities-2.html (accessed 4 November 2019).

5   Not impossible

Working with the Deafblind community to develop a more inclusive world

Alana Roy, Beth R. Crisp and Keith McVilly

Introduction

Deafblindness has been recognised by the European Parliament (2004) as a 'separate and distinct disability' and not simply the addition of vision and hearing impairments. Although Deafblindness impacts all aspects of life (Lee-Foster 2010), the capacity of people who are Deafblind to communicate and fully participate in society is compromised 'to such a degree that society is required to facilitate specific services, environmental alterations and or technology' (Nordic Centre for Social Welfare and Social Issues 2019).

Deafblind people experience marginalisation, exclusion, and oppression from professionals, family members, carers, deaf, and mainstream communities. Their experience of social exclusion typifies the explanation of Taket et al. (2009: 15) who explain social exclusion being the result of 'multiple deprivations . . . and mutually reinforcing effects of reduced participation, consumption, mobility access, integration, influence and recognition' which result in 'marginalising, silencing, rejecting, isolating, segregation and disenfranchising'. A small survey of Deafblind individuals from the UK found that that only three out of the ten participants had met another Deafblind person, only one of whom had regular contact with another Deafblind person (Barnett 2001).

The complexity and idiosyncratic nature of Deafblind communication needs are also influenced by a multiplicity of factors such as the age of onset of the dual sensory loss; the degree, type, and cause of the impairment; education; socioeconomic status; additional disabilities; exposure to communication modalities and supports; cultural and social networks; and differences in age, gender, ethnicity, religion, and culture (Brennan 2003; Brennan and Bally 2007; Mathos et al. 2011). Furthermore, Deafblind people utilise a variety of communication methods and do not share a common language. Touch to express thoughts, feelings, and language was identified as being a unique characteristic of Deafblind interactions (Barnett 2001).

Deafblind interpreting includes a range of approaches, many of which are forms of communication unique to the Deafblind community (Deafblind UK 2019; Frankel 2002; Grassick 2001; Reed et al. 1989; Rodriguez-Gil and Belote 2005). In addition to enabling the transmission of messages to and from people who are Deafblind, some forms of interpreting also facilitate a Deafblind person's sense of orientation, which refers to a person's ability to use their senses to know where they are positioned in their environment. Deafblind interpreting can also assist mobility, which refers to a person's capability to move within their environment. Methods utilised by Deafblind interpreters include:

- lip reading;
- sign language;
- signed English;
- key word signing;
- Deafblind manual alphabet;
- tadoma (Deafblind person places their thumb on the speaker's lips and their fingers along the jawline);
- co-active signing (taking the Deafblind person's hands and, in a respectful way, moulding signs and helping the Deafblind person to feel the signs);
- visual frame signing (signs are produced in a confined space depending on client needs); hard return close vision (the interpreter sits very close to the Deafblind person);
- tracking (client holds onto the wrists of the interpreter to ensure signs are kept within their field of vision);
- tactile signing (the Deafblind person accesses signs through hand-over-hand touch);
- haptics (touch used in social communication, e.g. to convey emotions, orientation in a room, or on a map);
- tactile fingerspelling (two-handed manual alphabet is produced onto the palm of the Deafblind person and shortcut signs (key signs produced on the palm of the clients hand to further support tactile sign); and
- voice-over interpreting in the ear of a Deafblind person who has residual hearing, gestures, body language, and facial expressions.

Many people refrain from communicating with Deafblind people due to the rigors of tactile signing (O'Brien and Steffen 1996), the need for touch, and close personal space to aid conversation (Brennan 2003; Brennan et al. 2005; Miner 1997). Consequently, Deafblind people are arguably one of the most socially isolated groups in the world. They are supported by a small group of specialist 'gatekeepers of knowledge' who typically advocate strongly for Deafblind people, often in relation to health concerns (Bodsworth et al. 2011). Frequently this occurs on the basis of their professional opinions rather than being based on consultation or engagement with the Deafblind community (Roy et al. 2018).

Research and consultation processes commonly rely on methodologies that assume participants have full use of all their senses and that they are part of a hearing and sighted world (Heine and Browning 2014). Much of what is known about the experience of being Deafblind comes not directly from people who are Deafblind but from the professionals who work with people who are Deafblind. Evidence of paternalistic attitudes and understanding of Deafblindness as a medical condition predominate in the associated literature (see Hersh 2013). Although it is essential to understand the challenges and needs of the Deafblind community, the literature typically describes Deafblind people in negative terms, i.e. as persons who have problems, particularly in respect of communication barriers and mental health issues, with little or no recognition of strengths (e.g. Jaiswal et al. 2018). As such, the Deafblind experience is often portrayed as something that needs to be rehabilitated; the Deafblind world is often described in terms of loss and vulnerability (Brennan et al. 2005; Simcock 2017; Simcock and Manthorpe 2014).

There is a growing imperative in research and policy development to shift the focus from conducting 'research on' or developing 'policy about' people who are Deafblind to a focus on research and policy development that is inclusive of people who are Deafblind (Selepak 2008). Although there is growing agreement among researchers and policymakers that people with the lived experience of disability, including those who are Deafblind, should be included in the formation of public policy, there is a dearth of literature to guide such practice (Bruce and Parker 2012; Mathos et al. 2011).

Consultation, research, and policy development has a history of 'doing research on people'. These processes began to shift in the 1940s to 1960s by attempting to 'engage and involve people'. Since the 1970s, various academic, public, and private domains have evolved with social movements and adopted the position of 'co-production and co-design' with employees, managers, partners, customers, citizens, end users, participants, and researchers (Bovaird and Loeffler 2010). Co-production as a process emerged as a way to engage communities in consultation, policy, and service delivery (Zarb 1992). Co-production seeks to engage stakeholders in dynamic and respectful communication with the goal of using lived experiences to address areas of policy, research, and service delivery.

Consistent with such approaches, in recent times there has been a rise in the use of 'community conversations' as a qualitative methodology to engage people with lived experiences in consultation, research, service, and policy development (Dutta et al. 2016). Despite being increasingly common for people living with other disabilities such as people with intellectual disabilities (Tanabe et al. 2018), people living with Autism (Milton 2014), and deaf communities (Barnett et al. 2011; Taylor 2010), to date, however, there has been little evidence of co-production with Deafblind people (Roy et al. 2018). One exception is a study conducted by Bruce and Parker (2012), who actively engaged young Deafblind adults aged 18–24 years in participatory research and co-production (with a focus on advocacy and self-determination). Not only did Deafblind participants contribute data about their lived experiences, but they were also actively involved in data analysis and generating key themes to inform policy and practice developments. Moreover, the work of Bruce and Parker provides an evidence base that attests to the capacity for Deafblind people to be active participants in the process of co-production of knowledge.

Although the Deafblind community struggles for inclusion and social recognition, recent advances in education, employment, leadership, and technology are enabling the Deafblind community to become more independent and connected.

For example, communication via Braille displays, iPhones, Skype, and email may be resulting in an increasingly more independent Deafblind culture, which is less reliant on outsiders for facilitating communication within the Deafblind community (Roy et al. 2019). These forms of communication are also facilitating new ways for Deafblind individuals to communicate with the wider societies in which they live, including participating in camps, international conferences, meetings, and cultural celebrations (Kowalski 2018; Mills 2019). The remainder of this chapter presents work undertaken by the authors to engage Deafblind people in community conversations, taking into account issues of language and communication, social inclusion, accessibility, and developments in assistive technology.

Developing a process for consultation

Engaging Deafblind people in consultative processes is a complex process due to the inherent power imbalances that exists between Deafblind people and the gate-keepers of knowledge in the community. Many Deafblind people rely on small group of professionals for communication and linguistic support, emotional and life skill guidance, orientation, and mobility support. Although gatekeepers of knowledge in the Deafblind community often seek to amplify the experiences, opinions, and expertise of Deafblind people, to date no one has actually asked Deafblind people what might constitute good practice approaches to consultation.

A first step in building a consultation process was for the first author to discuss, with service providers, including interpreters, the logistics of conducting a group consultation with the Deafblind community. One of the key issues that emerged was the likely need for interpreters for every Deafblind participant. As there are a relatively small number of interpreters qualified to work with the Deafblind community, a proposed date for a consultation was set well in advance to ensure all the interpreters in the State of Victoria were available on that day. Other con-siderations raised at this time included suitable spaces that might be available and the need to brief interpreters on what was expected of them at such an event. The possibility that a consultative event with the Deafblind community took the form of a World Café was also explored at this time.

World Café methodology is an adapted form of a focus group which draws upon appreciative inquiry (Cooperrider and Whitney 1999), an approach to research that asks 'what currently works', 'what form might it take if it was to be better than it currently is', and 'how might we achieve this enhanced/improved experience?' In particular, World Café provides a systematised method for implementing a series of small group discussions among large groups of people. World Café is designed to 'get people interacting', as a means of data generation. As such, small group discussions support people with specific (lived) experience in the topic of inquiry to interact and formulate solutions and future directions in response to a research question or topic of inquiry (Sheridan et al. 2010). World Café methodology has been utilised across a range of academic settings, business, community, and nongovernment settings with diverse groups of people (Brown et al. 2005; Fouché and Light 2011).

World Café methodology differs from a traditional focus group in that the overall environment should attempt to resemble a café-style atmosphere (e.g. food, coffee and tea, waiters, and decorative table settings). This attention to the environment is asserted to enhance the quality of the discussion. Furthermore, the World Café typically consists of three rounds of research questions, between which people move from one group to another to promote the sharing and cross-pollination of ideas. However, one participant from each group remains at a table to 'host' the next group and share the insights that were generated from the previous round (Brown et al. 2005).

Due to the inherent complexities conducting a World Café with Deafblind people, a World Café expert was consulted in regard to how to make World Café methodology accessible to this population. Traditionally World Café should consist of 12 or more people with tables of at least four. However, the World Café expert acknowledged the small sample sizes that Deafblind studies typically yield and suggested that tables of three would also be appropriate. Moreover, it was deemed appropriate, but notably challenging, to also accommodate and allow for the interactions of additional support people (e.g. support workers and interpreters). The World Café expert recommended using stories to help set up the context and encouraged the host to be aware of the language used, for example,

> I would find the language that spoke to my specific group. So, it might be in that case "what are you noticing?" or "what are you aware of?" Or you know, just changing the language so that it fits the needs of who you are with.

Furthermore, she acknowledged that consulting with professionals in the field of Deafblindness and educating them on Deafblind World Café methodology would be key to the delivery of the methodology.

One of the adaptations which was made to the World Café format was that participants initially formed a single large group and were given an introduction regarding the key principles of appreciative inquiry, together with World Café principles and etiquette (Brown et al. 2005; Vogt 2005). It was also explained that familiar support staff would be available during the day to provide support to individual participants, including assisting in the logistics of moving between groups. The World Café event was specifically scheduled for five hours, which is considerably longer than the traditional length of three hours. Given the complexities of sign language and tactile interpreting, it was anticipated that the participants and supporting professionals would need this additional time during the consultation process.

Participants engaged in three rounds of questioning. Each round took approximately 50 minutes. After each round, one participant from each table was asked to 'host' and provide a summary of the findings from the previous round of questions. All three rounds of research questions included the used of mixed communication modalities at each table (e.g. Australian Sign Language which is usually referred to as 'Auslan', tactile, and spoken language). Professional note takers were situated at each table, and throughout the World Café, they recorded participants' contributions to the conversation, including the communication type (e.g. Auslan, tactile, or spoken English).

Deafblind research participants are classified as 'vulnerable', according to Australia's *National Statement on the Ethical Conduct of Human Research* (National Health and Medical Research Council et al. 2018). Hence, a range of precautions was taken when recruiting participants for the World Cafés. A specialist provider of services to the Deafblind population contacted potential participants on behalf of the first author. Participants were able to provide independent, informed consent and told that they could withdraw from the World Café at any time and that withdrawing would not impact on any ongoing professional relationships or service delivery. In addition, the Plain Language and Consent forms were produced in Auslan and Braille-accessible PDF form. Furthermore, all documentation was made into a video with an interpreter who communicated in both spoken English and Auslan. The video also included yellow subtitles to maximise accessibility. Documentation was also provided in a Microsoft Word document accessible via Braille displays and voice-over computer technology.

World Café 1

Our first World Café involved 15 Deafblind participants (10 female and 5 male) all of whom were recruited via specialist service providers for the Deafblind. Three participants used tactile sign language, five used Auslan sign language within a close visual frame, and six used spoken language. Most participants were born with various levels of hearing loss and acquired Deafblindness as a result of Ushers Syndrome, but participants also included two who acquired Deafblindness during early adulthood due to chronic pain conditions and one who was born with congenital Deafblindness due to rubella. This sample is typically representative of the current adult Deafblind Australian community (Dyke 2013).

The aim of this first World Café was to enable Deafblind individuals to provide feedback on their experiences of being consulted. In the first round, participants discussed questions about times when they had been asked their opinions about policies, procedures, and services. Participants identified complex communication and social barriers and experiences of oppression and marginalisation that they believe have become deeply entrenched within the Deafblind community. As one participant commented, 'there are a lot of Deafblind people who just take what they are given and don't speak out' (Auslan). This is particularly so, when processes for consulting are undertaken by outsiders who have good intentions but who lack the cultural and linguistic literacy needed to successfully engage this complex and diverse community (Brennan et al. 2005; Brennan and Bally 2007). In particular, Deafblind people are often silenced or oppressed by accidental audism and ableism (Barnett et al. 2011; Taylor 2010). Hence, Deafblind people need to trust, understand, and develop relationships with researchers and in their community to ensure 'that the people who make policies know the perspective of Deafblind people' (Auslan).

In the second round, participants were asked to review the 'Personal Wellbeing Index' (International Wellbeing Group 2013). This is widely used internationally in studies across different populations, including with people who experience a range of disabling circumstances. The seven-item Likert scale is generally considered relatively accessible and a format representative of the type of measures commonly used in research and policy consultation processes. Yet the experience of people who are Deafblind is that the construction of questionnaires or scales typically assume that the respondent had vision and hearing and spoke English. Participants recognised that there are linguistic, cultural and technological challenges of designing tools that can be translated from a spoken language into a visual language and again into a tactile language. They further understood how these factors negatively impact their answers when attempting to complete a questionnaire with numbered or categorised scales, both on their own and with the support of an interpreter. Moreover, if questionnaires with scales have to be used, then they need to be individually tailored to meet the needs of each Deafblind person. For example, 'a full braille document with lots of time to read and consider', 'very simple English with large font and large pictures to match the scale, technology to enlarge everything online'. Not one of the 15 Deafblind participants reported a positive or successful experience of completing a questionnaire with scales (categories or numbers), suggesting that validity is likely to be an issue when using this form of data collection. Instead there was consensus that the Deafblind community favoured 'face-to-face interactions with people who we can communicate with' (tactile) and struggled to share their opinions over the phone or via email— 'sharing in person is important with Deafblind people' (Auslan).

In the third round, the participants were asked to give their opinions of what they would like researchers and the general community to know about the Deafblind community. They identified the importance of fully accessible consultation processes (e.g. interpreters, technology, and cultural sensitivities) so that Deafblind people are given information, know their rights, and have opportunities to 'understand where we are in the world, we need to be encouraged to make decisions on our values and beliefs' (Auslan). For Deafblind people, all research, consultation, policy, and procedural information 'needs to be translated in braille, audio format and simple English'. Furthermore, Deafblind communication needs to be interpreted from English into Auslan, which is a visual language, and then into tactile sign language. Deafblind people value highly specialised communication, professionals, and researchers who have a positive attitude, are flexible, and willing to build strong and long-term working relationships.

Participants reported enjoying the rare opportunity to express their lived experiences with a diverse range of communication modes. However, they suggested that research and consultation methodologies, including the World Café methodology, should establish 'key terms and key signs' (Auslan) to help the both the Deafblind person and their interpreter. It was also suggested that being provided with examples and scenarios, as well as opportunities for them to share their life experiences, helped Deafblind people to absorb the information, unpack the meaning, and then provide their own opinions. Furthermore, it was acknowledged that this requires a significant amount of time but overcomes issues of interpreter errors, communication breakdowns, or the inaccessibility of complex jargon.

The venue chosen for the Deafblind World Cafè was a known Deafblind cultural hub that all the participants had previously attended; many Deafblind people could travel independently and feel comfortable with the orientation and mobility of this site. However, the size of the room resulted in difficulties that occurred when attempting to move Deafblind people and their supports around the room. (More than 30 people participated in the event as every participant required their own interpreter.) This meant that it was not possible to take full advantage of the World Café methodology which recommends participants move from table to table to increase the number of interactions among participants (and consequently the richness of the data) throughout the course of the discussion process.

World Café 2

A second World Café was convened which recruited 15 individuals (11 female and 4 male) who worked providing professional services to people who were Deafblind. These included people known to the research team or recommended via industry experts. Participants included three professionals who were themselves Deafblind (one who utilised Auslan within a close visual frame, one who utilised spoken English, and one who utilised both Auslan and spoken English) and four deaf participants who utilised Auslan. There were also eight participants who were hearing and sighted professionals who utilised spoken English as their primary mode of communication, all of whom had some training in Auslan.

The professionals World Café followed a similar format to the first World Café involving people living with Deafblindness. The professionals were asked similar questions and asked to consider and respond to the data that was generated via group consensus from the Deafblind community.

Initially the 'gatekeepers of knowledge', the professionals in the field of Deafblindness were surprised to learn that Deafblind people did not feel that they had adequately been included or consulted in policy and service development. Furthermore, after the Deafblind professionals discussed the findings of the Deafblind World Cafè, there was a shift in group consensus toward recognising the need to challenge current practices and learn new ways to engage Deafblind people. There appeared to be general agreement that one-to-one interviews, forums, and online surveys were the easiest and most common ways to engage Deafblind people in conversations. Nevertheless, the professionals noted that new frameworks and methodologies such as World Café would be helpful in seeking the lived experience of Deafblind people. Such frameworks can address the power imbalances inherent in individual interviews, given that World Café can bring peers together to discuss issues of mutual importance and concern. However, facilitating multiple rounds of mixed communication with Deafblind people (who use Auslan, tactile sign, and English) is a new challenge for Deafblind professionals as historically Deafblind people are often grouped in forums (e.g. one person speaks at a time) or placed into groups of matched communication.

Professionals in the field of Deafblindness have the challenging task of bringing together one of the most heterogenous groups known to researchers and policymakers, and these gatekeepers generally have little to no formal training or experience in research or policy development within a socially inclusive framework. However, these gatekeepers are the essential players in policy development and service delivery for the Deafblind community (Mathos et al. 2011). Professionals who provide services to the Deafblind community need to be supported in the development of their theoretical and methodological skills as they play a key role in facilitating the involvement of Deafblind people in research and policy contexts.

There was a lack of consensus among the professionals providing services to the Deafblind community as to the suitability of using surveys and standardised scales to gain the perspectives of Deafblind people. Whereas in the previous World Café, Deafblind people expressed the desire to be involved in consultation processes involving face-to-face conversations, professionals in the field of Deafblindness were concerned with the challenges to co-production, including lack of consultation, access to funding for such endeavours, and attitudinal barriers in the professional, academic, and community sectors. Furthermore, it was noted that Deafblind people are not just a culturally and linguistically diverse group but can experience additional disabilities and mental health challenges.

Conclusion

Research and consultation do not by themselves lead to social inclusion but are a critical component of policy development that leads to sustained social inclusion. Although the United Nation's (2015) Social Development Goals (SDGs) propose that no one should be left behind, there are groups of people who researchers and policymakers have historically regarded as being too difficult to consult with. This includes people who are Deafblind. Yet given the opportunity, people who are Deafblind are wanting to and capable of making their views known, even if the professionals who are gatekeepers to this community are less convinced this is feasible, except in special events such as those reported in this chapter.

Deafblind people want to be included and ultimately drive the Deafblind research agenda. They are already connecting and uniting, both within Australia and around the world, despite their differences and complex barriers. The Deafblind participants were united in their view that meaningful consultations, research, and policy development that leads to sustainable social inclusion needs to engage with the lived experience of those who are Deafblind. As one participant stated, 'we are Deafblind, step into our world' (Auslan user). Their stories and conversations echo the 'nothing about us without us' slogan, which has become a catch-cry for people with disability (Tanabe et al. 2018).

The professional gatekeepers of knowledge are those whose involvement with the Deafblind community tends to be as providers of health, welfare, and interpreting services. In developing the consultation process, their insights were nevertheless valuable, as they provided practical advice for best practice approaches to working with groups that are sensitive to Deafblind cultural, linguistic, and accessibility issues. However, professionals who have expertise in Deafblindness and sign language require support to develop their capacity to facilitate research and consultation processes. The first author is developing a toolkit that includes guidelines for research and consultation that honours the diversity, culture, and community of Deafblind people.

Government, researchers, and policymakers alike can learn a lot from the Deafblind community, as this group teaches us a lot about sustaining social inclusion in respect of technology, transport, and communication. Furthermore, the Deafblind community is a microcosm of diversity and complexity, which should be celebrated with pride. Not only do Deafblind people experience every expression of the human form, e.g. gender, race, age, ethnicity, sexual orientation, socioeconomic status, etc.; they do so with limited sight and hearing. Much can be learnt about creating an inclusive world by listening to Deafblind people and the professionals who support them. A society that is accessible to those who cannot hear and see will be making a more inclusive society for all.

Although this chapter explores the process of consulting with people who are Deafblind, our work to date, suggests the World Café format has potential for working with people with a range of complex communication, orientation, and mobility support needs to explore their subjective insights and experiences. However, reasonable adjustments to research and consultation processes need to be made to suit each context. This involves specialist communications supports being available and recognising that for some groups, research and consultation methodologies that involved standardised questionnaires may be impossible for participants to engage with.

References

Barnett, S. (2001) 'Deafblind culture in the UK', *DbI Review*, 29: 7–11.

Barnett, S., Klein, J.D., Pollard, R.Q., Samar, V., Schlehofer, D. Starr, M., Sutter, E., Yang, H. and Pearson, T.A. (2011) 'Community participatory research with deaf sign language users to identify health inequities', *American Journal of Public Health*, 101: 2235–8.

Bodsworth, S.M., Clare, I.C.H. and Simblett, S.K. (2011) 'Deafblindness and mental health: psychological distress and unmet need among adults with dual sensory impairment', *British Journal of Visual Impairment*, 29: 6–26.

Bovaird, T. and Loeffler, E. (2010) 'User and community co-production of public services and public policies through collective decision-making: the role of emerging technologies', in T. Brandsen and M. Holzer (eds) *The Future of Governance*, Newark: National Center for Public Performance.

Brennan, M. (2003) 'Impairment of both vision and hearing among older adults: prevalence and impact on quality of life', *Generations*, 27(1): 52–6.

Brennan, M. and Bally, S.J. (2007) 'Psychosocial adaptations to dual sensory loss in middle and late adulthood', *Trends in Amplification*, 11: 281–300.

Brennan, M., Horowitz, A. and Su, Y-P. (2005) 'Dual sensory loss and its impact on everyday competence', *Gerontologist*, 4: 337–46.

Brown, J., Isaacs, D. and The World Café Community (2005) *The World Café*, San Francisco: Berrett-Koehler Publishers.

Bruce, M.S. and Parker, T.A. (2012) 'Young deafblind adults in action: becoming self-determined change agents through advocacy', *American Annals of the Deaf*, 157(1): 16–26.

Cooperrider, D.L. and Whitney, D. (1999) 'A positive revolution in change: appreciative inquir', in P. Holman and T. Devane (eds) *The Change Handbook*, San Francisco: Berrett-Koehler.

Deafblind UK (2019) 'Communication'. Online. Available at https://deafblind.org.uk/information-advice/living-with-deafblindness/communication/ (accessed 19 September 2019).

Dutta, A., Kundu, M.M., Johnson, E., Chan, F., Trainor, A., Blake, R. and Christy, R. (2016) 'Community conversations: engaging stakeholders to improve employment-related transition services for youth with emotional and behavioral disabilities', *Journal of Vocational Rehabilitation*, 45(1): 43–51.

Dyke, P. (2013) 'Identifying Australians who live with deaf blindness and dual sensory loss'. Online. Available at www.senses.org.au/wp-content/uploads/2016/01/a-clear-view—senses-australia.pdf?sfvrsn=6 (accessed 19 September 2019).

European Parliament (2004) 'Declaration of the European parliament on the rights of deafblind people'. Online. Available at www.europarl.europa.eu/sides/getDoc.do?pubRef=-//EP//TEXT+TA+P5-TA-2004-0277+0+DOC+XML+V0//EN (accessed 18 September 2019).

Fouché, C. and Light, G. (2011) 'An invitation to dialogue: "the World Café" in social work research', *Qualitative Social Work*, 10: 28–48.

Frankel, M.A. (2002) 'Deaf-blind interpreting: interpreters' use of negation in Tactile American sign language', *Sign Language Studies*, 2: 169–80.

Grassick, S.B. (2001) 'Interpreter guide'. Online. Available at www.deafblind.org.au/deafblind-information/communication/interpreter-guide/ (accessed 19 September 2019).

Heine, C. and Browning, C.J. (2014) 'Mental health and dual sensory loss in older adults: a systematic review', *Frontiers in Aging Neuroscience*, 6: 83.

Hersh, M. (2013) 'Deafblind people, communication, independence, and isolation', *The Journal of Deaf Studies and Deaf Education*, 18: 446–63.

International Wellbeing Group (2013) *Personal Wellbeing Index, 5th Edition*. Deakin University, Melbourne. Online. Available at http://www.acqol.com.au/uploads/pwi-a/pwi-a-english.pdf (accessed 10 February 2020).

Jaiswal, A., Aldersey, H., Wittich, W., Mirza, M. and Finlayson, M. (2018) 'Participation experiences of people with deafblindness or dual sensory loss: a scoping review of global deafblind literature', *PLoS One*, 13(9): e0203772.

Kowalski, K. (2018) 'New tech helps deaf-blind people "watch" TV'. Online. Available at www.sciencenewsforstudents.org/article/new-tech-helps-deaf-blind-people-watch-tv (accessed 19 September 2019).

Lee-Foster, A. (2010) 'Capacity to communicate: sense's three-year project training independent mental capacity advocates in communication skills', *Journal of Adult Protection*, 12(1): 32–42.

Mathos, K.K., Lokar, F. and Post, E. (2011) 'Gathering perceptions about current mental health services and collecting ideas for improved service delivery for persons who are deaf, deafblind and hard of hearing', *Journal of the American Deafness and Rehabilitation Association*, 44: 134–52.

Mills, N. (2019) 'Device that converts iPhone screen into braille a "lifeline" for deaf-blind people'. Online. Available at www.abc.net.au/news/2019-02-09/gadget-turns-iphone-screens-into-braille-to-help-deaf-and-blind/10732100 (accessed 19 September 2019).

Milton, D.E. (2014) 'Autistic expertise: a critical reflection on the production of knowledge in autism studies', *Autism*, 18: 794–802.

Miner, I.D. (1997) 'People with Usher syndrome Type II: issues and adaptations', *Journal of Visual Impairment and Blindness*, 91: 579–89.

National Health and Medical Research Council [NHMRC], the Australian Research Council and Universities Australia (2018) 'National statement on ethical conduct in human research 2007 (Updated 2018)'. Online. Available at www.nhmrc.gov.au/about-us/publications/national-statement-ethical-conduct-human-research-2007-updated-2018 (accessed 19 September 2019).

Nordic Centre for Social Welfare and Social Issues (2019) *Nordic Definition of Deafblindness*. Online. Available at https://nordicwelfare.org/wp-content/uploads/2018/03/nordic-definition-of-deafblindness.pdf (accessed 19 September 2019).

O'Brien, S. and Steffen, C. (1996) 'Tactile ASL: ASL as used by deaf-blind persons', *Gallaudet University Communication Forum*, vol. 5. Washington, DC: Gallaudet University Press.

Reed, C.M., Durlach, N.I., Braida, L.D. and Schultz, M.C. (1989) 'Analytic study of the Tadoma method: effects of hand position on segmental speech perception', *Journal of Speech, Language, and Hearing Research*, 32: 921–9.

Rodriguez-Gil, G. and Belote, M. (2005) 'Coactive and tactile signing', *California Deafblind Services reSources*, 11(5): 1–3. Online. Available at http://files.cadbs.org/200000037-3e6333f5d3/Spring05.pdf (accessed 19 September 2019).

Roy, A., McVilly, K.R. and Crisp, B.R. (2018) 'Preparing for inclusive consultation, research and policy development: insights from the field of Deafblindness', *Journal of Social Inclusion*, 9(1): 71–88.

Roy, A., McVilly, K.R. and Crisp, B.R. (2019) 'Working with Deafblind people to develop a good practice approach to consultation and research activities', *Journal of Social Work*, DOI: 10.1177/1468017319860216.

Selepak, L. (2008) *Challenges Facing People with Disabilities from Culturally and Linguistically Diverse Backgrounds (CaLD) Monograph*, Perth: Disability Services Commission WA. Online. Available at www.disability.wa.gov.au/Global/Publications/About%20us/Count%20me%20in/Research/cald.doc (accessed 19 September 2019).

Sheridan, K., Adams-Eaton, F., Trimble, A., Renton, A. and Bertotti, M. (2010) 'Community engagement using World Café: the Well London experience', *Groupwork*, 20(3): 32–50.

Simcock, P. (2017) 'One of society's most vulnerable groups? A systematically conducted literature review exploring the vulnerability of deafblind people', *Health and Social Care in the Community*, 25: 813–39.

Simcock, P. and Manthorpe, J. (2014) 'Deafblind and neglected or deafblindness neglected? Revisiting the case of Beverley Lewis', *British Journal of Social Work*, 44: 2325–41.

Taket, A., Crisp, B.R., Nevill, A., Lamaro, G., Graham, M. and Barter-Godfrey, S. (2009) *Theorising Social Exclusion*, London: Routledge.

Tanabe, M., Pearce, E. and Krause, S.K. (2018) ' "Nothing about us, without us": conducting participatory action research among and with persons with disabilities in humanitarian settings', *Action Research*, 16: 280–98.

Taylor, G. (2010) 'Empowerment, identity, and participatory research: using social action research to challenge isolation for deaf and hard of hearing people from minority ethnic communities', *Disability and Society*, 14: 369–84.

United Nations (2015) 'Transforming our world: the 2030 agenda for sustainable development'. Online. Available at https://sustainabledevelopment.un.org/post2015/transformingourworld/publication (accessed 16 September 2019).

Vogt, E. (2005) 'The World Cafe hosting guide', in J. Brown and D. Isaacs (eds) *The World Cafe: Shaping our Futures through Conversations that Matter,* San Francisco: Berrett-Koehler.

Zarb, G. (1992) 'On the road to Damascus: first steps towards changing the relations of disability research production', *Disability, Handicap and Society*, 7: 125–38.

Part 3

Sustaining programmes which support social inclusion

6   Opening doors

Creating and sustaining community leadership for promoting social inclusion

Ann Taket, Alex Mills, Sally-Ann Nadj and Ronda Held

Introduction

> Opening Doors gave me a platform to work towards the goals that I wanted to achieve in my life. That was to create happiness amongst people, to join them together and probably fill the gap in their life that they had formed as a result of either isolation or their circumstances they were in.
>
> (2015 graduate, quoted in Naccarella 2016: 26)

This quote, taken from a recent external evaluation of the *Opening Doors* programme, encapsulates the programme's aim, preparing community leaders to stimulate positive community change. Social exclusion, with its well-recognised negative health impacts (Popay et al. 2008), has been a priority concern of public health practitioners when addressing the social determinants of health (Brooks and Kendall 2013; Ottmann et al. 2006). This has led to establishment of asset-based community development (ABCD) approaches to promote social inclusion (Brooks 2009). One such programme is the *Opening Doors* programme, initiated in 2009 by organisations in the Inner East Primary Care Partnership (IEPCP). The IEPCP is one of Victoria's 28 primary-care partnerships which were established in 2002. It includes the inner Eastern Metropolitan Region of Melbourne comprising the local government areas of the cities of Boroondara, Monash, Manningham, and Whitehorse. In 2007, IEPCP recognised social exclusion in older people as its priority health concern since many people in the catchment of inner Eastern Metropolitan Region of Melbourne were identified as being isolated due to frailty, disability, low income, or cultural background and depression had the largest burden of disease in the catchment's population profile. There was a deliberate choice at this point to take a leadership and capacity-building approach rather than fund short-term projects for specific groups. The aim was to build grassroots leadership. In order to combat social isolation, *Opening Doors* Community Leadership Programme was launched in 2009 under the Inner East Social Inclusion Initiative. In later years, the scope of the programme broadened to focus on other groups in the community who were experiencing social exclusion. The leadership programme runs annually and is currently delivered as one of the ongoing programmes offered by Link Health and Community, a community health provider in Melbourne, Australia.

The recruitment stage, discussed under key elements later, is crucial—aiming to engage with grassroots leaders not necessarily agency workers, although their participation in small numbers has also been valuable. The programme itself is delivered over six months. It begins with a three-day intensive retreat (delivered in partnership with Global Leadership Foundation, based in Melbourne). This focuses on raising participants' awareness about their own leadership styles, introducing strengths-based community development approaches, and maintaining emotional health. During the programme, participants learn how to plan, fund, and implement initiatives to promote social inclusion. They also learn about barriers to inclusion, creating consensus and co-designing, managing challenging behaviours, self-care, social media, advocacy, public speaking, effective promotion strategies, and sustainability. They start work on a community initiative that plays to their own particular background and passions. The programme content is progressively developed over the years with input from community members and graduates.

As at the beginning of 2018, over 100 community initiatives to promote social inclusion have been led by the 190 graduates of the programme, leading to over 15,000 community members who are now engaged with their communities in new and positive ways and a network of over 150 different organisations, businesses, and groups supporting the *Opening Doors* Program. The *Opening Doors* graduates represent more than 50 cultural and religious backgrounds and bring passions as diverse as mental health, disability, LGBTIQ rights, positive aging, interfaith dialogue, and many, many more. The initiatives are extremely diverse, including,

- Universities of the Third Age (U3A)—three have commenced thus far;
- TransFamily—a peer support group for parents, siblings, extended family, and friends of trans people;
- The Black Dog community art exhibition—exploring the lived experiences and stigmas of mental health in our community;
- Pathways for Carers—monthly walks which connect people in caring roles with each other and services which can better support them (now running across six local government areas);
- Numerous new community associations, including Bangladeshi Senior Citizens Victoria, Afghan Women's Welfare Association, and Rohingya Women's Association;
- Bringing together groups of people with a shared interest to produce books (e.g. 'Good for you: celebrating the stories of our Chinese Seniors' and 'With The Light' promoting understanding and awareness of autism in the Chinese community through a graphic novel series);
- Bene Connect: Bringing people of all faiths (and none) together to connect, collaborate, and discuss important issues in the Manningham community, supported by Benevolence Australia;

- Different journeys: monthly dinners for teens and young adults with Autism Spectrum Disorder (ASD), their families, friends, and carers;
- The Respect Community Soccer Tournament: Bringing youth from all major faith and cultural groups in Manningham together to promote respect for diversity and inclusion through sport; and
- Grow: A social enterprise bringing women from diverse backgrounds together to collaborate, creating art, craft, clothing, and other garments and empowering them to share their stories.

In this chapter, the origins of the programme are first explored followed by a discussion of the impact and outcomes from the programme, exploring both overall programme achievements and the achievements of the community initiatives started by programme graduates. The chapter then considers the key elements in the *Opening Doors* model. Throughout we discuss the key elements in the *Opening Doors* model that underlie its success as a sustainable model for promoting social inclusion.

Origins

The Inner East Social Inclusion Initiative (IESII) partnership developed in 2006 with a shared vision to reduce social isolation for older residents in the four municipalities of the Inner East Metropolitan Region of Melbourne: Boorondara, Monash, Manningham, and Whitehorse (Held 2011b). A literature review was commissioned (Ottmann et al. 2006). This proposed a 'three tiered approach to health promotion, that not only integrates the personal, relational as well as collective sphere but is also capable of drawing on the benefits of a strength-based methodology' (Ottmann et al. 2006: 44) and discussed the benefit of ABCD in this context. In 2007, a group of key strategic partners came together under this initiative to examine and address the issue of social isolation in the creation of the Inner-East Social Inclusion Initiative working group. In 2009, following extensive consultation and best practice research, the *Opening Doors* Community Leadership Programme was born as one of two programmes of the Inner East Social Inclusion Initiative aimed at tackling social isolation in the community. The programme was modelled on the successful Leadership Victoria 'Williamson Program' (Held 2011a).

   In 2009, *Opening Doors* focussed on potentially isolated older people and then in 2010 broadened its scope to include other vulnerable groups, such as people with disabilities, young mothers, youth, and people on low incomes (Held 2011a). Initially the programme attempted to focus its participant recruitment on areas of disadvantage as identified by Australian Bureau of Statistics (ABS) data; however this produced limited success, so recruitment used a wider range of methods to reach out through the whole of the four local government areas. The original aim was to have a mixture of people from the community, local agencies, and businesses so the resources could be pooled to support projects. However, recruitment of those from the private sector was lacking and also problematic where businesses were seeking to use the engagement as an opportunity to promote themselves rather than sponsoring projects or sharing resources.

The Inner East Social Inclusion Initiative was externally evaluated in 2009 (Teshuva and Reid 2010) which examined the first year of the *Opening Doors* programme. Two internal evaluations of the *Opening Doors* programme were produced based on its first two years. One examined the impact of the programme on its graduates and the community projects generated (Held 2011a), and the other focussed on the lessons learnt about successful partnerships for promoting health (Held 2011b). A further external evaluation of *Opening Doors* was undertaken in 2015–2016 (Naccarella 2016). The impact of two of the projects initiated by *Opening Doors* graduates was examined in a master's thesis undertaken by a Deakin University student (Asghar 2017). This last study is the only one based on the views of the participants in the initiatives started by *Opening Doors* graduates.

Outcomes and impacts

Through the various evaluations, both internal and external, efforts have been made to document the outcomes and impact of the *Opening Doors* programme. It is important to acknowledge that only a partial picture can be presented, only some of the outcomes and impacts on programme participants, their communities, and beyond have been documented. In this section, we consider first the programme participants themselves and then the various initiatives that they led.

Building community leadership capacity

> Opening Doors gave me insight into how I can contribute. It helped me to focus on my strengths and see a different way to attract people to become involved.
>
> (2009 graduate, quoted in Held 2011a: 19)

The first type of outcomes and impacts from the programme were the effects on the participants themselves. The external evaluation carried out of the first year of programme delivery (Teshuva and Reid 2010) as well as the internal evaluation carried out on the first two years of programme delivery (Held 2011a) demonstrated the success of the programme in building leadership capacity in its participants and graduates. Using both quantitative and qualitative measures, participants' leadership knowledge, skills, and confidence all increased. Some quotes from the graduates in the first two years of the programme illustrate what was achieved.

> There were a lot of ordinary people passionate about what they wanted to do. Once we knew where to go and how to network things happened, it all came together.
>
> (2010 graduate, quoted in Held 2011a: 32)

The program changed the way I think about myself, I learnt that ordinary people can do extraordinary things.

>   (2010 graduate, quoted in Held 2011a: 32)

The program made me more aware of how important community leaders are, to empower and inspire others, to lead by example, to delegate and to step back and encourage others to take a more active role.

>   (2010 graduate, quoted in Held 2011a: 35)

I learnt a lot from that program, most importantly how to listen.

>   (2010 graduate, quoted in Held 2011a: 35)

The course helped me to put a finger on what I could do. I am now taking leadership and loving it.

>   (2010 graduate, quoted in Held 2011a: 36)

I learnt that a leader can be anyone who responds to the need of the community—they don't have to be known as a leader. . . . The Community Leadership program provided the self-management skills as well as diverse pathways for social inclusion for myself and community around me. The program developed the clear transition from self-isolation to social inclusion that has created the self-confidence.

>   (recent migrant and 2010 graduate, quoted in Held 2011a: 36)

As these quotes also illustrate, the graduates considered they gained a lot personally from the programme. One graduate from the first programme talked about the most important aspect being 'learning that we can all be leaders' (graduate 2009, quoted in Held 2011a: 26). These early findings have been reinforced in later years of programme delivery and are echoed in the findings of Naccarella's external evaluation (Naccarella 2016). One 2015 graduate expressed it as follows:

> Opening Doors was a safe environment. They nurtured my confidence and my strengths. The strengths-based teaching was really significant for me and I've used that with my clients. I do work on that way. It's had a real ripple effect on my clients. So it's built their confidence. I didn't know I could publicly speak until I . . . was on the course.
>
>   (Naccarella 2016: 26)

The leadership skills gained by the graduates and their use of these skills are also evident in the recognition received by graduates, for example, Nopporn Ganthavee's 2015 award as Boroondara Young Citizen of The Year, following her graduation from *Opening Doors* in 2014. 2011 graduate Krishna Aurora received an Order of Australia Medal in 2013. Judy Cox, who graduated from Opening Doors in 2013, received accolades at the Victorian Premier's Volunteer Awards in 2017 for her founding of the Wheeler's Hill University of the Third Age (U3A).

In 2014, Opening Doors coordinator Alex Mills was one of four Australians shortlisted for the Tony Fitzgerald Memorial Community Award by the Australian Human Rights Commission.

Initiatives that make a difference

The second important set of outcomes and impacts arises in different communities through the community initiatives that graduates led, contributing to increased social inclusion. With over 100 community initiatives started since 2009, it is obviously impossible to document them each in detail. Instead, first we draw on the one study (Asghar 2017) that has talked directly to participants in two of the initiatives: U3As, one long-standing, created as a result of the first year of the programme in 2009, and the other set up more recently in 2015. Following that, we bring together in tabular presentation some examples of different initiatives, their impacts, and outcomes into the community, drawing on Naccarella (2016) and the different bulletins produced by the programme coordinator.

Asghar (2017) interviewed 21 participants in two U3As: ten from Wheelers Hill, launched in 2015, and eleven from Deepdene, launched in 2009. The older U3A, Deepdene, has a larger membership and more programmes on offer than the younger U3A. Despite these differences, the impacts of involvement as perceived by the participants in the two U3As were similar and fell under the same four themes: keeping active (both physically and mentally); lifelong learning; social connections; and sense of belonging.

Participants in both U3As identified physical and mental stimulation as a major benefit of involvement in their U3A. Participants from both the U3As have been involved in classes aimed at improving physical health in an engaging environment such as strength training, yoga, and dancing classes. Participants commented on the physical courses being an opportunity to get involved in physical activity at a much cheaper price than the local gyms. The walking programmes have been attended by many participants in both the U3As and have been identified as not only promoting physical activity but also providing a prospective hub of social interaction where they can leave their homes and walk around historic places or parks and carry out conversations with other members while enjoying the surrounding environment. Participants from both the U3As recognise the benefit of walking groups as both physically and mentally stimulating and conducive to healthy ageing because of social as well as health benefits.

Lifelong learning was identified by majority of participants from both the U3As as their motivation for joining U3A, and the huge wealth of knowledge possessed by U3A members was considered an invaluable asset. Learning through peer-supported and peer-led programmes was identified as particularly helpful in learning new skills such as use of smart phones, playing guitar, or learning patchwork and knitting. When such learning is carried out in supportive groups, as in the U3A, there is an additional benefit of social engagement because there is a non-competitive environment aimed at learning for self-fulfilment rather than formal qualification.

Both the U3As promoted social connections through diverse avenues including physical training and peer-education groups. The majority of participants from both the U3As, men and women alike, recognised U3A as a platform that has enabled them to connect with like-minded people from their local community which they would not have had a chance to meet otherwise because of the differences in their ethnic and professional backgrounds. Participants particularly perceive U3As as all-embracing and welcoming of sociocultural differences and includes people from all walks of life based on their similarities of vision, their interests of pursuing knowledge, their need to find purpose, and their desire to engage in meaningful activities. This all-inclusive framework of U3As is perceived as an enabler in engaging older people who feel lonely and isolated facing retirement or bereavement due to loss of friends or family, which is commonly seen among older adults. One Deepdene member explained,

> My husband passed away and . . . then it was that U3A figured into my life . . . because there was just this huge void . . . it was just my husband and me, and I needed to have structure to my day and to, I think, build more of a social network . . . it just provided such a fulfilling part of my life after such a traumatic change.
>
> (Deepdene U3A member, quoted in Asghar 2017: 31)

The majority of Deepdene U3A participants had been associated with their U3A for longer duration and reported a sense of belonging to their U3A, while in Wheelers Hill U3A, with shorter lengths of association, this was reported by a few, for example:

> As a group of ladies that dance together, we do yoga together I feel a sisterhood. I feel warm, I feel friendship . . . I feel I'm not lonely because I don't have any family, any friends here. I live(d) in the States for 41 years, all my friends, my kids are there and I'm alone here but when I go to U3A I don't feel that way.
>
> (Wheelers Hill U3A member, quoted in Asghar 2017: 36)

The participants identified U3A as the place where they feel genuinely welcomed, where they know people and are known by them. They are aware that although they do not share very close friendships with all the other members, there are people who are willing to lend a listening ear and support if they ask for it, that is, being supportive in a non-intrusive way. Some of the retirees regarded U3A as an important constituent of their lives, which allowed them to contribute back to the community in a way where their volunteering was not only beneficial for the community but also for themselves, as they gained the physical and psychosocial benefits of involvement in a diverse range of activities and at the same time felt being part of the wider multicultural community.

The repetition of these impacts among participants from both the U3As suggest that these two community-based initiatives have been able to engage older people from diverse backgrounds in activities that not only promote social connectedness but also promote healthy and active ageing as perceived by the participants. The inclusive nature of these groups can be linked to insights gained as part of the *Opening Doors* programme.

Turning now to some of the other community initiatives led by *Opening Doors* graduates, Table 6.1 summarises important outcomes and impacts as reported by the graduates.

Table 6.1 Community initiatives, their outcomes, and impacts

Initiative	Effects on participants	Wider community effects
Broadband access for Seniors programme	Improved access to computers for older residents	Increased respect for elders Increased confidence of community members Shared stories Increased networks and connections to address social isolation
Celebrate the stories of Chinese seniors in our communities	Empowerment for individuals in relating stories	Wider appreciation of different immigrant journeys and experiences
Established parent support groups	Increased connections amongst parents who may be at risk of social isolation	Increased networks and connections to address social isolation
Black Dog Community Art Exhibition	Empowered and increased self-esteem of people with anxiety and depression to be heard, informed, and have a voice	Empowered and inspired people with anxiety and depression through art Reduced stigma for people with mental ill health Built leadership capacity, empowering people living with anxiety and depression Increased opportunities to employment for people living with anxiety and depression
Welcome dinners for migrants and refugees	Connected newly arrived migrants and refugees with established Australians	Increased connections between migrants and refugees and Australians in the local community Increased awareness of local community leaders about the value of welcome dinners as a way to promote social inclusion
Created a neighbourhood information resource about local services and businesses	Increased knowledge of new families about how to access local services and businesses	Increasing local community know-how about accessing local community services and businesses Increased feeling of belonging in the local community

Initiative	Effects on participants	Wider community effects
Facilitated Indian Senior Citizens Association to connect and work more collaboratively to promote social inclusion	Increased awareness amongst Indian Senior Citizens about social isolation and ways to promote social inclusion Increased knowledge and connections between the Indian Senior Citizens Association and other senior organisations from other cultures Built connections amongst a community of like-minded people who are passionate about social inclusion	Built networks and connections between local community organisations Creating opportunities to connect Senior organisations from all cultures Increased knowledge and skills
Working with those affected by gambling, using multiple methods: dancing groups, a drumming circle, creating mandalas and other crafts, storytelling, and performing scenes	Healing individuals from the harms caused by gambling Empowering people to find their voice on the journey to recovery and to become advocates for change	An increase in the depth of understanding of the risks of gambling, as well as the challenges and stigmas faced by those who have experienced harm from pokies
'Different Journeys' ASD (autism spectrum disorder) support group Parent support group	Empower young people with ASD (by providing them with a social platform that fosters an environment for them to create positive connections and feeling of inclusion Linking families with services and support.	Increased knowledge, understanding and acceptance of parent of children with ASD and carer issues Empowered parents of children with Autism Spectrum Disorder (ASD) and carers Gave parents of children with Autism Spectrum Disorder (ASD) hope Increased volunteering in the community Existing and emerging community leaders feel empowered, educated, and connected

Sources: Derived from Naccarella (2016) and Opening Doors Bulletins November 2014, August 2015, December 2017

The table illustrates the diversity of initiatives led by graduates and the breadth of their influence. Naccarella (2016: 35) summarises this in terms of eight different domains of change in the broader community:

1   Increasing the awareness and knowledge of factors that contribute to social isolation, social exclusion, and those factors that promote social inclusion;

2   Increasing the quality and number of relationships, connections, networks, and collaborations;
3   Increasing ideas, viewpoints, mind-sets, and ways of thinking about social inclusion using asset-based community development approaches;
4   Increasing the leadership capabilities—increased empowerment, confidence, and advocacy;
5   Increasing the level of participation and engagement of marginalised local communities;
6   Increasing the level of respect and acceptance of people who are marginalised and socially excluded from society;
7   Increasing the level of belonging and decreasing the level of loneliness of marginalised communities; and
8   Increasing the level of volunteering, generosity, goodwill, and benevolence—giving back to others.

Key elements in the *Opening Doors* model

Naccarella (2016) identified three different 'key ingredients for success'. The first of these was a particular type of programme coordinator: benevolent; non-judgmental; honest; open; goodwill; reliable; accepting and personable; well-connected; and with lived experience of both the *Opening Doors* programme and using ABCD. The second of these was in terms of features of the programme itself: free; structured; pragmatic and practical content, especially ABCD; supported, both financially and in other ways, and authorised by a diversity of health, human, and social service organisations; and its focus on building community leaders and leadership. The third ingredient was the post-programme strategy to support graduates with social and skill-based opportunities. Six features instrumental in these results are expanded on below using information from all the different evaluations.

Interview process

A key component of the selection process for the *Opening Doors* programme is a group interview. Three to five applicants participated in each interview which was structured as a discussion with the programme coordinator, a Steering Committee representative, and an independent stakeholder when possible. The discussion was constructed to promote conversations as opposed to strict question-and-answer format. Relevant topics such as: teamwork, leadership, and personal strengths were explored, and this provided opportunity for applicants to demonstrate their ability to engage with others and to meet with potential fellow group participants. A visioning exercise was also included using Baker's (2004) picture book *Belonging* as an example of how a socially inclusive community can develop over time. Applicants were encouraged to draw or describe the transformation of their own local community to a socially inclusive one and then to explore the commonalities of their vision with the other group members. People were finally selected based on their passion and ability to work with others in the programme.

Opening retreat

Evaluations from the 2010 programme (Held 2011a) for the initial live-in retreat emphasises its importance in the leadership journey, and this was reinforced by Naccarella (2016) as one important aspect of the programme's structure, providing a safe environment for building relationships. Expansion in the length of the retreat, from two to three days, early on in the life of the programme was important in ensuring this outcome. Here's how one of the graduates expressed their views:

> I have so many strong memories. The opening retreat was a wonderful experience; to be able to come together and get to know such an amazing group of people. Formalising past learnings was excellent too.
>
> (graduate 2013 quoted in December 2106 *Bulletin*)

ABCD—Asset-Based Community Development

The programme has a core focus on ABCD, a strengths-based approach to community development. Following the opening retreat, the first two full-day sessions of the programme are dedicated to exploring this approach. Participants are provided with a theoretical framework as well as many tangible examples of the approach in practice. Distinctions are drawn between a 'needs based' approach—seeing people as clients in a service system with problems to be solved—and the asset-based approach, which sees all individuals as equal and participating members of their community, with gifts, talents, and assets to be shared. Participants are strongly encouraged to think about individuals and groups who have been 'needs assessed out of community', defined by their challenges and deficits. These sessions emphasise the important of working from an ABCD framework as the most effective and sustainable way to bring about lasting change in communities and to empower new and emerging community leaders. The ABCD approach also explicitly challenges models which reinforce entrenched notions of dependency—communities which are free from reliance on external 'experts' will thrive and achieve self-determination in contrast to needs and charity-based models of intervention.

The Asset Based Community Development approach underpinning the *Opening Doors* model was first outlined by John P. Kretzmann and John L. McKnight (1993) in their book *Building Communities From The Inside Out: a path towards finding and mobilising a community's assets*. These principles were further explored in Robert Putnam's (2000) *Bowling Alone: the collapse and revival of American community* and *ABCD: when people care enough to act* (Green et al. 2006).

*Opening Door*s has worked closely with global leaders active in the ABCD field, including Peter Kenyon (Bank of Ideas, Australia), Cormac Russell (Nurture Development, Ireland), Jim Diers (Neighbour Power, USA), and Ted Smeaton (Australia), the latter two of which have delivered several workshops directly to Opening Doors participants and alumni.

From the earliest years of the programme, graduates talked of the value of ABCD to them:

> Exposure to ABCD theory in the program cemented my ability to identify community resources and the strengths of individuals in the implementation of a project. Exposure to different spaces in the community laid down the foundation to explore community resources as well.
>
> (graduate 2009, quoted in Held 2011a: 18)

Naccarella (2016) reports that *Opening Doors* graduates overwhelmingly valued the ABCD approach to community development, regarding it as a key enabler to the success of *Opening Doors*.

Peer support

From the initial interview process through the intensive opening retreat of the programme and then through the interactive workshops during the rest of the programme, a web of strong and enduring supportive relationships are built between programme participants and also includes the programme coordinator. These nurture participants through the design and implementation of their project, both throughout the programme and after their graduation from it when they continue to work on their community initiatives as alumni. In discussing peer support, graduates often mention gaining from the diversity in the programme participants.

> Never have I been part of such a diverse group of individuals. This eclectic mix of culture, age, gender, faith and interest has created a community that is incredibly honest and supportive. I will hold onto the lessons from this community for the rest of my life.
>
> (graduate 2015, from reflection delivered at graduation ceremony)

Intersectional learning

Beyond the individual session content, a key strength of the *Opening Doors* model is the opportunity to bring leaders from diverse backgrounds and lived experiences together. Through sharing exercises and informal interactions, participants are frequently exposed to perspectives, cultures, religions, and lived experiences they may not have encountered outside of the programme environment. In addition to deepening the learning experience for participants, this also leads to collaboration opportunities beyond the participants' existing networks and/or community. Leaders from new and emerging cultural communities are exposed to issues facing the LGBTIQ community, whilst leaders from senior citizens groups are connected with younger disability advocates. This formal and informal sharing of knowledge and lived experiences greatly enriches the learning environment and enables participants to share this knowledge with peers in their own communities. As one participant put it,

> I was exposed to so many new perspectives and experiences. . . . People who I never would have met outside of the program. To be sharing this journey with people who have just arrived in Australia, through to LGBTQ advocates . . . People in their 20s through to their 70s. It's so rare to learn and grow in an environment where everyone's lived experiences are honoured and valued, and we are all richer for it.
>
> (graduate, 2017, from reflection delivered at graduation ceremony)

Network of linked organisations

The extensive network of organisations linked to the programme provides participants and alumni with access to resources to individuals with specific expertise, to venues, to funding or suggestions as to funding sources, and to support in gaining them. The importance of this was emphasised in both external evaluations (Naccarella 2016; Teshuva and Reid 2010) and the internal evaluation (Held 2011b). The role of the programme coordinator is key here in linking people out to other organisations, but the participants themselves also play an important role in linking their peers out to their own contacts and networks. As one programme graduate expressed it,

> it's the networking processes which have really stuck with me. I think sometimes it might take people a while for that to sink in . . . But it's so critical. When something works because you know someone, that's incredible. It was also really powerful to visit the different locations at each session. It was great to visit Monash and Manningham Councils, the Blackburn Sikh Temple, Mulgrave Neighbourhood House . . . The whole experience was just incredible. It's opened so many new pathways for me, and honestly, it's one of the best models for community engagement and leadership I've ever encountered.
>
> (2013 graduate, quoted in December 2016 bulletin)

Building sustainability

Looking around the world, all of the best practice examples show communities building on their strengths: starting with what is strong and the things that are assets and continuing to build from there. With the support of Global Leadership Foundation, Leadership Victoria, and a group of passionate social and community health agencies, it was in this spirit that the *Opening Doors Leadership Programme* was born. By the time of writing in 2018, *Opening Doors* has a vibrant and thriving alumni group, with its graduates mobilising to organise workshops, social events, and opportunities to further their leadership journeys and ultimately support each other in their visions. The programme looks forward to welcoming future graduates into this ever-growing community and continuing to promote a society which is socially inclusive for all.

The financial sustainability of programmes that produce significant positive social outcomes, that cannot always be quantified, is always difficult to achieve. Link Health and Community supports the programme over and above the funding made available through grants, as it sees it as a worthy and justifiable component of its community charter within a social model of health. However, the constant struggle to find more and more funds means that the project coordination role has to contend with spending time finding appropriate funding, and writing applications, rather than working directly on the programme. In 2011, a prospectus was developed to elicit corporate sponsorship; however it was not successful. Additionally other strategies have included connecting with fundraising organisations, which again has not elicited much funding. The difficulty, as always with poorly funded programmes, is managing the competing demands of needing to find new funding all the time, managing the expectations of the current funders, along with managing the day-to-day operations of the programme annually. Additionally, maintaining a salary level that is commensurate with the skills and expertise of the project coordinator is also fundamental to sustaining and stabilising the project. By Link Health and Community taking on the programme as one of its 'standing' programmes means that at least there is back-end support for the role and more opportunities for exposure to the communities of interest.

References

Asghar, B.U.A. (2017) '*Opening Doors* into community: evaluating the impacts of *Opening Doors* projects aimed at social inclusion in Inner East Melbourne', unpublished Master of Public Health thesis, Deakin University, Australia.

Baker, J. (2004) *Belonging*, London: Walker Books.

Brooks, D. (2009) 'Easy as ABCD: making social inclusion happen', *Drug Action NSW Community Drug Strategies Newsletter* (Spring), 4.

Brooks, F. and Kendall, S. (2013) 'Making sense of assets: what can an assets based approach offer public health?' *Critical Public Health*, 23: 127–30.

Green, M., Moore, H. and O'Brien, J. (2006) *ABCD: When People Care Enough to Act*, Toronto: Inclusion Press.

Held, R. (2011a) *Inner East Social Inclusion Initiative, Opening Doors, a Community Leadership Program for Social Inclusion: Evaluation Report*, Melbourne: Inner East Primary Care Partnership.

Held, R. (2011b) *Inner East Social Inclusion Initiative, Opening Doors, a Community Leadership Program for Social Inclusion: Partnership Report*, Melbourne: Inner East Primary Care Partnership.

Kretzmann, J.P. and McKnight, J.L. (1993) *Building Communities from the Inside Out: A Path Towards Finding and Mobilising a Community's Assets*, Evanston, IL: Center for Urban Affairs and Policy Research, Northwestern University.

Naccarella, L. (2016) *Impact Evaluation of the Opening Doors Community Leadership Program for Social Inclusion: Final Report*, Melbourne: Inner East Primary Care Partnership and Melbourne School of Population and Global Health, The University of Melbourne.

Ottmann, G., Dickson, J. and Wright, P (2006) *Social Connectedness and Health: A Literature Review*, Bundoora: La Trobe University.

Popay, J., Escorel, S., Hernández, M., Johnston, H., Mathieson, J. and Rispel, L. (2008) *Understanding and tackling social exclusion. Final report to the WHO commission on social determinants of health from the social exclusion knowledge Network, February 2008*. Online. Available at www.who.int/social_determinants/knowledge_net works/final_reports/sekn_final%20report_042008.pdf (accessed 24 November 2019).

Putnam, R. (2000) *Bowling Alone: The Collapse and Revival of American Community*, New York: Simon and Schuster.

Teshuva, K. and Reid, K. (2010) *Evaluation of the Inner East Social Inclusion Initiative: Final Report February 2010*, Bundoora: Australian Institute for Primary Care, La Trobe University.

7 Responding to hunger in Australia

The role of traditional and emerging food distribution measures in addressing food insecurity

Fiona H. McKay

Introduction

Over the past two decades, Australia has experienced strong economic growth and an increase in household wealth. While many have benefited from this growth, inequality has also increased, related to an increase in the cost of living, energy prices, cost of education and healthcare, and low wage growth. According to a report published by the Australian Council of Social Service [ACOSS] (Dorsch et al. 2016), an estimated 2.9 million people or 13.3 per cent of the Australian population live below the poverty line (A$433 per week for a single adult). Approximately one third of those living below the poverty line receive wages as their main source of income, while over half report relying on Social Security as their main source of income—with many Social Security payments themselves falling below the poverty line.

Research shows that for households already facing financial stress, any increase in the cost of living, related to increase in utility cost or interest rates, can have a flow-on effect that leaves households unable to pay bills or to purchase sufficient quality or quantity of food (Dorsch et al. 2016). While official data suggests that Australia is a food-secure nation with enough high-quality, nutritionally adequate food for all, there is food insecurity in Australia (Lawrence et al. 2013). Foodbank Australia (2017) reports that 3.6 million Australians have experienced food insecurity at least once in the last 12 months, with almost 650,000 Australians having sought food relief each month in 2017, an increase of 10 per cent over the previous year. This increasing need for food relief has resulted in an increased demand on services, with over 65,000 people unable to have their charitable food needs met each month. The increasing number of people seeking food relief has put a strain on charitable organisations whose mandate it is to service this need. Due to this increased demand, many of these agencies have described turning people away or limiting the frequency with which clients can receive assistance (McKay and McKenzie 2017). Given the strain emergency food relief is under and with need unlikely to decrease, other responses to food need have emerged over recent years. This chapter will introduce and explore responses to food insecurity in Australia, including charitable emergency food relief, prepared meal programmes, safety net programmes, community gardens, and social enterprise.

Food insecurity and the right to food

The Food and Agriculture Organization (FAO) of the United Nations is the agency responsible for efforts to defeat hunger. Within its mandate, the FAO defines four pillars of food insecurity that act upon an individual's ability to procure sufficient quality and quantity of food: availability, access, utilisation, and stability. *Availability* refers to the physical availability of food from farms, markets, or through donation. *Access* refers to one's ability to produce or acquire food, necessitating adequate infrastructure and financial resources. *Utilisation* requires adequate knowledge, social structures, and cooking facilities. Finally in order to truly achieve food security, these parameters must also be *Stable* over time (Renzaho and Mellor 2010).

Ongoing, secure, sustainable access to food is recognised as a basic human right under the *International Covenant on Economic Social and Cultural Rights* (ICESCR), ratified by Australia in 1975. The right to food enshrined in the *ICESCR* implies that individuals have sufficient access to food and that the food available is culturally and nutritionally appropriate, protecting an individual from hunger, food insecurity, and malnutrition. A right to food recognises that dignity comes from feeding oneself, not from being fed (Raponi 2017), and is only realised when an individual can independently and culturally appropriately achieve food security. While Australia has ratified several key documents that outline the right to food and, as such, has agreed to take measures to ensure the progressive realisation of the right to food, many of these international human rights documents have not been incorporated into Australian domestic law (Booth 2014). Furthermore, as Australia has no Bill of Rights and these instruments are not declared under the *Human Rights Commission Act*, there is little recourse for hunger or a lack of food in Australia.

Responding to food insecurity

High-income counties typically employ a combination of both public and private responses to food insecurity and hunger. First and foremost is the provision of food aid directly to those in need (through food banks or pantries); however, increasingly this approach is recognised as unable to meet the needs of those chronically hungry. Alternatives to emergency food aid are becoming more common and include community-supported gardens (Loopstra and Tarasuk 2013), local food hubs (Levkoe and Wakefield 2011), and mobile produce markets that visit low-income neighbourhoods (Haines et al. 2018). These responses have a range of strengths and weaknesses showing varying levels of success at reducing food insecurity and hunger.

At the centre of emergency food relief efforts are food bank programmes. The term 'food bank' can refer to one of two types of service: a large redistributor of rescued or surplus food to smaller charities that provide cooked and/or uncooked food to food-insecure populations or a service that provides grocery items directly to clients (Kicinski 2012). Unless otherwise stated, focus here is on the latter. While food banks (sometimes called food pantries) and other forms of food aid have traditionally been seen as a source of supplemental food for people experiencing short-term need and not a solution to achieving food security (Handforth et al. 2013), there is increasing evidence to suggest that some people are coming to rely on food banks as their only source of food (Holmes et al. 2018).

Food banks first appeared in high-income countries at times of economic decline or recession, implemented in response to reduction in state welfare expenditure alongside increasing need (Daponte and Bade 2006). In Australia, food banks were introduced in the 1970s (Lindberg et al. 2015). While they were originally seen as a temporary measure to address an immediate need, food banks, and pantries now form a staple in Australia's response to food insecurity.

Food banks in Australia are typically operated by the charity sector, staffed largely by volunteers operating out of churches and community centres. These organisations generally work by supplying free groceries—mostly that which is market surplus and provided via the national Food Bank programme (a programme that collects and redistributes surplus foods) or goods that have been donated by the public—to individuals vulnerable to or experiencing food insecurity and hunger. High demand for assistance means that food banks may limit the frequency with which clients can visit, impose means testing, or require proof of receipt of social assistance (McKenzie and McKay 2017). Given their reliance on donations, food banks have little control over the types and quality of food they provide and often report receiving surplus or expired packaged foods, low-quality perishable items, or foods that have little nutritional quality (Wilson et al. 2012). A typical food bank will provide clients with a pre-prepared parcel of food, designed to feed the recipient for up to three days.

While food banks play an important role in responding to a food emergency, it is becoming clear that only a small proportion of food-insecure households ever access these services (Loopstra and Tarasuk 2015). Many people only visit a food bank as a last resort, due to feelings of shame, stigma, and embarrassment (Garthwaite 2016). Overwhelmingly, the literature suggests that food banks are not a socially acceptable way to obtain food, with many clients describing feelings of shame most strongly upon the first food bank visit (Tarasuk and Beaton 1999), a feeling that can mean people in need cease accessing the service (McKay et al. 2018a). This is true for a range of users of food banks, including low-income parents, older people, and asylum seekers and refugees (Piwowarczyk et al. 2008). Culturally and linguistically diverse groups have also reported difficulty communicating with staff and an absence of culturally appropriate foods at food banks (Bazerghi et al. 2016). In seeking to address this stigma experienced by users of food banks, some services have implemented alternative models that give clients greater agency, promote social capital, or include other on-site services (Mukoya et al. 2017).

Playing an important role in emergency food relief in addition to food banks are community meals provided through community kitchens, soup vans, and breakfast programmes. These programmes are typically run in conjunction with food banks or other charities and can be available to clients daily (as in the case of a soup van or breakfast programme) or weekly (as in the case of a community kitchen).

Community kitchens, often attached to a food bank, include community-based cooking programmes in which small groups of individuals regularly come together to prepare one or more meals which may be taken home for later consumption or consumed together. These kitchens have been found to employ community development and health promotion strategies and draw on community resources to enhance self-help and social support (Tarasuk 2001).

Soup vans have been operating in Australia for several decades to feed those experiencing homeless, social isolation, and unemployment. Those who visit soup vans can access a hot, nutritious meal, fruit, and drinks and are often able to access non-food items such as blankets, clothing and food vouchers, donated books, and referrals. Soup van users are typically those who will not access other forms of food relief as the formality of other services can feel uncomfortable (McKay and McKenzie 2017). While responding to an acute need, soup vans are not able to resolve food insecurity for the many hundreds of people who rely on them for emergency meals.

Children are not immune from the experience of food insecurity and hunger. According to Foodbank Australia (2015), two thirds of Australian teachers report having a child come to school hungry, with estimates suggesting that students can lose two hours of class time each day due to hunger. In Australia, school breakfast clubs were set up under the Disadvantaged Schools Program during the late 1970s. Despite changes in funding over this time, many schools continue to operate breakfast clubs to meet the needs of hungry students. These breakfast clubs provide students with a simple meal at the beginning of each school day; some schools also provide students with a packed lunch (Engels and Boys 2008).

Despite their central role in providing emergency food relief for acute periods of hunger, food banks, and other types of emergency relief have been found to have little tangible impact on alleviating long-term food insecurity (Bazerghi et al. 2016; Lindberg et al. 2015). Research suggests that food provided by food banks is typically high in sodium and fat, with few fresh fruits or vegetables, an inadequate supply of foods containing important micro and macro nutrients, and an insufficient caloric intake to maintain an active life (Mukoya et al. 2017). The foods provided by emergency food relief, at best, can provide short-term relief from hunger but cannot meet client need in the long term (McIntyre et al. 2016).

Alternatives to traditional food aid

A growing acceptance of food insecurity as an ongoing rather than acute need for many, combined with the increasing realisation that food banks are unable to meet the needs of the hungry and food insecure, has led to the creation of several alternative responses. These responses to food insecurity and hunger are designed with empowerment goals in mind and seek to provide food via mutual support strategies, not just through passive giving and receiving (Tarasuk 2001).

The alternatives to food banks described here enjoy many of the same defining features as food banks. Like food banks, these initiatives have tended to be ad hoc and community based, and they have typically retained a strong emphasis on food and food-related behaviours. Importantly, however, they reflect a very different understanding of the problems that give rise to food insecurity and the form that effective community response should take. While these alternatives do seek to provide those in need with food, food insecurity is often seen as an issue of food production, social isolation, and poverty rather than acquisition. While these alternative responses do seek to address the social issues related to food insecurity, they do not in themselves seek to address food insecurity as a primary objective. These programmes are both targeted and seek to address hunger in low-income groups and community-wide responses that seek to address broader issues of food access and utilisation.

Social safety net programmes

Public policies and programmes that provide support for low-income individuals and families play an important role in reducing and preventing food insecurity for a very large number of people. The Supplemental Nutrition Assistance Program (SNAP) in the USA is the largest public response to food insecurity. Originally termed the Food Stamp Program, the programme in its initial form allowed people to purchase an orange stamp with money they would ordinarily use for food, and as a bonus, they would receive 50 cents worth of blue stamps for every dollar spent. Any food could be purchased with the orange stamps, which could be supplemented with additional cash, with the blue stamps then used to purchase surplus foods, at the time mostly eggs, butter, and beans. The programme had the dual purposes of 1) allowing low-income people to purchase greater quantities of food and therefore relieve some of the burden on food banks and 2) allowing US farmers to sell their surplus food to the government.

Since its introduction, the Food Stamp programme has gone through several changes in scope and eligibility, resulting in an increase in the number of participants. The current programme has tight eligibility requirements, including means testing and time limits on access to the programme, with average benefits of approximately $500 per month for a family of three from one month to three years. SNAP benefits can be used to purchase foods for the household to eat, and in some areas, restaurants can accept SNAP benefits from those experiencing homelessness and the elderly or disabled in exchange for low-cost meals. SNAP benefits cannot be used to buy alcohol, tobacco, or any non-food items.

While food subsidies can increase food access and facilitate choice, under this programme, this right is only fulfilled intermittently and not for all individuals. However, with over 40 million Americans currently on SNAP (Cragg and Stiglitz 2017), it has been called 'the cornerstone of the nation's nutrition safety net' (USDA 2017), and reflecting high costs of living and low incomes, the majority of SNAP benefits are distributed to working families with children (Wilde 2012). While many recipients report difficulties in meeting nutrient requirements on the amount of money provided through SNAP, with some participants accessing community food pantries and other services to secure sufficient food (Dharod et al. 2011), there are positive results of the programme including improvements in school performance and health of children, increasing food sales, and creating employment (Tiehen et al. 2012).

Community gardens

Community gardens, while still evolving as a response to food insecurity, are some of the most well-established community-based food initiatives. Community gardens work by providing a plot of land, often land that was formerly vacant, for individuals to cultivate their own food in a community setting. There is a large body of literature highlighting the positive outcomes of engagement in community gardens, particularly in their role as 'third places' or as a location that allows individuals or groups a place to meet beyond home and work (Veen et al. 2016). By acting as a third place, community gardens can enhance social life in urban neighbourhoods, allowing residents the opportunity and space to get to know each other and to develop a sense of community (Bellows et al. 2004). By allowing community members the opportunity to be involved in the production of their own food, they also provide a space for some to resist the commodification of food (Bailey et al. 2018). Community gardens can also enhance social cohesion by contributing to 'place attachment', with many community gardeners maintaining their plots and the communities around them for decades (Hale et al. 2011).

Most of the work investigating community gardens has focused on their role as a setting for health promotion, with limited literature exploring the role of community gardens in increasing food security (McCormack et al. 2010). While having the potential to provide a supplemental source of fresh produce, often through a bartering system or through the exchange of free foods (Bailey et al. 2018), due to the requirement for space, involvement is limited, and much of the research suggests that those who are engaging in community gardens are those who would seek out fresh produce anyway (McCormack et al. 2010). Community gardens cannot be seen as a sustainable solution for all families; those who lack the skill, interest, or access will continue to be isolated from community gardens (Loopstra and Tarasuk 2013). However, the strength of community gardens is that they have the potential to provide a source of culturally appropriate foods and to act as a positive social setting by providing a space for gathering (Gichunge and Kidwaro 2014).

Social enterprises

While still new, social enterprises have begun to enter the food relief space. A social enterprise is characterised by the use of business solutions to solve social problems. Social enterprises are typically underpinned by a clear social purpose that can be addressed through trade in which profits or surplus are reinvested to fulfil a specific mission (Barraket et al. 2016). Social entrepreneurs tie their activities to actions they deem to have the greatest positive social impact, with many social enterprises playing a role in addressing health inequities (Roy et al. 2014). Social enterprises have emerged in recognition that government provided social support or support provided through charity is limited and, more importantly, is not meeting public need. While there are some who question the ability of the social enterprise to combat long-term food insecurity and to affect change within the broader food system (Shannon 2016), proponents of social enterprises argue that they provide an 'additional tier of support' in the food security space aside from the role of charitable organisations and government assistance (Popielarski and Cotugna 2010). This is supported by some literature that has explored the ability of social enterprises to address food insecurity or to act as an additional provider of food and nutrition. Three examples are specifically addressed here: The Stop, The Food Justice Truck, and the Intervale Centre.

Emerging from food banks and other forms of emergency relief are neighbourhood hubs, allowing individuals the opportunity to come together to grow, cook, and share food. The Stop Community Food Centre, Toronto Canada, is one example of a successful community food hub that also operates as a social enterprise. The Stop was developed to respond to an increase in local residents who were seeking food relief from the local church (Russell 2002). With increasing need and a recognition that to respond to food insecurity, more than emergency food relief would be needed, The Stop began to incorporate political and social initiatives, such as advocating for renters' rights and assisting with employment services in addition to traditional food relief (Levkoe 2003). The centre provides community meals, a community garden, drop-in centre, food bank, and a range of programs for individuals of different ages, providing both social connection and fresh produce, alongside capacity-building and education and training programmes (Levkoe and Wakefield 2011).

The Food Justice Truck (FJT) is another example of a food-based social enterprise. The FJT was established by the Asylum Seeker Resource Centre (ASRC) in Melbourne, Australia, in March 2015 to complement their cleaning and catering social enterprises, with the aim of providing subsidised fresh produce for asylum seekers vulnerable to food insecurity. Unlike the on-site food bank at the ASRC, the FJT purchases foods from low-cost suppliers and operates less like a food charity and more like an enterprise. The FJT operates as a mobile fresh produce market, designed to overcome the transport barriers faced by many people seeking asylum by going directly to the populations in need. The FJT trades as a social enterprise by selling fruits, vegetables, rice, and legumes and offering a 60–75 per cent discount for asylum seekers, while maintaining full prices for the public. The FJT has been found to have the potential to promote social connection by providing customers with a third place to meet and get to know other people seeking asylum and volunteers and overall eliciting positive experiences for customers (McKay et al. 2018b). As a response to food insecurity, the FJT has also been found to provide increased low-cost food to those in need, with users of the FJT found to have lower rates of food insecurity than other studies with people seeking asylum (Haines et al. 2018). Customers of the FJT also reported experiencing lower stigma when using the FJT than has been reported by users of other sources of food aid and are more engaged and comfortable with, and able to use, non-aid food providers including commercial providers (Haines et al. 2018).

The Intervale Centre takes a different approach again by seeking to strengthen the food system through agricultural initiatives, including community-supported agriculture, large-scale composting, food hubs, and farm incubators. The Intervale Centre operates out of Burlington, Vermont, in the USA and sits on 700 acres of reclaimed land that supports several social enterprises. The farm incubation enterprise makes land, storage, and equipment available to small and new farmers, with opportunities for chefs, food writers, and apiarists also available. These activities produce a number of employment opportunities and at the same time result in hundreds of tonnes of fresh produce, and through food rescue and gleaning, the Centre has fed hundreds of families (Intervale Centre 2019; Rose 2017). These activities allow the Centre to generate income and to employ farm-led income practice where prices are set so that farmers are paid a fair price for their goods. The income generated also allows the Centre to reinvest in social justice projects, including subsidies for low-income households (Schmidt et al. 2011). This model allows the Intervale Centre to employ innovative strategies, so food can be made available for anyone who wants it (Intervale Centre 2019).

Conclusions

Emergency relief strategies such as food banks, soup vans, and prepared meals programs play a vital role in addressing acute food insecurity. However, limited resources mean that these programs have little effect on systematic, long-term, food insecurity and hunger. Focusing on emergency food relief only may deflect attention from the structural causes of poverty, ignoring community solutions to food insecurity and hunger. To make systemic changes to the food landscape and to achieve food security for all, alternative initiatives that engage community members in a range of activities and cater food security and hunger needs must be adopted. Alternative food initiatives which are emerging are addressing the long-term, structural challenges confronting the food system that lead to chronic food insecurity in an integrated and comprehensive way. Confronting food insecurity challenges will required dynamic, interdisciplinary, and multisectoral strategies that include antipoverty efforts, food, and community building that work with all aspects of the food system.

References

Bailey, S., Hendrick, A. and Palmer, M. (2018) 'Eco-social work in action: a place for community gardens', *Australian Social Work*, 71: 98–110.

Barraket, J., Mason, C. and Blain, B. (2016) *Finding Australia's social enterprise sector 2016: Final Report*. Online. Available at www.socialtraders.com.au/wp-content/uploads/2016/07/FASES-2016-full-report-final.pdf (accessed 13 March 2019).

Bazerghi, C., McKay, F.H. and Dunn, M. (2016) 'The role of food banks in addressing food insecurity: a systematic review', *Journal of Community Health*, 41: 732–40.

Bellows, A.C., Brown, K. and Smit, J. (2004) *Health Benefits of Urban Agriculture*, Portland, OR: Community Food Security Coalition's North American Initiative on Urban Agriculture. Online. Available at https://community-wealth.org/content/health-benefits-urban-agriculture (accessed 13 March 2019).

Booth, S (2014) 'Food banks in Australia: discouraging the right to food', in G. Riches and T. Silvasti (eds) *First World Hunger Revisited: Food Charity or the Right to Food*, London: Springer.

Cragg, M. and Stiglitz, J.E. (2017) 'The economists' voice: special issue on nutrition and poverty introduction', *The Economists' Voice*, 14(1).

Daponte, B.O. and Bade, S. (2006) 'How the private food assistance network evolved: interactions between public and private responses to hunger', *Nonprofit and Voluntary Sector Quarterly*, 35: 668–90.

Dharod, J.M., Croom, J., Sady, C.G. and Morrell, D. (2011) 'Dietary intake, food security, and acculturation among Somali refugees in the United States: results of a pilot study', *Journal of Immigrant and Refugee Studies*, 9: 82–97.

Dorsch, P., Phillips, J. and Crowe, C. (2016) *Poverty in Australia 2016*, Strawberry Hills, NSW: ACOSS. Online. Available at www.acoss.org.au/wp-content/uploads/2016/10/Poverty-in-Australia-2016.pdf (accessed 13 March 2019).

Engels, B. and Boys, P. (2008) 'Food insecurity and children: an investigation of school breakfast clubs in Melbourne, Victoria', *Just Policy*, 48: 4–15.

Foodbank Australia (2015) *Hunger in the Classroom*. North Ryde: Foodbank Australia. Online. Available at www.foodbank.org.au/wp-content/uploads/2015/05/Foodbank-Hunger-in-the-Classroom-Report-May-2015.pdf (accessed 15 September 2018).

Foodbank Australia (2017) *Foodbank Hunger Report*. Online. Available at www.foodbank.org.au/wp-content/uploads/2017/10/Foodbank-Hunger-Report-2017.pdf (accessed 13 March 2019).

Garthwaite, K. (2016) 'Stigma, shame and "people like us": an ethnographic study of food-bank use in the UK', *Journal of Poverty and Social Justice*, 24: 277–89.

Gichunge, C. and Kidwaro, F. (2014) 'Utamu wa A frika (the sweet taste of Africa): the vegetable garden as part of resettled African refugees' food environment', *Nutrition and Dietetics*, 71: 270–5.

Haines, B.C., McKay, F.H., Dunn, M. and Lippi, K. (2018) 'The role of social enterprise in food insecurity among asylum seekers', *Health and Social Care in the Community*, 26: 829–38.

Hale, J., Knapp, C., Bardwell, L., Buchenau, M., Marshall, J., Sancar, F. and Litt, J.S. (2011) 'Connecting food environments and health through the relational nature of aesthetics: gaining insight through the community gardening experience', *Social Science and Medicine*, 72: 1853–63.

Handforth, B., Hennink, M. and Schwartz, M.B. (2013) 'A qualitative study of nutrition-based initiatives at selected food banks in the feeding America network', *Journal of the Academy of Nutrition and Dietetics*, 113: 411–15.

Holmes, E., Black, J.L., Heckelman, A., Lear, S.A., Seto, D., Fowokan, A. and Wittman, H. (2018) ' "Nothing is going to change three months from now": a mixed methods characterization of food bank use in Greater Vancouver', *Social Science and Medicine*, 200: 129–36.

Intervale Centre (2019) 'Programs'. Online. Available at www.intervale.org/programs (accessed 21 February 2019).

Kicinski, L.R. (2012) 'Characteristics of short and long-term food pantry users', *Michigan Sociological Review*, 26: 58–74.

Lawrence, G., Richards, C. and Lyons, K. (2013) 'Food security in Australia in an era of neoliberalism, productivism and climate change', *Journal of Rural Studies*, 29: 30–9.

Levkoe, C.Z. (2003) 'Widening the approach to food insecurity: the stop community food centre', *Canadian Review of Social Policy*, 52: 128–32.

Levkoe, C.Z. and Wakefield, S. (2011) 'The community food centre: creating space for a just, sustainable, and healthy food system', *Journal of Agriculture, Food Systems and Community Development*, 2: 249–68.

Lindberg, R., Whelan, J., Lawrence, M., Gold, L. and Friel, S. (2015) 'Still serving hot soup? Two hundred years of a charitable food sector in Australia: a narrative review', *Australian and New Zealand Journal of Public Health*, 39: 358–65.

Loopstra, R. and Tarasuk, V. (2013) 'Perspectives on community gardens, community kitchens and the good food box program in a community-based sample of low-income families', *Canadian Journal of Public Health*, 104(1): e55–9.

Loopstra, R. and Tarasuk, V. (2015) 'Food bank usage is a poor indicator of food insecurity: insights from Canada', *Social Policy and Society*, 14: 443–55.

McCormack, L.A., Laska, M.N., Larson, N.I. and Story, M. (2010) 'Review of the nutritional implications of farmers' markets and community gardens: a call for evaluation and research efforts', *Journal of the American Dietetic Association*, 110: 399–408.

McIntyre, L., Patterson, P.B., Anderson, L.C. and Mah, C.L. (2016) 'Household food insecurity in Canada: problem definition and potential solutions in the public policy domain', *Canadian Public Policy*, 42: 83–93.

McKay, F.H., Bugden, M., Dunn, M. and Bazerghi, C. (2018a) 'Experiences of food access for asylum seekers who have ceased using a food bank in Melbourne, Australia', *British Food Journal*, 120: 1708–21.

McKay, F.H., Lippi, K., Dunn, M., Haines, B.C. and Lindberg, R. (2018b) 'Food-based social enterprises and asylum seekers: the food justice truck', *Nutrients*, 10: 756.

McKay, F.H. and McKenzie, H. (2017) 'Food aid provision in metropolitan Melbourne: a mixed methods study', *Journal of Hunger and Environmental Nutrition*, 12: 11–25.

McKenzie, H.J. and McKay, F.H. (2017) 'Food as a discretionary item: the impact of welfare payment changes on low-income single mother's food choices and strategies', *Journal of Poverty and Social Justice*, 25: 35–48.

Mukoya, M.N., McKay, F.H. and Dunn, M. (2017) 'Can giving clients a choice in food selection help to meet their nutritional needs? Investigating a novel food bank approach for asylum seekers', *Journal of International Migration and Integration*, 18: 981–91.

Piwowarczyk, L., Keane, T.M. and Lincoln, A. (2008) 'Hunger: the silent epidemic among asylum seekers and resettled refugees', *International Migration*, 46: 59–77.

Popielarski, J.A. and Cotugna, N. (2010) 'Fighting hunger through innovation: evaluation of a food bank's social enterprise venture', *Journal of Hunger and Environmental Nutrition*, 5: 56–69.

Raponi, S. (2017) 'A defense of the human right to adequate food', *Res Publica*, 23: 99–115.

Renzaho, A.M.N. and Mellor, D. (2010) 'Food security measurement in cultural pluralism: missing the point or conceptual misunderstanding?' *Nutrition*, 26: 1–9.

Rose, N. (2017) 'Community food hubs: an economic and social justice model for regional Australia?' *Rural Society*, 26: 225–37.

Roy, M.J., Donaldson, C., Baker, R. and Kerr, S (2014) 'The potential of social enterprise to enhance health and well-being: a model and systematic review', *Social Science and Medicine*, 123: 182–93.

Russell, C. (2002) 'In the beginning', *The Stop News*, 2.

Schmidt, M.C., Kolodinsky, J.M., DeSisto, T.P. and Conte, F.C. (2011) 'Increasing farm income and local food access: a case study of a collaborative aggregation, marketing, and distribution strategy that links farmers to markets', *Journal of Agriculture, Food Systems, and Community Development*, 1: 157–75.

Shannon, D. (2016) 'Food justice, direct action, and the human rights enterprise', *Critical Sociology*, 42: 799–814.

Tarasuk, V.S. (2001) 'A critical examination of community-based responses to household food insecurity in Canada', *Health Education and Behavior*, 28: 487–99.

Tarasuk, V.S. and Beaton, G.H. (1999) 'Household food insecurity and hunger among families using food banks', *Canadian Journal of Public Health*, 90: 109–13.

Tiehen, L., Jolliffe, D. and Gunderson, C. (2012) *Alleviating Poverty in the United States: The Critical Role of SNAP Benefits*, Washington, DC: US Department of Agriculture, Economic Research Service. Online. Available at https://ideas.repec.org/p/ags/uersrr/262233.html (accessed 24 November 2019).

USDA (2017) 'Outreach grants'. Online. Available at www.fns.usda.gov/outreach/out reach-grants (accessed 15 September 2018).

Veen, E.J., Bock, B.B., Van den Berg, W., Visser, A.J. and Wiskerke, J.S. (2016) 'Community gardening and social cohesion: different designs, different motivations', *Local Environment*, 21: 1271–87.

Wilde, P.E. (2012) 'The new normal: the supplemental nutrition assistance program (SNAP)', *American Journal of Agricultural Economics*, 95: 325–31.

Wilson, A., Szwed, N. and Renzaho, A. (2012) 'Developing nutrition guidelines for recycled food to improve food security among homeless, asylum seekers, and refugees in Victoria, Australia', *Journal of Hunger and Environmental Nutrition*, 7: 239–52.

8 Developing inclusion in a small-town food service

Rohena Duncombe, Joe Fay, Gwen Gould,
Charlie Fay, Malcolm Fay, Julia Harrington,
Kuatarina Mount, Brian Neale and
Suzanne Arnold

Introduction

In preparing this chapter, we have taken the opportunity to reflect on and deepen our own engagement with inclusion and sustainability in a regional coastal town's food programme, a weekly breakfast. We hope to contribute to interest in building inclusion when working in food security with volunteers, arguing that inclusion can be developed incrementally. The breakfast programme serves a population of people living homeless and others who have food affordability issues. These people often have a history of abuse that can result in psycho-emotional disorders, which in turn can present self-management problems for them and risk management issues for those around them. Risk management and inclusion need to be carefully balanced.

We have used a cooperative inquiry approach to collect, develop, and share our understandings. The co-authors were both the research participants and the researchers. Our research questions were:

- What are the elements of inclusivity in the breakfast programme?
- What factors contribute to its sustainability?

Through this inquiry, we have identified key factors that have sustained our programme over its 15 years: qualities of leadership, integrating other providers (place-based servicing), a family model (inclusivity), and minimal resource dependency. During that time, our commitment to inclusion has been maintained by the idea of developing a supportive welcoming atmosphere and progressing inclusion incrementally. Developing this chapter has led us to consider new ways to develop both sustainability and inclusivity.

We conclude that inclusivity can contribute to sustainability, that sustainability is about more than secure funding, and that inclusion can be developed incrementally in food security delivery, enabling a shift from charity to solidarity.

Background

Internationally inequality is accompanied by exclusion, and inequality itself is increasing in many countries (Stiglitz 2012; Wilkinson and Pickett 2010).

Exclusion exacerbates, among other things, physical, social, and psycho-emotional health issues at community and individual levels (Taket et al. 2009; Wilkinson and Pickett 2010, 2018). Inequity and exclusion are closely linked to homelessness and food insecurity (Ortiz-Ospina and Roser 2018).

A number of high-income countries, including the United States, Italy, the United Kingdom, and Germany, have growing populations of people living with inadequate food supplies (The Economist Intelligence Unit 2015). Food inequality itself constitutes a form of exclusion, i.e. exclusion from a food supply that is reliable, adequate, and affordable. This in turn has implications for social and physical well-being. In Australia, inequality increased from the mid-1980s (ABS 2017; Wilkinson and Pickett 2010), stabilising at higher levels between 2013 and 2016 (Wilkins and Wooden 2017). Australian census data indicate a 4.6 per cent increase in the population of people living homeless between 2011 and 2016. Homelessness Australia reports the Australian rate of homelessness as 49 people per 10,000, with New South Wales (NSW) the worst affected (Homelessness Australia 2018). Within NSW, the coastal town that hosts the breakfast has 12 times the NSW homelessness rate (Black 2016).

Although food insecurity in Australia is not rising (The Economist Intelligence Unit 2015), 3.7 per cent of the Australian population reported having run out of food and been unable to buy more during the previous 12 months. This is much more likely in remote areas and for Indigenous Australians (ABS 2018b). Others cite the charitable food sector in Australia as feeding up to 8 per cent of the population in 2015 (Brooke 2016; Lindberg et al. 2015), with around 4,000 food services presently operating (Pollard et al. 2016). The role of volunteers in addressing food insecurity is significant. However, this dependence on charity can perpetuate hierarchical 'doing for' rather than 'doing with' relationships that fail to address exclusion (Poppendieck 1999).

The growing scale of the charitable food sector since the mid-1990s highlights the inequality between the food rich and the food poor. This is despite Australia being a net food exporter and producing 90 per cent of our domestic food requirements (Brooke 2016). Growth in the charitable food sector in Australia is associated with stagnant Social Security benefits fixed at below poverty-line levels (ACOSS 2018) that have also contributed to homelessness. It could be expected that this would be an embarrassment for a rich country that might trigger a robust government response, but it is the charitable sector through volunteers and philanthropists who take much of the responsibility for this significant health problem (Lindberg et al. 2015).

The charitable sector is, however, not designed to sustain regular supply of a basic human right, food. Some organisations in the sector are dependent on donations of food waste, which can make good nutrition difficult to ensure (Thomas 2004). The sector is also fragmented with multiple providers not necessarily knowing about each other and many without government or other secure funding. There is no coherent overarching approach, so some areas are very well served and others not provided for at all.

People volunteer in the sector with a desire to help but often without an understanding of how hierarchical relationships, doing 'for' rather than 'with', can perpetuate marginalisation. The dependence on charity for food services means they tend to be provided beyond the reach and influence of professional expertise and research evidence. Volunteers, though motivated and genuine, may be unfamiliar with concepts related to inclusion. Food provision that remains in the 'service to' as against 'service with' modality will miss the opportunity for inclusive practice that can contribute to wellbeing. This is as much a challenge for the breakfast programme as for any other volunteer-led community initiative.

In addition, some people living homeless may not want to be more participatory for a range of reasons (see later 'mistakes are made') and may not welcome what they might perceive as excessive encouragement to participate. A 'Pre-treatment' approach advises the necessity of forming a working alliance before wider inclusion can be possible (Conolly 2017). In relation to identity, Johnson et al. (2008) found that some people actively resist identifying as homeless, quite likely because of the poor social status associated with it, and this might contribute to a reluctance to participate in a 'homeless' activity. Ultimately, what is needed, argue Lindberg et al. (2016), is for the underlying causes of food insecurity to be addressed in a national policy of poverty reduction and indexed Social Security payments. In the meantime, programmes such as the one described in this paper play a role in ameliorating food insecurity.

The breakfast

The Homeless and Community Breakfast is located on the east coast of NSW, Australia, in a town with a population of 9,000 at the 2016 Census (ABS 2018a). The breakfast was one of few food services in the town when it started. There were two other meals per week. There is now food available most days including free groceries and cooked lunches but no other cooked breakfast. No food services in the town have government funding. The breakfast helps support people with the least resources and does this at a local level, outside of local, state, or federal government policy or service provision.

We have been fortunate to have fresh food purchased and donated locally to provide a nutritious and substantial cooked breakfast once a week. It comprises coffee, a range of teas, toast, porridge and cereals, fresh fruit, omelette and fried eggs, sausages, bacon, stir-fried vegetables, sliced tomatoes, and fried onion. People living homeless do not generally have food storage, preparation, or cooking facilities. Food provided to them needs to be able to be eaten in situ or provided in take-away form. Our programme does not collect any details of the people using it and so is characterised as 'anonymous' according to Herzfeld's (2010) characterisation of models of food relief. Herzfeld also has an 'empowerment' category, which we meet to the extent that our inclusive and place-based approach adds some capacity beyond simply food provision as described later.

A cooperative inquiry

Our reflections and investigations in preparing this chapter have been undertaken in the form of a cooperative inquiry. This is an experiential research approach that facilitates the involvement of non-researchers and values reflexivity, reflection, and lived experience (Reason 2002; Short and Healy 2017). We worked together as co-researchers and co-subjects reflecting on both our achievements and short-comings to date and developing ideas for the further development of both inclusion and sustainability for the breakfast.

The process of undertaking this approach has involved cycling through four phases of reflection and action (Reason 2002). Rohena initiated the inquiry inviting Gwen, the breakfast initiator, and Joe, a volunteer who is an experienced international community developer, to join her. Joe initiated widening the group to invite all the breakfast volunteers so that we were all thinking and talking about inclusion and sustainability and our ideas for furthering these. As he said at the time, 'I can't see us going into inclusion without having the whole team on board'. As a result, a further six of our volunteers participated in discussions and were kept in touch with the writing as it progressed.

Our parameters were set by this book section, sustaining programmes which promote social inclusion. We wanted to explore the degree of inclusivity we have attained and how we could further develop this. We also reflected on what had contributed to our sustainability over 15 years and how we could further ensure our sustainability into the future.

We have undertaken this through a series of audio recorded face-to-face discussions and through email exchanges. Rohena has led the writing, and Joe and Gwen both engaged with and contested that writing as well as being active in identifying and developing ideas. Other members of the team have participated in conversations and commented on the emerging manuscript. This has enabled us to look at the breakfast, our endeavours, and its possibilities through new eyes (Reason 2002). In the fourth and final phase of the inquiry, we have come to new understandings of the breakfast programme and of opportunities for action on inclusion and sustainability.

Inclusion

Conversations about language

Our discussions tackled the issue of language. We were aware of the role of language in setting a tone of inclusion, exclusion, and hierarchy. Rohena was using the word 'participants' to refer to the people who live homeless and come to breakfast. In precis, the discussion went:

Joe: When you say 'participants', who do you mean? I use the term, I don't like, 'clients'. We need to be clear who we are talking about.
Gwen: I have never thought of them as clients. I think of them as people.

Rohena:	The people who come for breakfast and the people who come to help.
Joe:	Well, why don't we just agree that when we say participants, there are people who come who may help out and there are the people who are living rough or are just. . .
Rohena:	We are talking about two things. The three of us agree that we should be referring to people as people. But the other thing we are discussing is the need sometimes to differentiate the roles people are in at particular times.

This discussion was not conclusive but did clarify the language problem and our understanding of each other. What we confirmed was that we do not like terms such as 'client' that inherently imply hierarchy.

The importance of talking about inclusion

The importance of talking about inclusion emerged. We realised we need to talk about our attitude toward inclusion and our knowledge of its benefits (Taket et al. 2014) within the breakfast community, with other homelessness services and with the wider community centre and its management. As not all our volunteers come with an understanding of inclusion, that idea needs to be introduced and explored. People are familiar with the idea of helping, of doing good—they know that they themselves are fortunate and so they can afford to give some of their time and efforts for people who are less so. This is a valid motivation, but inclusion can value-add to the provision of food, communicating acceptance and acknowledgement of people's intelligence and capabilities and so be somewhat more strengths-based in style (Saleebey 2002). Just as inclusion is best introduced gradually to the people who are homeless, we find this is also true for our volunteers. We need to introduce the idea and allow time for them to become comfortable with the concept.

Talking about inclusion promotes the idea of 'solidarity with' rather than 'charity for' and can draw attention to the exclusion and imbalance in power and silencing of people who are living homeless. Talking about inclusion helps counter the unconscious 'othering' of people caught up in the effects of below poverty line 'social security' payments and unaffordable accommodation.

Warm and welcoming

Our first principle of inclusion is a warm welcome. For Gwen, who initiated the food service, inclusion is about nurturing a family atmosphere.

> The way I approached it—part of what I did was, I'm a real family person and I didn't have family near me at the time, and I sort of made this my family so, that's how you define inclusive. They weren't just people out there they were people that you cared about.

Making people welcome is a crucial element in working with those living homeless (Wen et al. 2007), and a warm welcome is important in setting the tone and lowering boundaries between people coming for breakfast and people who come to help. A warm welcome is an element of both inclusion and of good service provision for vulnerable populations.

From its inception, there were elements of inclusion in our service design: the family welcome and the sharing of space. Gwen fought for the sharing of space within our host organisation, the community centre. A new food service that was to work from the same space as us wanted to reformat the breakfast space so that all volunteers were behind service counters. This was inconsistent with what we were doing, but the new service was providing the funds for the refurbishment. Taket et al. (2014), in discussing inclusive environments, note that separated zones are implicitly stigmatising and so foster exclusion. Keeping the volunteers in separate zones reifies the underlying 'us and them' assumption and the implicit message that 'they' are dangerous. Physical barriers would hinder our efforts to encourage interaction and create a more homelike atmosphere.

Sustaining spatial inclusion has been maintained for the present but remains a point of vulnerability that we need address by sharing ideas of inclusion within the wider homelessness service setting. Mingling in the space doesn't of itself remove social boundaries. It is supported by our commitment to forming relationships with the people who come for breakfast in a friendly, low-key manner. These relationships, for a number of the volunteers, extend beyond the breakfast into the streets and onto the beaches. When we stop and speak with people outside the breakfast environment, we are telegraphing a degree of inclusion in the wider town community beyond the breakfast environment. Challenging social status boundaries in this way can have people feel welcome, to belong and connect in the wider community.

Similarly it is important for us to not wear badges or team tee shirts, not to differentiate ourselves. We converse and develop relationships with the people who come to breakfast. Sometimes we celebrate birthdays. We send cards to people in jail and hospital. We have also advocated for people with the housing agencies, provide court support, and support people going into rehabilitation programmes. We become involved in their lives, and to some extent, they become involved in ours. Some of the volunteers have had people stay in their homes or have employed them in trade work they were qualified for. Broaching the usual social barriers effectively telegraphs an acknowledgement of people beyond their situation of homelessness.

Involvement in breakfast

We like to involve people attending for breakfast in the preparation, delivery, and pack-up of the meal. As Gwen said,

> We used to open the doors at 7:30, everyone would pile in, homeless and everything and they would be part of the set-up to get it going and I think that was a big barrier breakdown where they were part of setting up the whole thing.

Involving people can require care and patience as each person needs a right time and a right task. Especially for long-term homeless, there is an issue of de-habilitation—a loss of confidence and a loss of familiarity with domestic skills. One person who was invited to help with food preparation initially declined but at a later date was happy to assist by tearing lengths of greaseproof paper. Social exclusion is related to status syndrome. As humans, we know where we are in a social hierarchy and may over time cease to challenge this or start to self-exclude, perhaps as a strategy for contesting that powerlessness or rejecting imposed separateness (Marmot 2004; Taket et al. 2014). The shift from de-skilled and discouraged to full participation can be a long-term one, and an initial refusal is not necessarily an indication of lack of interest. We must continually invite participation.

There are issues of power and agency. Inclusion involves the opening of opportunity and movement toward more equal power relations, in this case social ones (not economic or political). The breakfast needs to be a safe place to begin to have the confidence and trust to risk social involvement. It needs to be a safe place to extend social networks, a crucial factor in being able to access public resources (Winkworth et al. 2010). Joe reflected on 'the terrible length of time that is needed' both to develop trust with individuals and within the wider group. Kuatarina and Gwen spoke about the importance of finding something for people to contribute as soon as they ask. Gwen said, 'what doesn't work, hasn't worked, if in the early part of the day when there's nothing to do you say, there's nothing to do can you come back later they don't'. Kuatarina elaborated, saying, 'you've got to get them on the spot. Like (someone) today said, "What else can I do?" As I turned around I saw the floor was really dirty, "Sweep the floor"'. Rohena further noted the need for all team members to be responding similarly, commenting that 'We need to be really careful not to say "no", we need to all be on the same page about that. We all know that people need encouragement, so if anyone offers, find something'.

The degree of inclusion we have achieved is still relatively low, probably at 'placation' on Arnstein's (1969) ladder of inclusivity, but with elements of participation. We have noted that it is necessary to begin subtly for some people. There are some, however, who have become members of the volunteer team. Four of our regular volunteers initially came to eat breakfast. One of these is now in our leadership team.

We do not have formal consultations with people living homeless, though some discussions do happen. The breakfast is not run by people living homeless, but four of our volunteers started by coming for breakfast. We are incrementally moving toward greater inclusion and to embedding inclusion in our service ethos (Taket et al. 2014).

Mistakes are made

Rohena reflected on her misguided attempts to include people living homeless on the electoral role to vote. The electoral office was very helpful with a special process for people without addresses, but the reality was that most did not have any faith in the system and some did not want to risk being located for outstanding fines or offences. This led Rohena to wonder whether it was self-exclusion as an assertion of agency in a context of limited opportunities, a rejection of the society that has rejected them, or simply common sense from their perspective.

Mistakes like these have made us experts by experience in our own environment.

Gwen: When we were looking at setting up a camp area for people . . . and they were like, 'no that wouldn't work for us, you can't put us all together'. Us on the outside looking to see how it would work and unless we included them in the decision it wasn't appropriate.

Joe: Yes, our experience, our expertise now is helping us to determine where we should go, what we should do.

Inclusion and risk management

We have started speaking about inclusion in the local meeting of homelessness service providers and with community centre management. While Rohena finds that this is often quickly accepted as relevant and important, it has come up against the concept of risk management. Our policy of tolerance and inclusion was seen as risky, and the community centre ceased allowing students to attend as part of their field education placements.

People who have been abused, have a mental illness, have had a head injury, or use substances often find emotional self-management a challenge (McLean and Foa 2017) Services may use a 'zero tolerance' approach to verbalised anger and disruptive behaviour with the aim of protecting both volunteers and other people who come for meals or groceries. This may be supported by a clear evacuation plan and clearly articulated strategies for managing and excluding people who contravene. While we appreciate the basis for this approach, we choose to differ. As Joe wrote,

> The risk management issue comes up at times during the breakfast and can be disruptive. For those who come regularly, we often know them well and there is a level of trust and respect that helps to defuse any sign of violence before it starts.

Some incidents will result in the individual being asked to leave and return when they are calm again. When the community centre has required us to bar someone, we have still been able to provide a service by serving them on a bench located just outside the centre. This is in a public space where many people congregated. Also we have had guest workshops on understanding the more common mental health issues. We have had similar workshops that present ways to respond to physical violence.

Although a formal debriefing process has not been developed, incidents are informally discussed during a regular coffee discussion after breakfast closes. These informal meetings have bonded the volunteers so that we understand each others' lives and are able to debrief and feel supported and included in the breakfast programme.

The breakfast feeds a population of people who have a reasonably high risk of aggression profile: severe situational stress, socioeconomic disadvantage, low social support, and a history of abuse and neglect. In addition, many have mental health and substance issues that arise from the former set of factors (Centrelink/ Comcare 2000). It is our observation that risk management can be approached with understanding, tolerance, and softer security strategies (Kavaliūnaitė 2011; Rasmusson and Jansson 1996). Softer security uses quiet and unobtrusive strategies. At the breakfast, this includes a trauma-informed understanding that much aggression stems from personal damage suffered by the person, in frustration, and by the knowledge that the wider community doesn't care. Some of our soft security strategies include not leaving knives around, having plenty of people in the shared space, having built personal relationships with regular attendees, and utilising our people skilled in de-escalating conversations. As Gwen noted, 'love and compassion with good boundaries. You can't have compassion without good boundaries, and you can't have good boundaries without compassion'.

Joe adds that we need to take into account the person and the atmosphere. Gwen specifies that she has always asked people to take their arguments away from the breakfast and been strict about not taking sides or becoming involved. She sees this as having contributed to our success. Gwen also built relationships with the police to ensure their support and response if we need it. We take an elastic tolerance approach rather than a zero-tolerance approach, encouraging considerate behaviour but understanding that people living with stress and trauma or head injuries can struggle with self-management. In response, we aim to be patient and understanding.

Sustainability

We suspect the family approach, its inclusiveness, and atmosphere have been a factor in our sustainability. Because the breakfast is a good gathering place for people living rough, it has recommended itself for place-based servicing. This, leadership, and the low cost of our programme are what we presently see as having helped our sustainability.

Leadership qualities

Gwen brought important personal qualities to her leadership. She is very hardworking, a great communicator, and more importantly a tireless negotiator who persisted through ongoing conflict to preserve our programme when there have been challenges to its survival. The challenge of sharing a space with a new food service has been referred to.

That food service is now a valuable and continuing service that we work well with. Initially, however, things were difficult; our equipment was moved or removed, and our provisions disappeared. That service too had a tenacious leader, and understandably the centre manager did not want to be involved in the conflict. This could be an example of how the lack of formalisation and the fragmentation of the human services sector can 'undermine its ability to work in a collaborative and integrated way' (Lindberg et al. 2015: 636). Gwen's tireless negotiation with both centre management and the then-leader of the new service sustained the breakfast programme and protected our commitment to sharing space.

Low cost

Gwen always wanted to keep the breakfast simple, and it may be that, and our low cost have been an advantage. We haven't had to raise significant sums of money, spend large amounts of time tendering for funds, develop fundraising strategies, or report to other agencies. Being a low-cost operation reduces our exposure but does not protect us completely. The loss of funding streams to our hosting community centre and the recent closure of our supporting green grocer have required us to look elsewhere which has been relatively easy with our low budget.

Our funding is presently comprised of: A\$25 a week fruit and vegetable supply from a major supermarket chain; the local hospital provision of milk, bread, sausages, tea, coffee, and sauce for five breakfasts every two months, also valued at around \$25 per week; and access to an annual charity of the day gate at the local monthly market valued at around A\$1500 per year. The significant support of the local hospital has been sustained by regularly informing managers about the programme and identifying the high needs of the population group. A number of us have used our personal and professional connections to sustain various sources of funds over the period.

Place-based servicing

Lindberg et al. (2015) refer to the strength of the inter-relationships in the charitable food sector including between primary care providers, hospitals, social services, food industry, welfare, business, and governments. This is certainly the case for the breakfast. Gwen attributes the support of Aboriginal health and social work staff for providing a solid foundation and transforming a food service to a service delivery venue. Now a participating community health nurse actively sustains our ongoing links with the local hospital. We see the breakfast as a site for improving service delivery for people who use the breakfast.

Gwen's desire to keep things simple was somewhat challenged by Rohena's persistent spotting of other opportunities; the most valuable has been to involve the community health nurse. The nurse provides initial consultations and much wound care. The community health nurses also introduced annual flu vaccinations for this vulnerable population.

Other services provided via the breakfast include bookings for showers, bookings for and transport to dental appointments, and secondhand clothes. Other personnel presently attending include a mental health team member, a Legal Aid solicitor, needle exchange staff, and Aboriginal Health. At other times Centrelink (an Australian government agency responsible for paying pensions and benefits) and homelessness service providers have attended. These people do not always have skills for community-based work and may need to be coached to integrate and not just chat among themselves. Gwen describes an interaction with a homelessness worker who came to breakfast.

> One girl said to me "oh I'm frightened". The way to do it is to make yourself a cup of tea, just go and sit down somewhere and chat to the person next to you and that way you start to break down the barriers.

This multiplicity of functions has networked us well into services for people living homeless and led to the breakfast being the place others come to access this community. Homelessness week activities are centred at the breakfast, and a local writers group produced a photo-story book with excerpts of peoples' lives with stunning photography, using the breakfast as the location to source their participants, as Rohena has also done for her homeless health research. In these ways, the place-based servicing has linked us well with other service providers, and this network assists our sustainability through the access to this population who are otherwise characterised as hard to reach. Place-based servicing is a preferred model for vulnerable groups generally and people living homeless in particular. Hwang et al.'s (2005) systematic review indicated that for health service delivery, coordinated treatment of mental health and substance use rather than stand-alone services were preferable and that services should be tailored to the homeless population. In particular service provision to people, living homeless should be warm and welcoming (Wen et al. 2007). We think our place-based approach addresses these criteria and contributes to our sustainability.

Initiatives resulting from this inquiry: strategies for action on inclusion and sustainability

An outcome of using a cooperative inquiry to prepare this chapter has been the development of strategies to further develop our inclusivity:

- Open discussion among key volunteer participants of adopting inclusion as an agreed approach: 'solidarity not charity';
- Discussion with wider group of participants, both breakfast attenders and volunteers about inclusion: forming relationships, sharing tasks, and inviting participation;
- Thinking together about risk management;
- Actively starting conversations with participants who live homeless about issues that arise and decisions we are making;
- Needing to reconnect with police now that a new inspector of police has been appointed; and
- Being explicit with new volunteers about our commitments to forming relationships as part of inclusivity.

Conclusion

We have used a cooperative inquiry to reflect on and deepen inclusion and sustainability in a small coastal food programme, the breakfast. We have built on our own commitment to and understanding of inclusion and hope this contributes to interest in the concept in the wider charitable food sector. We are arguing that the development of inclusion and sustainability can be incremental. We have come to think that inclusion might contribute to sustainability and to risk management.

The elements of our inclusivity are a warm welcome and family atmosphere, creating opportunities for participation, forming relationships that extend beyond the breakfast, and emphasising inclusion within our own group and in our wider sector.

The factors that have sustained our programme over its 15 years are qualities of leadership, integration with other providers (place-based servicing), inclusivity, and minimal resource dependency. During that time, our commitment to inclusion has been maintained by the idea of developing a supportive welcoming atmosphere and progressing incrementally. Developing this chapter has led us to consider new ways we will be able to develop both our sustainability and inclusivity.

During this project, we have begun speaking more about inclusion, acknowledging that we have different understandings of that but having it as an agreed commitment. We have concluded that sustainability is about more than secure funding and that both inclusion and sustainability can be developed incrementally as we move from charity to solidarity.

References

Arnstein, S.R. (1969) 'A ladder of citizen participation', *Journal of the American Institute of Planners*, 35: 216–24.

Australian Bureau of Statistics [ABS] (2017) 'Inequality stable since 2013–14'. Online. Available at www.abs.gov.au/ausstats/abs@.nsf/Lookup/by%20Subject/6523.0~2015-16~Media%20Release~Inequality%20stable%20since%202013-14%20%20(Media%20Release)~103 (accessed 20 June 2018).

Australian Bureau of Statistics [ABS] (2018a) '2016 Census Quick Stats'. Online. Available at http://quickstats.censusdata.abs.gov.au/census_services/getproduct/census/2016/quickstat/UCL114003?opendocument (accessed 11 January 2019).

Australian Bureau of Statistics [ABS] (2018b) 'Australian aboriginal and Torres strait islander health survey: nutrition results—food and nutrients, 2012–13', Online. Available at www.abs.gov.au/ausstats/abs@.nsf/Lookup/by%20Subject/4727.0.55.005~2012-13~Main%20Features~Food%20Security~36 (accessed 27 June 2018).

Australian Council of Social Service [ACOSS] (2018) *Budget Priorities Statement: Federal Budget 2018–19*, Strawberry Hills, NSW: Australian Council of Social Service. Online. Available at www.acoss.org.au/wp-content/uploads/2018/02/ACOSS-Budget-Priorities-Statement-2018-19_FINAL.pdf (accessed 11 January 2019).

Black, C. (2016) *Street Life in Byron: Project Report*, Byron Bay: Byron Bay Community Centre.

Brooke, F. (2016) *Food Security and Health in Rural and Remote Australia*, Wagga Wagga: National Rural Health Alliance and Rural Industries Research Development Corporation.

Centrelink and Comcare (2000) *Applying Best Practice Principles to the Prevention and Management of Customer Aggression: A Risk Management Guide for Customer Service Providers*, Canberra: Centrelink and Comcare.

Conolly, J. (2017) 'Pre-treatment therapy: a central London counselling service's enhanced response to complex needs homelessness', in J.S. Levy and R. Johnson (eds) *Cross-cultural Dialogues on Homelessness*, Ann Arbor: Loving Healing Press.

The Economist Intelligence Unit (2015) *Global Food Security Index 2015: An Annual Measure of the State of Global Food Security*. Online. Available at https://foodsecurityindex.eiu.com/Home/DownloadResource?fileName=EIU%20Global%20Food%20Security%20Index%20-%202015%20Findings%20%26%20Methodology.pdf (accessed 8 October 2018).

Herzfeld, M (2010) *The Intersection of Emergency Food Relief and Food Security*, Hobart: Tasmanian Council of Social Service (TasCOSS).

Homelessness Australia (2018) 'Homelessness statistics'. Online. Available at www.home lessnessaustralia.org.au/about/homelessness-statistics (accessed 8 October 2018).

Hwang, S., Tolomiczenko, G., Kouyoumdjian, F. and Garner, R. (2005) 'Interventions to improve the health of the homeless: a systematic review', *American Journal of Preventative Medicine*, 29: 311–19.

Johnson, G., Gronda, H. and Coutts, S. (2008) *On the Outside: Pathways in and Out of Homelessness*, North Melbourne: Australian Scholarly Publishing.

Kavaliūnaitė, S. (2011) 'Comparative analysis of concepts "soft security" and "soft power" in EU legislation', *Public Policy and Administration*, 10: 231–46.

Lindberg, R., Kleve, S., Barbour, L., Booth, S. and Gallegos, D. (2016) 'Introduction beyond emergency food: responding to food insecurity and homelessness', *Parity*, 29(2): 4–6.

Lindberg, R., Whelan, J., Lawrence, M., Gold, L. and Friel, S. (2015) 'Still serving hot soup? Two hundred years of a charitable food sector in Australia: a narrative review', *Australian and New Zealand Journal of Public Health*, 39: 358–65.

Marmot, M. (2004) 'Status syndrome', *Significance*, 1: 150–4.

McLean, C.P. and Foa, E.B. (2017) 'Emotions and emotion regulation in posttraumatic stress disorder', *Current Opinion in Psychology*, 4: 72–7.

Ortiz-Ospina, E. and Roser, M. (2018) 'Homelessness'. Online. Available at https://our-worldindata.org/homelessness (accessed 24 September 2018).

Pollard, C., Begley, A., Kerr, D., Mackintosh, B., Jancey, J., Campbell, C., Whelan, J., Milligan, R., Berg, J., Fisher, B., Halliday, K. and Caraher, M. (2016) 'Working in partnership with the charitable food sector to better meet the food needs of people in Perth', *Parity*, 29(2): 39–40.

Poppendieck, J. (1999) *Sweet Charity? Emergency Food and the End of Entitlement*, New York: Penguin.

Rasmusson, L. and Jansson, S. (1996) 'Simulated social control for secure internet commerce', in C. Meadows (ed) *Proceedings of the 1996 New Security Paradigms Workshop*. Online. Available at http://citeseerx.ist.psu.edu/viewdoc/download?doi=10.1.1.36 4.7464&rep=rep1&type=pdf (accessed 8 October 2018).

Reason, P. (2002) 'The practice of co-operative inquiry', *Systematic Practice and Action Research*, 15: 169–76.

Saleebey, D. (2002) *The Strengths Perspective in Social Work Practice*, 3rd edn, Boston: Allyn and Bacon.

Short, M. and Healy, J. (2017) 'Writing "with" not "about": examples in co-operative inquiry', in S. Gair and A.V. Luyun (eds) *Sharing Qualitative Research: Showing Lived Experience and Community Narratives*, London: Routledge.

Stiglitz, J. (2012) *The Price of Inequality: How Today's Divided Society Endangers Our Future*, trans A. Goldhammer. New York: Norton.

Taket, A., Crisp, B.R., Graham, M., Hanna, L. and Goldingay, S. (2014) 'Scoping social inclusion practice', in A. Taket, B.R. Crisp, M. Graham, L. Hanna, S. Goldingay and L. Wilson (eds) *Practising Social Inclusion*, London: Routledge.

Taket, A., Crisp, B.R., Nevill, A., Lamaro, G., Graham, M. and Barter-Godfrey, S. (2009) *Theorising Social Exclusion*, London: Routledge.

Thomas, P. (2004) 'Homelessness food relief', *Parity*, 17(3): 18.

Wen, C.K., Hudak, P.L. and Hwang, S.W. (2007) 'Homeless people's perceptions of welcomeness and unwelcomeness in healthcare encounters', *Journal of General Internal Medicine*, 22: 1011–7.

Wilkins, R. and Wooden, M. (2017) 'What 17 years of data tells us about Australia'. Online. Available at https://pursuit.unimelb.edu.au/articles/what-17-years-of-data-tells-us-about-australia (accessed 8 October 2018).

Wilkinson, R. and Pickett, K. (2010) *The Spirit Level: Why Equality Is Better for Everyone*, London: Penguin.

Wilkinson, R. and Pickett, K. (2018) *The Inner Level: How More Equal Societies Reduce Stress, Restore Sanity and Improve Everyone's Well-being*, London: Penguin.

Winkworth, G., McArthur, M., Layton, M., Thomson, L and Wilson, F. (2010) 'Opportunities lost: why some parents of young children are not well-connected to the service systems designed to assist them', *Australian Social Work*, 63: 431–44.

Part 4

Sustaining organisations which promote social inclusion

9 How to imagine and make good universities[1]

Raewyn Connell

Dr Pangloss and the League Tables

A few years ago, the Australian Vice-Chancellors' Committee (AVCC) re-badged itself as 'Universities Australia', and since then, the assembled vice-chancellors have presented themselves as 'The voice of Australia's universities'. That's what their website says, and this is undoubtedly a rich mine of corporate wisdom (Universities Australia 2018).

'Australia's universities', the website tells us, 'offer a unique educational experience that fosters self-belief, rewards independent thought and fuels inquiring minds'. Universities Australia (2013) has a 'vision for a smarter Australia', which will be achieved if more students, grants, and fees come into universities. But of course, growth 'will not be at the expense of quality. Universities have, and will continue to maintain, robust internal quality assurance mechanisms and processes' (Universities Australia 2018).

This robust declaration is of course written by the Universities Australia' advertising people, but it undoubtedly reflects the vice-chancellors' corporate view. They have excellent reasons to be pleased with progress. Their annual salaries *averaged* A$835 000 each (including the bonuses) in 2014. If Universities Australia's lobbying for unrestricted fee increases eventually bears fruit, they will get even more. For each current vice-chancellor, we could get a dozen tutors, research associates, and administrative officers.

A few years ago, one of their number, Glyn Davis of The University of Melbourne, delivered the ABC's Boyer Lectures, subsequently published as a book called *The Republic of Learning* (Davis 2010). This is the most widely circulated Australian text ever written about higher education, so it's worth taking note. It's an excellent guide to the ruling mentality, and you can still find it in good second-hand bookshops.

In genial style, *The Republic of Learning* takes the listener/reader through the fascinating world of universities. Davis speaks of old and new achievements in teaching, research, and academic life, with many powerful insights. 'Much needs to be done that is new—but much needs to be preserved' (Davis 2010: 29). In universities, 'Authority is held collectively by the academic body, represented through an academic board or senate' (Davis 2010: 97). The system has dilemmas but faces the future with confidence. 'Each public university, determined to make its way in the world, will invent the future that makes sense for it and its communities' (Davis 2010: 123). And so on.

Davis starts and finishes by invoking the great sixteenth-century scholar Erasmus of Rotterdam. It's a brave choice. That sardonic and embattled writer was a noted enemy of complacency, clichés, and intellectual sloppiness.

Davis succeeds, through his six lectures, in conveying a truly Panglossian picture: all is for the best in the best of all possible worlds. Trust us! It's a verbal version of the imagery now found on all Australian university websites: sunny skies and flowering jacarandas, happy students on manicured lawns, contented staff, brilliant breakthroughs in laboratories, and glimpses of wise chancellors conferring well-earned awards.

Easy to laugh at, when you know the reality at the coal face. But the logic of misrepresentation has now been built into a technology of policymaking, which has very real effects. A striking feature of the neoliberal era is the proliferation of 'metrics' for outcomes. This has grown into a system of ranking scales, informally known as League Tables, that imply an unending competition of excellence—between journals, papers, individual academics, departments, and whole universities.

The system now has, in fact, an institutionalised definition of the good university. It takes the form of widely publicised international rankings, before which even vice-chancellors tremble. Every year, as the rankings in the *Times Higher Education* or the Academic Ranking of World Universities (also known as the Shanghai Ranking) are published, there is a flurry of media releases from Australian universities, boasting of their rank or—should the overall score unhappily have slipped—finding a sub-ranking they can boast about. There is now a small industry supplying many different kinds of rankings (new universities, technical universities, regional rankings, discipline rankings, etc.) so the market can get what it wants.

And each year, to no one's surprise, the top universities on the main global scoreboards turn out to be Harvard, MIT, Chicago, Stanford, Caltech, Cambridge . . . the well-known, wealthy, highly selective, private, or more-or-less-private, elite institutions of the Global North. Basically, the metrics of excellence are measuring how far all the other universities in the world resemble the most economically, socially, and politically privileged. The paradigm of the good university, the best of the best of all possible worlds, is there at the top of the table—in Harvard, MIT, Chicago.

Actually these are horrible institutions. I've spent a year each at two of them (one as a post-doc and the other as a visiting professor) and have seen how destructive their privilege and arrogance are for the engagement and trust that create real quality in higher education. Yes, the Ivy League and Friends have wonderful libraries, astonishing computers, elegant buildings, great art collections, and low student/staff ratios. They have these because they have wealth skimmed from the corporate economy that has relentlessly degraded the global environment for the rest of humanity. And their wonderful Nobel Prize–winning research? Well, much of it depended on military or corporate funding, and these universities played a major role in the creation of atomic weapons and almost equally destructive 'conventional' armaments, not to mention the neoliberal economy itself.

The League Table definitions of excellence, nevertheless, are deeply embedded in corporate ideology and practice and have been taken up by governments. That monument of neoliberal policy orthodoxy, the 2012 white paper *Australia in the Asian Century*, formulated this as a National Objective: 'By 2025, 10 of Australia's universities will be in the world's top 100' (Australian Government 2012: 16). Since no neoliberal government, Labor or Coalition, is going to put tax money into even one Australian university on a scale that would make it look much like Harvard, the real effect of the League Table rhetoric is to provide a permanent justification for the vice-chancellors to increase fees and trawl for corporate money.

Defining the good: five approaches

For those who do not swallow the official wisdom, it becomes important to find other ways of defining a good university. This is not easy to do, if we want the result to have a grip on the practical situation in universities, but let us try. There are five ways of approaching the job.

The first is to compile a wish list. That was what I did when the 2013 strike at University of Sydney showed the shocking gulf between what management was trying to do and what universities actually needed. This is what my list looked like at the time (Connell 2014).

Good universities would be:

1 Educationally confident;
2 Socially inclusive;
3 Good places to work;
4 Democratic as organisations;
5 Epistemologically multiple;
6 Modest in demeanour; and
7 Intellectually ambitious.

Such an exercise can be done collectively and perhaps should be. A collective list was attempted by the 2015 conference from which this chapter was originally produced, producing a declaration that has a more generous 24 points (see The Brisbane Declaration 2016). They overlap my seven, introducing new themes but also dropping a couple.

The problem with wish lists is obvious: they are arbitrary in coverage and can be incoherent. They are not constrained by organisational limits, budgets, or the need to persuade constituencies. Yet the exercise is genuinely useful, especially at a time when neoliberal universities are steadily shutting down their internal forums for debate. Trying to formulate a wish list is jarring: it pushes you out of the every day and obliges you to think in a long time frame. Everyone working in universities should try it—and circulate the results.

Second, there's the classic academic method: compile a reading list and study the authorities. Those who do this are likely to find John Henry Newman's (1852/1873) *The Idea of a University* and Clark Kerr's (1963) *The Uses of the University*. If they look a little harder, they will find the economist Thorstein Veblen's splendid and highly relevant 1918 (1918/1957) book *The Higher Learning in America: a memorandum on the conduct of universities by business men.*

From the classics we can certainly get stimulating ideas, but we always have to consider them in context. Newman, for instance, wrote his famous text when he was brought from England to Ireland to help the church set up a new Catholic university. The difficulty was that the bishops insisted on having control, but in that case, the Protestant-dominated government would not pay, so the project died. Newman's eloquent 'University Teaching Considered in Nine Discourses' was thus a design for an imaginary university. Its central concern was to justify having theology in the curriculum.

Newman had a critique of utilitarianism that applies to neoliberalism too: 'it aimed low, but it has fulfilled its aim' (ouch!). But he was utterly opposed to the model of the research university, new at the time, that was emerging from Germany. Newman declared on the first page of his preface that the object of a university

> is the diffusion and extension of knowledge rather than the advancement. If its object were scientific and philosophical discovery, I do not see why a University should have students.
>
> (Newman 1852/1873: ix)

(Ouch again!) Research should be left to scientific academies. The proper role of universities was to be places for liberal education, gardens for 'the cultivation of the intellect'.

Newman didn't understand research, but he did know a lot about teaching. He showed how a profusion of topics or curriculum detail would distract students from deeper understanding, wrestling with principles and developing a sense of Universal Knowledge. No lectures at all would be better than too many. But this admirable idea of undergraduate life was designed for one social group, the gentry, specifically the gentlemen. It wouldn't meet our diversity KPI.

Nor, of course, do existing elite universities. There are some indications indeed that universities at the top of the international League Tables have become *less* diverse in the last decade or so, consistent with the trend of growing social inequalities under neoliberal regimes.

This points to a third approach to defining the good university rather more grounded than the wish lists. This is the procedure we might call the horror list: examining the ghastliest features of the University of Melbourne and designing a good university by antithesis. (To be strictly fair, I would examine the University of Sydney too. I'm a graduate of both.) Antitheses can readily be drawn up from the critical literature about contemporary Australian universities. On my reading, the main themes that emerge from this literature are:

1   *The relentless commercialisation that has gone on since the Dawkins policy changes of the late 1980s.* The re-introduction of fees was the trigger, but the effects have ramified. Lucrative teaching programmes have been expanded, and the least vocational areas (such as philosophy) declined. There is growing dependence on a flow of full-fee-paying students, who demand returns on their personal or family investment. The public face of universities has been turning into a giant corporate PR exercise. The antithesis approach would define a good university as one that taught without fees, that maintained non-commercial courses, and that did informative outreach with honesty.

2   *The relentless centralisation of power in the hands of a managerial elite, increasingly modelled on for-profit corporate management.* This trend has overwhelmed the moves toward democratisation that were made from the 1960s to the 1980s. Most often this is pictured as a loss of autonomy by academics, but the trend has also wiped out student power and industrial democracy involving non-academic staff. The antithesis approach would define a good university as a democratic workplace, devolving power rather than centralising it, and finding ways to have much wider participation in all levels of organisational decision-making.

3   In consequence of trends 1 and 2, *the flattening of university culture*. Formulaic teaching is encouraged by intrusive online templates; forums for serious debate and dissent shrink or are closed; and staff and students alike are overworked and preoccupied with ticking boxes, doing tests, and filling in audit statements. With this side of the critique, antithesis is less clearly defined. Broadly, however, it suggests that a good university will be a place rich in coffee shops, with the coffee shops rich in passionate argument, intense thought, and exotic projects. It certainly implies that staff and students must have *time* for the passionate arguments, not to mention the coffee.

The wish list, classics, and horror list approaches all yield material for defining a good university. But this material lacks either coherence or direct relevance to the situation we find ourselves in. Can we get an approach that hangs together better and speaks to what is practically possible? The two remaining approaches offer this possibility.

The fourth approach is illustrated by a remarkable text from the early days of the Dawkins policies. In 1994 Ian Lowe published a short book in the UNSW Press's 'Frontlines' series, called *Our Universities are Turning Us into the 'Ignorant Country'*. It was an impressive account of a university system in change. Lowe laughed at the attempt to impose an entrepreneurial culture, but also at the rigidities of academic culture. He diagnosed early the inequalities produced by the Hawke government's attempt to get an expanded university system on the cheap. Positively, Lowe developed an agenda of modernisation without commercialisation. His model emphasised social knowledge and responsibility; engaged, face-to-face teaching; and a diversity of institutions of modest size (rejecting orthodox ideas about economies of scale).

A later attempt at synthesis was the *Charter for Australia's Public Universities* produced by the National Alliance for Public Universities (2014). This was based on an economic analysis emphasising that higher education and knowledge production are public goods in constant tension with government policies of commercialisation and reinforcement of inequality. The document pictured a good university as an institution working fully in the public interest, internally pluralistic, and marked by continuous debate and negotiation among its communities. It sounds strenuous!

These two texts attempt to think about the university sector as a whole. They aim to be realistic about its everyday working and to generate alternatives from possibilities that exist in the current situation. It may sound a little pretentious, but I'd call that a *structural* approach to developing ideas of the good university.

The fifth approach seems the simplest of all: find working examples of better universities. But there is a catch. The neoliberal policy regime has forced all mainstream universities to converge on the neoliberal model. The diversity that existed a generation or two ago, for instance, the innovative curricula and degree structures of the greenfields universities of the 1960s and 1970s (Pellew 2014 on the UK case), has been sharply reined in.

Nevertheless, if we open the lens wider, there is a great deal of relevant thinking and experience. Progressive education in schools, for instance, has been undertaken in very difficult conditions while innovating in teaching method and curriculum. The Freedom Schools of the civil rights movement in the United States are a striking example (Perlstein 1990).

Sometimes these initiatives led to innovation in higher education, as with Rabindranath Tagore's Patha Bhavana school and Visva-Bharati college (later university). This college rejected both top-down pedagogy and colonial control and tried to create flexible and what we would now call multicultural programmes.

Perhaps the most amazing story of bold thinking and action is the Flying University in Warsaw, set up under the Russian empire in the late nineteenth century. It was illegal, co-educational, and very seriously intellectual. It was called 'Flying' because it had to change location to avoid detection by the authorities. And it lasted for years, finally becoming legal. The tradition was revived under the repressive Communist regime in the 1970s (Buczynska-Garewicz 1985).

In capitalist countries, the university system is strongly shaped by social and economic exclusions, and there have been attempts to build working-class alternatives, notably labour colleges in many countries. One offshoot is the current Global Labour University (2018), a network backed by ILO. Another strategy is followed by the interesting Freedom University in Atlanta, USA, which functions as a point of access to existing higher education for students, mostly from ethnic minorities, who are prevented from entering Georgia's public universities because they lack documentation (Muñoz et al. 2014).

An important new development is online activism around universities. In response to the big publishers' use of paywalls to commodify the knowledge produced by university research, there have been many attempts to provide open access. The *PLOS* online journals are the most celebrated, though their publication model requires the authors to pay. An extraordinary website has been set up by the Russian neuroscientist Alexandra Elbakyan, apparently giving free access to millions of research papers (Sci-Hub 2018). Elsevier is taking her to court, and her response is that these publishers are breaking Article 27 of the *Universal Declaration of Human Rights* (United Nations 1948), saying, 'everyone has the right freely to participate in the cultural life of the community, to enjoy the arts and to share in scientific advancement and its benefits'.

The history of universities and the history of education more generally is a source of ideas, practical examples, and inspiration. But because circumstances change, this approach needs to be combined with the others to develop agendas for our own situation. A good place to start that synthesis is the work universities do.

The work and the workforce

The main practical business of universities is intellectual labour of several kinds: teaching and learning at advanced levels, doing research, and circulating knowledge that is the product of research. I emphasise that these are forms of *labour*. Research is not done by magical inspiration; nor is teaching done by bolts of lightning. The university is a workplace, the people in it are a workforce, and the university gets its results by patient, time-consuming labour.

Though our cultural images of intellectual work still invoke isolated geniuses— Dr Faustus and his pentagram, Dr Freud and his cigar, Professor Einstein and his hair—the production of knowledge has become more collectivised over time. This involves more than the fact that as researchers, teachers, and learners, we stand on the shoulders of giants—a humbling truth we all have to recognise, as Newton did. It's also the fact that more and more of us are standing on their shoulders at the same time.

Contemporary research, with *very* few exceptions, now involves the coordinated effort of a variety of specialist workers—including those who supply the services (clerical, financial, technical, maintenance, and transport) without which the people who have their names on the scientific papers could not operate at all. The same goes for teaching. Much of this coordination exists before any particular research team is assembled, grant received, or course authorised. There has to be a library, an ICT service, a teaching space, a flow of students, or a journal for the publication to go into—and other universities, where there are other researchers, other students, and other libraries.

There is, in fact, a profound institutionalisation of the intellectual labour process, a collectivisation that has become the necessary condition for every performance that the metrics purport to measure.

The metrics then focus on what is most superficial about intellectual labour, and I think university staff sense that, hence their usual scepticism about the ranking game that so excites university managers, publicists, and ministers of education. But this divergence of opinion also points to an important dimension of what makes good universities. It's the well-being of the labour force *as a whole* and the design of the institutions to maximise *cooperation* across the institutions and workers involved.

The institutionalisation of knowledge production and circulation is worldwide. There is a global economy of knowledge, with a definite structure. As the philosopher Paulin Hountondji (1997) points out, the global periphery, the majority world, mainly serves as a source of data. In fields ranging from climate change and epidemiology to gender studies and linguistics, a flood of information streams to the main world centres. In the knowledge institutions of the Global North, especially the elite ones, data are accumulated, processed, and theorised. Concepts, methodologies, models, and causal analyses are mainly produced in the global metropole.

As a result of this structure, universities in the periphery are in a situation that has been called 'academic dependency' (Alatas 2003). Universities Australia boasts that Australia produces nearly 3 per cent of the world's academic publications, punching above our weight as usual. It would have been more informative to say that we are obliged to import 97 per cent. Overwhelmingly, Australian universities import from Western Europe and the USA the theories, research paradigms, and disciplinary frameworks that organise their curricula and research.

What the output calculations miss is the fact that the mainstream economy, as currently organised, excludes other knowledge formations. On a world scale, other knowledge formations are very substantial indeed. They include Indigenous knowledges, very much alive (Odora Hoppers 2002); alternative universalisms, such as the intellectual traditions of Islam; and the knowledge formations I have called 'Southern theory', generated in the colonial encounter and from the experience of postcolonial societies (Connell 2007).

The Islamic tradition of great learning centres is at least as old as the European university tradition, and across the Muslim world are many examples of interweaving the two. Local Indigenous knowledges may seem harder to combine with university teaching, but there is no lack of experimentation. The Kaupapa Maori project in Aotearoa New Zealand, is known internationally and has given rise to a classic text, *Decolonizing Methodologies*, by Linda Tuhiwai Smith (2012). The revival of Indigenous culture in the Andean countries of South America is now represented in higher education by several institutions. One is the Indigenous University of Bolivia founded under the Morales government, with three campuses, which awarded their first degrees in 2014 (Mandepora 2011).

Universities in the periphery, far more than those at the top of the international League Tables, have the opportunity for a great cultural enrichment of organised knowledge and higher education. A good university will surely take such an opportunity. Australian moves so far have been timid.

Universities are expensive institutions, and a university system on the modern scale involves a major commitment of social resources. The way funding is organised matters. The model of wholly private 'for-profit universities', which has aroused some excitement in neoliberal circles, is well established in the United States, Latin America, and some other regions. Basically these institutions sell vocational training, with guarantees of subsequent employment; not surprisingly, they have recruited employers to help plan the curriculum (Tierney and Hentschke 2007). Australian universities have moved in this direction to scoop up fee-paying students. We can see the chaos and corruption implicit in this logic from the disastrous privatisation of TAFE in Australia over the last twenty years.

Any alternative to the instability and opportunism of the current funding system rests on achieving some social compact about the role, value, and resource level for the university sector. This would explicitly recognise that we cannot get a good university in isolation; we get a good university sector or nothing.

A compact will not be easy to get, as the donnybrook around the Gonski plan for Australian schools funding shows: the privileged defend their privileges. But a compact is still something to aim for. It can shift discussion forward to questions about professional knowledge requirements, knowledge formations, and just how much glitz a university really needs. Above all, it will require us to think long term about the knowledge workforce.

Recent university management has followed two remarkably destructive workforce strategies: outsourcing of non-academic work and casualisation of academic work (not just in Australia: see Schwartz 2014). The complex coordination of a differentiated labour process is best achieved when the workers know each other and can develop working relationships over considerable periods of time. Outsourcing of services and rapid turnover wreck this cooperation.

Further, as casualisation has become an entrenched organisational strategy, a damaging split has opened between a primary and secondary academic labour force. Tutoring, once rationalised as a limited period with the flavour of apprenticeship, is turning into a mass experience of long-term insecurity and exploitation. It is not too much to say that the long-term sustainability of the academic workforce is now under threat.

However, the generation most affected by precarious employment has been involved in a wave of imaginative alternative-university work, some of it connected with the Occupy movement. The Free University of NYC (2018), for instance, uses public spaces through the city to conduct free educational activities and draws on the Freedom Schools tradition. In Australia, there are Free U projects in Melbourne (Melbourne Free University 2018) and Brisbane (Brisbane Free University 2018). The Brisbane project runs classes in a carpark, produces podcasts, and has a good set of links to similar projects. Many more examples can be found on the web, such as the impressive Social Science Centre in Lincoln UK (Social Science Centre Lincoln 2018), a not-for-profit co-operative.

A good university and a good university system will be concerned with the sustainability of its workforce. This means thinking not one budget ahead, but a generation ahead. Universities need to be places where people feel valued, find scope, aren't pushed about, and want to stay. Career structures need to offer, not spectacular rewards for a minority, but decent conditions and security for the workforce as a whole. Organisational structures need to create space for cooperation, learning, and decision-making from below. We already know how to do this. It's not rocket science.

In conclusion

In writing this chapter, I did not want to define the good university by picturing my utopia. There has never been a golden age in universities, and there may never be one. We will probably need a range of new types of university, as the domain of knowledge becomes more complex. We certainly need the habit of thinking for ourselves and generating ideas from our own situations and problems. We should be sceptical of distant palaces, on earth or in heaven.

For all the madness of the neoliberal regime, the current workforce does a tremendous amount of good work in teaching, in administration, in research, and in services. That's what keeps the universities going! And there are programmes that expand the episteme with Indigenous knowledge and multiple cultures; there are departments with some participatory decision-making; there are many experiments with student-directed learning. It is important to document, share, and reflect on this experience.

I cannot predict how that discussion will go, but I am confident about some principles. It isn't enough to imagine a good university; we need to plan a good university system. Quality doesn't come from privilege or from an elite; quality concerns a whole workforce and the working of a whole institution. Working conditions and workplace relations matter for the intellectual project. We need to think about sustainability in a much longer frame than the policymakers and managers generally do. And we have many starting points now for doing something more intellectually exciting, more socially valuable, and more globally significant than Australian universities have yet managed.

Acknowledgments

I'm grateful to all participants in the 'Where To, Enterprise U?' workshops during the enterprise bargaining campaign at University of Sydney in 2013. Particular thanks to Dr Nour Dados for her engagement and creative intellectual labour.

Note

1 An earlier version of this chapter was published as Connell, R. (2016) 'What are good universities?', *Australian Universities' Review*, 58(2): 67–73, and is published here with the permission of the author, Raewyn Connell, and *Australian Universities' Review*.

References

Alatas, S.F. (2003) 'Academic dependency and the global division of labour in the social sciences', *Current Sociology*, 51: 599–613.

Australian Government (2012) *Australia in the Asian Century*. Online. Available at www. defence.gov.au/whitepaper/2013/docs/australia_in_the_asian_century_white_paper.pdf (accessed 29 September 2018).

The Brisbane Declaration (2016) *Australian Universities' Review*, 58(2): 8.

Brisbane Free University (2018) 'Brisbane Free University'. Online. Available at https:// brisbanefreeuniversity.org/ (accessed 8 October 2018).

Buczynska-Garewicz, H. (1985) 'The flying university in Poland, 1978–1980', *Harvard Educational Review*, 55: 20–34.

Connell, R. (2007) *Southern Theory: The Global Dynamics of Knowledge in Social Science*, Sydney: Allen & Unwin.

Connell, R. (2014) 'Love, fear and learning in the market university', *Australian Universities Review*, 56(2): 56–63.

Davis, G. (2010) *The Republic of Learning: Higher Education Transforms Australia*, Sydney: HarperCollins.

Free University of NYC (2018) 'The Free University of NYC'. Online. Available at https:// freeuniversitynyc.org/ (accessed 8 October 2018).

Global Labour University (2018) 'About the global university'. Online. Available at www. global-labour-university.org/341.html (accessed 8 October 2018).

Hountondji, P. (ed) (1997) *Endogenous Knowledge: Research Trails*, Dakar: CODESRIA.

Kerr, C. (1963) *The Uses of the University*, Cambridge, MA: Harvard University Press.

Lowe, I. (1994) *Our Universities are Turning Us Into the "Ignorant Country"*, Sydney: University of New South Wales Press.

Mandepora, M. (2011) 'Bolivia's indigenous universities', *ReVista: Harvard Review of Latin America*, 11(1): 68–9.

Melbourne Free University (2018) 'Melbourne free university'. Online. Available at www. facebook.com/MelbourneFreeUni/ (accessed 8 October 2018).

Muñoz, S, Espino, M.M. and Antrop-González, R. (2014) 'Creating counter-spaces of resistance and sanctuaries of learning and teaching: an analysis of Freedom University', *Teachers College Record*, 116(7): 1–32.

National Alliance for Public Universities (2014) *A Charter for Australia's Public Universities*. Online. Available at https://napuaustralia.files.wordpress.com/2014/10/napu-a_charter_for_australias_public_universities.pdf (accessed 26 September 2018).

Newman, J.H. (1852/1873) *The Idea of a University: Defined and Illustrated*, London: Basil Montagu Pickering.

Odora Hoppers, C.A. (ed) (2002) *Indigenous Knowledge and the Integration of Knowledge Systems: Towards a Philosophy of Articulation*, Claremont: New Africa Books.

Pellew, J. (2014) '"Utopian" universities: a 50-year retrospective', *Past and Future* (Institute of Historical Research, University of London), 15: 10–11.

Perlstein, D. (1990) 'Teaching freedom: SNCC and the creation of the Mississippi freedom schools', *History of Education Quarterly*, 30: 297–324.

Schwartz, J.M. (2014) 'Resisting the exploitation of contingent faculty labor in the neoliberal university: the challenge of building solidarity between tenured and non-tenured faculty', *New Political Science*, 36: 504–22.

Sci-Hub (2018) 'Sci-Hub: to remove all barriers in the way of science'. Online. Available at https://sci-hub.tw/ (accessed 8 October 2018).

Smith, L.T. (2012) *Decolonizing Methodologies: Research and Indigenous Peoples*, 2nd edn, London: Zed Books.

Social Science Centre Lincoln (2018) 'The social science centre, Lincoln: free co-operative higher education'. Online. Available at www.socialsciencecentre.org.uk/ (accessed 8 October 2018.

Tierney, W.G. and Hentschke, G.C. (2007) *New Players, Different Game: Understanding the Rise of For-profit Colleges and Universities*, Baltimore: Johns Hopkins University Press.

United Nations (1948) 'Universal declaration of human rights'. Online. Available at www. refworld.org/docid/3ae6b3712c.html (accessed 4 November 2019).

Universities Australia (2013) *A Smarter Australia: Policy Advice for an Incoming Government 2013–2016*. Online. Available at www.universitiesaustralia.edu.au%2FArticleDo cuments%2F209%2FPolicy%2520advice%2520for%2520an%2520incoming%2520go vernment%25202013.pdf.aspx&usg=AOvVaw0o_u5jsPy0ymiYCFxwUaHG (accessed 26 September 2018).

Universities Australia (2018) 'University participation & quality'. Online. Available at www. universitiesaustralia.edu.au/uni-participation-quality (accessed 26 September 2018).

Veblen, T. (1918/1957) *The Higher Learning in America: A Memorandum on the Conduct of Universities by Business Men*, New York: Sagamore Press.

10 Four decades plus of promoting inclusion to higher education

Beth R. Crisp

Introduction

Since its founding in 1974, Deakin University has had making access to higher education as a university priority. How it has sustained this vision over more than four decades is the focus of this chapter. However, the context of higher education in Australia has changed enormously in that time, and it is worth first considering the context from which this inclusive priority emerged.

As a school student in the 1970s in metropolitan Melbourne, it was not the norm to complete secondary schooling in the government school I attended. Starting with 150 students in Year 7 in 1975, there were approximately 100 students in Year 11 and 60 of us in Year 12 in 1980. I do not have the data on how many of those 60 went on to higher education, but I would think it not higher than 20–30 at the most. This was an era in which many students could go straight to employment without higher education or without even completing school. Many of those who left school early were academically competent who would have had the intellectual capacity to undertake further studies but either chose to leave or were encouraged to do so (Ross and Gray 2005). With the official retention rate to Year 12 for all of Australia being 34.5 per cent (Department of Employment, Education and Training [DEET] 1991), the 40 per cent retention rate in my school was above the national average. By 1990, retention to Year 12 had increased to 64.0 per cent (DEET 1991), whereas by 2017 84.8 per cent of Australian students were completing their final year of schooling (Australian Bureau of Statistics [ABS] 2018a).

In an era in which the majority of Australians did complete schooling, higher education was a bastion to which few could ever hope to gain admittance as an enrolled student. Until student fees for university students were abolished in 1974, higher education was available only to those who could afford the fees or who were awarded a scholarship. With many scholarships offered to prospective teachers, the choice of courses for those reliant on them could be limited by the requirements of the particular scholarship they held. This was certainly the line of some of the more candid teachers whom I encountered during my secondary schooling.

In the mid-1970s, there was also very little access to university education in rural and regional Australia. Although there were three other universities in the

State of Victoria when Deakin was established, all were in Melbourne, making Deakin the first university in the state outside the state capital and only the third in Australia. While there were several colleges of advanced education (similar to polytechnics in the UK) and teachers' colleges in rural Australia which subsequently combined to form universities in the late 1980s and 1990s, these tended to offer a restricted range of courses and, despite often having good reputations in their local communities, lacked the status of being a university.

Australia's geography was another contributing contextual factor which influenced how Deakin University was established in what is the country with the sixth-largest landmass on the planet (Australian Government 2018a) but with the lowest population density of just 2 persons per square kilometre now (Australian Government 2018b) and even lower in the 1970s. In 1970, almost two thirds of Australians lived in the state and territory capitals (ABS 2018b), but those who did not could have lived hundreds or even thousands of kilometres from a major population centre.

Even if one lived near a university, higher education offerings also privileged those who did not have employment or caring commitments which precluded them from attending daytime classes, often on a full-time basis. In the late 1980s when I decided to return to university to complete a social work degree, my inquiries to the four universities which then offered this qualification in Victoria suggested that part-time enrolment was only a possibility if a student had exceptional circumstances, with the need to earn a living unlikely to be accepted as a reason for studying part time.

The need for more flexible forms of learning had long been recognised with the need to provide university education to those living outside Australia's capital cities first recognised in the early years of the twentieth century (Evans 1995). However, prior to the mid-1970s, the offerings available to students studying by distance education modes were extremely limited, and distance students comprised approximately 6 per cent of all students enrolled in Australian higher education institutions in 1975 (Northcott 1986). However, the establishment of the Open University in the UK in the early 1970s gave rise to a new model of university education. More than 42,000 Britons, many of whom did not meet the traditional requirement for university entry, applied for the initial 25,000 places available at the Open University in its first intake in 1970 (Open University 2018). This new model of a university was viewed with considerable interest from Australia. In particular, it was suggested that the Open University 'added a much needed academic respectability to distance education, lending moral support and confidence to teaching staff and administrators involved in distance education, to students using the mode, and the community to have the confidence in the product' (Smith 1985 in Northcott 1986: 33).

Values

When Deakin University was established in 1974, it not only brought university education to regional Victoria with its base in the regional city of Geelong, but from the beginning of its operations, a distance education programme was integral to the model of the university. Between 1975 and 1982, the percentage of higher education students enrolled in distance education programs across Australia doubled (Northcott 1986), with the establishment of Deakin University one of the major contributors to this expansion. Since its founding, Deakin has understood part of its mission as providing opportunities to obtain university-level qualifications not only to secondary school graduates but also to school non-completers who can demonstrate their capacity for undertaking higher education by alternate means (Watson 2013). For example, the basis of admission was completion of secondary schooling for just 11 per cent of Deakin's Bachelor of Social Work students in 2017, compared to 44 per cent of all students entering the same degree in Australian universities. Not surprisingly, Deakin social work students were much older with 29 per cent aged under 25 compared to 76 per cent of students nationally. Deakin social work students were also more likely to come from rural and remote areas, live in areas which have a low socioeconomic status, have a disability, and be an Indigenous Australian (Crisp 2018).

Unlike universities dedicated to distance education which were established in other countries at this time, including the Open University (Zawacki-Richter and Naidu 2016), Deakin has always had a mix of on- and off-campus courses (Crisp 2018). For courses which are taught in both on- and off-campus modes, students undertake the same courses and must meet the same requirements for the award of a degree. Not only is this a matter of academic integrity, but given there have always been sceptics as to the quality of distance education courses (Crisp 2017; Northcott 1986; Shale 1988), the enrolment in and awarding the same degrees to students, irrespective of their mode of enrolment (Holt and Thompson 1995), remains an important signifier as to the university's stance that students studying at a distance have not earnt an inferior degree to those studying on campus (Pelech et al. 2013). That over 14,000 students were enrolled in Deakin's Cloud Campus in 2018 (Deakin University 2018a) attests to a demand from students for study options which can take account of their personal circumstances, including location, employment, and/or caring responsibilities.

With approximately one quarter of all students enrolled in the Cloud Campus (Deakin University 2018a), cynics could suggest that offering courses in distance mode just reflects identifying a need in the market and providing options which seek to meet that need. A university which was only concerned with the business case may well decide to limit its offerings to high-demand courses which are most profitable. However, an organisation which identifies its values as 'Inclusive' as well as 'Excellent', 'Ethical', and 'Sustainable' (Deakin University 2018b) may be more inclined not only to be more inclusive but also be seen to be more inclusive. Importantly, the need for an inclusive approach to higher education is strongly held by the current vice chancellor, the most senior member of university staff, for whom her experience of being an impoverished student who was first in her family to attend university, influences her views on the need for a university which actively promotes inclusivity (Clarke 2011). Shortly after becoming vice chancellor of Deakin in 2010, Professor Jane den Hollander said,

> If we accept students, we have obligations to make sure that we get them up to speed on their preparedness for a robust higher education experience quickly. I don't think we should lower the standards, I think we should bring them up to standard. If we accept someone, we have an obligation to say, "All things being equal, we believe you can graduate". And if there are interventions required to ensure that that happens, at least in the first year—then we should do them. Often, these are expensive interventions but we must do this in order to . . . widen participation properly so that people do end up with a qualification which does help them transform their lives for themselves and for their families and future generations.
>
> (Clarke 2011: 4)

In an organisation with thousands of staff (Deakin University 2018a), it is important that it is not only the most senior members of an organisation who seek to promote social inclusion, but that this permeates throughout the organisation. As the leader of an academic discipline, I have occasionally been surprised by job applicants who at interview have suggested that distance education is not appropriate, despite having applied for a position in a programme in which the majority of students are enrolled in Deakin's Cloud Campus. Yet such individuals play a valuable role in reminding us of why it is important to recruit staff who at least accept, if not are enthused by the institution's values, including the need for widening participation. Notwithstanding the importance of having staff committed to widening participation in education, Deakin's establishment and its continuing to value approaches which promote social inclusion have been supported by many government policies over the last four decades which also encouraged this (Gale and Tranter 2011). As such Deakin's founding is consistent with the view that

> "Widening participation" in higher education and "social inclusion" more generally are seen as possible only in periods of expansion. That is, the vision of social justice has tended to be distributive rather than re-distributive. Equalising opportunities for social groups to participate in higher education by redistributing existing opportunities (from the advantaged to the less advantaged) has not been a palatable option.
>
> (Gale and Tranter 2011: 42)

In other words, it may be easier for a new university to establish policies and procedures which would enable it to attract groups underrepresented in higher education, including people from rural and remote areas, people who were socio-economically disadvantaged, people with disabilities, and Indigenous Australians, than it would be for established university to change its priorities and widen their student base (Gale and Tranter 2011).

Change

Sustaining an organisational ethos which prioritises an inclusive approach to higher education does not equate with a lack of change. If anything, continuing to provide educational offerings which are relevant to students as well as technological advances which have the capacity to improve the learning environment for students not studying on campus means that change is a constant (Crisp 2018). Early in the twenty-first century, it was noted by Deakin academics that

> In response to the forces of globalization, societies and organizations of all types have had to adapt and even proactively transform themselves. . . . Universities have had to recognize the value of forms of practical working knowledge developed in workplace settings beyond university domains, and promote the value of academic forms of knowledge making to the practical concerns of everyday learning, life and work. It is within this broader systems view that strategic action taken by universities needs to be understood.
>
> (Segrave and Holt 2003: 14)

One of the most obvious changes since Deakin was established was the way in which off-campus learning is delivered, support is provided to students, and mechanisms for communication with students, including the processes of submitting and returning assignments. Distance education students in the twentieth century would be mailed a package of learning resources prior to the commencement of each semester, along with details of assessment tasks and information about administrative procedures and how to access various university services, including the library. The learning resources tended to be print-based and often 'rivalled the production quality of commercial textbooks' (Crisp 2018: 720). Indeed it was not unheard of for study materials to subsequently form the basis of commercially published texts (e.g. D'Cruz and Jones 2004; Fook 2002). For many students, their only other contact with the university about a unit of study would be the mailing of a product they had created (e.g. written assignment, video, or audio tape) which would be marked and then mailed back to the student with comments.

Online learning management systems were initially developed in 1995 at the University of British Colombia in Canada, as a means for distributing content (University of British Columbia 2004). While there was much interest at Deakin as to the potential applications of such systems (Bottomley et al. 1999; Segrave and Holt 2003), it was not until 2004 that there was a requirement that all teaching units would have at least a minimal online presence on Deakin's learning management system. With the move to delivering courses to off-campus students online and the reality that many 'distance' students actually lived relatively close to the university, the terms 'distance education' and 'off-campus' were eventually replaced by the notion of students enrolling in the 'Cloud Campus' rather than at one of Deakin's several physical campuses located in different parts of Victoria.

While some individuals and groups of teaching staff moved quickly to embrace the new opportunities which this technology enabled, some parts of the university essentially remained reliant on print technologies and used the online systems for supplementary materials, particularly those who were heavily invested in print production (Bottomley et al. 1999). For example, in social work, where we have a number of students living in remote areas with inadequate internet access, in 2004 it was argued that 'print technologies were felt to have served the programme well and it was argued by some staff that with many students having inadequate access to the internet, online delivery would disadvantage many students' (Crisp 2018: 721). Such arguments were still being put forward in 2012 when the university decided to cease producing print materials and move the provision of learning materials fully online (Crisp 2018).

It is interesting that many of the debates about moving or not moving to online learning in the first years of the twenty-first century were framed in terms of social inclusion, although it has been suggested that those opposing online teaching may have been doing so as a way of hiding their lack of competence or confidence to work in the online environment (Crisp 2018). In contrast to opponents who argued that some students would be disenfranchised, an alternate view was that print-only teaching isolated students who often had no contact with one another, whereas online technologies enabled students to develop relationships with each other and not just with teaching staff. In particular, it enabled students who were 'geographically scattered . . . to still participate in collective and collaborative learning encounters' (Maidment 2006: 48). Initially such encounters were by discussion boards in which students posted messages which could be read by others whenever they logged on. While asynchronous discussion boards continue to be used, the development of virtual classroom software has for more than a decade enabled geographically disparate students to engage in real-time synchronous discussions with groups, including other students and staff (Pelech et al. 2013). Initially an option which staff could choose to provide, there is now an expectation that all units offered in the Cloud Campus will provide opportunities for synchronous contact. However, with the exception of units in which online interaction with peers has been made compulsory, some students do not take advantage of the opportunity to be in contact with others in the class (Goldingay and Land 2014). While for some students this may reflect a preference, for many of the students I work with, family or employment commitments make it impossible to participate in synchronous contact sessions, and they not only rely on, but value, opportunities for asynchronous contact with both staff and other students.

Deakin's Cloud Campus is only one example of how the university has sought to promote social inclusion over the past four decades. In 1980 Deakin was the first university in Australia to appoint a disability resource officer to support students with disabilities. In 1986, it developed an innovative programme to provide university education to Indigenous Australians while enabling them to remain living in their own communities. This award-winning programme, known as the Institute for Koorie Education, continues to this day to be a major provider of higher education to Aboriginal and Torres Strait Islander peoples. In terms of promoting social inclusion for staff, while it was not until 1988 that the first female professor was appointed at Deakin, the university has since had two female vice chancellors: Sally Walker (2003–2010) and Jane den Hollander (2010–2019) (Deakin University 2018c).

Challenges

It is important not to underestimate just how difficult it is for a university to retain a commitment to social inclusion. Although assisted by a range of policies seeking to widen participation to higher education in recent decades, expectations as to which students universities should be recruiting, and by what means, are continually changing (Pitman 2017). While these policies have tended to encourage participation from groups which Deakin was already engaging, policy priorities change, and it is possible that widening participation will at some point in the future no longer be a government priority, or the funds provided to encourage widening participation will shift in a direction away from Deakin's traditional student base (Department of Education and Training [DET] 2018).

Widening participation is just one of a myriad of policy and procedural requirements which the twenty-first-century university must juggle. The reputation of universities depends on the quality of its research and teaching. In the highly competitive university rankings, Deakin has been ranked among the top 2 per cent of universities internationally (Deakin University 2018d), suggesting that valuing social inclusion and being a quality university can be complementary rather than alternate priorities. However, as in other universities which teach online (Dodo-Balu 2017), on a day-to-day basis the teaching staff with which Cloud students have direct contact are often junior academics, many of whom are employed on a sessional basis. Moreover, while the commitment of such staff to assisting students succeed in their studies means they often work far more hours than they are paid for, the marginalisation experienced by casual staff does not bode well for staff retention (Dodo-Balu 2017).

A further challenge for a large university with more than 4,000 staff (Deakin University 2018a) is ensuring all staff are aware of university priorities. As indicated previously, direct contact with students disproportionately is undertaken by those staff who are furthest from the processes of university policymaking. Widening access to higher education may be straightforward in theory, but in practice it often brings requests from students seeking adaptations in course requirements, ranging from a request for an extension on a due date for an assignment on the basis that a student has only just received a book mailed from the university library to students requesting exemptions from course requirements or alternate assessment tasks on the basis of a disability. Although agreement to some requests requires approval of a course director or committee, some requests do need to be actioned by the staff directly involved in teaching a unit. As such, each staff member in effect acts as what is known as a 'street-level bureaucrat' when it comes to responding to the discretionary requests from students.

The work of street-level bureaucrats is multifaceted and of a contradictory nature. Demands and expectations are imposed on them from a variety of sources. . . . Their tasks entail making decisions based on the needs of the individual within the confines of prevailing policy. They are forced to make necessary prioritisations when they must bring into alignment public objectives and the individual's need for assistance and support with available resources.

(Dunér and Nordström 2006: 426)

One of the difficulties of having many individuals making discretionary decisions is the lack of consensus, particularly if the staff making decisions do not have a good understanding of the organisation's ethos and values which underpin policies and procedures. A further difficulty is that students for whom discretionary measures may be most appropriate are not necessarily those who have enough knowledge and confidence to request modifications to their study requirements (Crisp 2009).

As well as challenges at the organisational level in sustaining an inclusive ethos, there are also challenges for individuals or groups of academic staff which need to be managed. While witnessing students, who would not otherwise have the opportunity of attending university, benefit from participating in online classes (Crisp 2018; Dodo-Balu 2017), those committed to online education may have to endure accusations that they are not providing a legitimate learning experience of sufficient quality to undertake the work expected of someone who holds a particular qualification. This is particularly the case with professional qualifications (Crisp 2017).

A further challenge to sustaining approaches which promote social inclusion is complacency. Developing policies and procedures which promote social inclusion is not a one-off event but something which a large organisation, such as a university, needs to be doing continually.

While we have remained responsive to student needs . . . this has required continual reflection . . . and being willing to innovate. . . . These same qualities will be required just as much in coming decades if we are to continue to be responsive to the changing needs of . . . students.

(Crisp 2018: 728)

Conclusion

Deakin University has led the promotion of social inclusion through widening participation to higher education for the more than four decades since it was founded. A founding ethos, support from staff at all levels of the organisation, and government policies which have encouraged the promotion of social inclusion have no doubt all contributed to this sustained focus on social inclusion. However, there are many challenges to sustaining social inclusion, and these need to be continually addressed, including ensuring the very large staff is not only aware of the organisational values but understand their role in enacting these in their interactions with students and the wider community. It is this enaction, rather than history, which will be critical in ensuring social inclusion continues to be sustained by Deakin University.

References

Australian Bureau of Statistics [ABS] (2018a) 'Schools, Australia 2017'. Online. Available at www.abs.gov.au/ausstats/abs@.nsf/0/9448F2F814FA0311CA2579C700118E2D?Opendocument (accessed 21 August 2018).

Australian Bureau of Statistics [ABS] (2018b) '25 million population milestone'. Online. Available at www.abs.gov.au/websitedbs/D3310114.nsf/home/25+Million+Population+Milestone (accessed 22 August 2018).

Australian Government (2018a) 'The Australian continent'. Online. Available at www.australia.gov.au/about-australia/our-country/the-australian-continent (accessed 22 August 2018).

Australian Government (2018b) 'Our people'. Online. Available at www.australia.gov.au/about-australia/our-country/our-people (accessed 22 August 2018).

Bottomley, J., Spratt, C. and Rice, M. (1999) 'Strategies for effecting strategic organisational change in teaching practices: case studies at Deakin University', *Interactive Learning Environments*, 7: 227–47.

Clarke, J.A. (2011) 'Interview with Jane den Hollander, Deakin University', *The International Journal of the First Year in Higher Education*, 2(1): 1–7.

Crisp, B.R. (2009) 'Professional discretion and social exclusion', in A. Taket, B.R. Crisp, A. Nevill, G. Lamaro, M. Graham and S. and Barter-Godfrey (eds) *Theorising Social Exclusion*, London: Routledge.

Crisp, B.R. (2017) 'Leadership and social work education in the online environment', *Advances in Social Work and Welfare Education*, 19: 80–91.

Crisp, B.R. (2018) 'From distance to online education: two decades of remaining responsive by one university social work programme', *Social Work Education*, 37: 718–30.

D'Cruz, H. and Jones, M. (2004) *Social Work Research: Ethical and Political Contexts*, London: Sage.

Deakin University (2018a) 'Deakin at a glance'. Online. Available at www.deakin.edu.au/__data/assets/pdf_file/0005/1363325/Brochure-Deakin-at-a-Glance-March-2018.pdf (accessed 22 August 2018).

Deakin University (2018b) 'The Deakin values'. Online. Available at www.deakin.edu.au/about-deakin/values (accessed 22 August 2018).

Deakin University (2018c) 'History'. Online. Available at www.deakin.edu.au/about-deakin/reputation/history (accessed 23 August 2018).

Deakin University (2018d) 'Reputation'. Online. Available at www.deakin.edu.au/about-deakin/reputation (accessed 24 August 2018).

Department of Education and Training [DET] (2018) 'Higher education participation and partnerships program (HEPPP)'. Online. Available at www.education.gov.au/higher-education-participation-and-partnerships-programme-heppp (accessed 24 August 2018).

Department of Employment, Education and Training [DEET] (1991) *Retention and Participation in Australian Schools 1967 to 1990*, Canberra: Australian Government Publishing Service.

Dodo-Balu, A. (2017) 'Students flourish and tutors wither: a study of participant experiences in a first-year online unit', *Australian Universities' Review*, 59(1): 4–13.

Dunér, A. and Nordström, M. (2006) 'The discretion and power of street-level bureaucrats: an example from Swedish municipal eldercare', *European Journal of Social Work*, 9: 425–44.

Evans, T. (1995) 'Distance education in Australia', *European Journal of Engineering Education*, 20: 233–4.

Fook, J. (2002) *Social Work: Critical Theory and Practice*, London: Sage.

Gale, T. and Tranter, D. (2011) 'Social justice in higher education policy: an historical and conceptual account of student participation', *Critical Studies in Education*, 52: 29–46.

Goldingay, S. and Land, C. (2014) 'Emotion: the "e" in engagement in online distance education in social work', *Journal of Open, Flexible and Distance Learning*, 18: 58–72.

Holt, D.M. and Thompson, D.J. (1995) 'Responding to the technological imperative: the experience of an open and distance education institution', *Distance Education*, 16: 43–64.

Maidment, J. (2006) 'Using on-line delivery to support students during practicum placements', *Australian Social Work*, 59: 47–55.

Northcott, P. (1986) 'Distance education for managers: an international perspective', *Open Learning*, 1(2): 33–41.

Open University (2018) 'First students and first graduates'. Online. Available at www.open.ac.uk/researchprojects/historyofou/story/first-students-and-first-graduates (accessed 22 August 2018).

Pelech, W., Wulff, D., Perrault, E., Ayala, J., Baynton, M., Williams, M., Crowder, R. and Shankar, J. (2013) 'Current challenges in social work distance education: responses from the Elluminati', *Journal of Teaching in Social Work*, 33: 393–407.

Pitman, T. (2017) 'Widening participation in higher education: a play in five acts', *Australian Universities' Review*, 59(1): 37–46.

Ross, S. and Gray, J. (2005) 'Transitions and re-engagement through second chance education', *The Australian Educational Researcher*, 32(3): 103–40.

Segrave, S. and Holt, D. (2003) 'Contemporary learning environments: designing e-learning for education in the professions', *Distance Education*, 24: 7–24.

Shale, D. (1988) 'Concepts: towards a reconceptualization of distance education', *American Journal of Distance Education*, 2(3): 25–35.

University of British Columbia (2004) 'UBC computer scientist wins $100,000 award for popular course software', *University of British Columbia News and Events*, 15 October. Online. Available at http://news.ubc.ca/ubcnewsdigest/2004/04oct15.html#4 (accessed 5 September 2018).

Watson, S. (2013) 'Tentatively exploring the learning potentialities of postgraduate distance learners' interactions with other people in their life contexts', *Distance Education*, 34: 175–88.

Zawacki-Richter, O. and Naidu, S. (2016) 'Mapping research trends from 35 years of publications in *Distance Education*', *Distance Education*, 37: 245–69.

11 Socially inclusive service development

A new expression of democracy for nongovernment organisations delivering social care

Sarah Pollock

Introduction

This chapter explores the democratic possibilities created when a rights-based approach to service development is operationalised in a nongovernment organisation (NGO) setting. It argues that a rights-based approach can offer opportunities for collective and sustainable action on systems for care to reduce suffering, suggested as an appropriate intent for our social institutions (Rorty 1989). The chapter draws on work to implement an inclusive approach to service development undertaken in a large, multisector NGO located in Melbourne, Australia, and on the author's PhD research on that initiative.

The context for rights-based approaches to service development

Traditionally, NGOs have played an important role in the development of policies and programmes that impact on the lives of vulnerable people, families, and communities through collaboration with policy actors and system decision-makers (Wilson et al. 2012). In doing this, they draw on their knowledge of the communities they work with, although these processes do not always directly involve the people from these communities. In the Australian context, despite widespread endorsement by all levels of government, service user participation largely remains restricted to input into decision-making on the mix of services that individuals receive at an operational level (Ottmann et al. 2009). This narrows the democratic role that NGOs play. Rather than offering people a say on the problems in their lives and how to address these, participation is reduced to having a say on how they receive predetermined services that they cannot shape. The relationship between purpose, mechanisms, and outcomes of inclusive endeavours is complex. Two broad categories of activity can be identified, each of which has different practical aims and theoretical underpinnings: consumerist and citizenship (Gustafsson and Driver 2005; Rose et al. 2003). The former is focused on the improvement of service delivery structures and processes, defined by accepted standards for those services. In the latter, service users define their own objectives and priorities for the development activity. These different aims may empirically incorporate elements from different points along a continuum from wholly practical/consumerist to wholly transformational/citizenship (Cousins and Whitmore 1998), although the weight given to the purpose of participation will impact on how the outcomes of an initiative are interpreted and how the effectiveness of the participatory aspect is understood (Newman et al. 2004).

Involving service users in the development of services offers an excellent opportunity to enhance people's rights at the same time as responding to their needs as consumers. Rights-based approaches to service development provide opportunities to incorporate principles of human rights and social justice (Singh 2010; Triggs 2013). Four principles underpin rights-based approaches: the responsibility that duty-bearers have (including NGOs) to respect, protect, and fulfil human rights; the recognition that every individual is a rights-holder regardless of their personal circumstances and should be able to access their rights without discrimination; the need to involve affected stakeholders and communities at every stage of policy and programme design and delivery; and the accountability that duty-bearers have towards rights-holders should be operationalised and adapted to local contexts (Gruskin et al. 2010). The right to participation is central to the application of rights-based approaches in the context of service delivery organisations (Potts 2010), and the opportunity to include individual voices in local decision-making is central to ensuring autonomy and dignity for all (Singh 2010). Whilst evidence supports the effectiveness of rights-based approaches in delivering improved health outcomes (Gaventa and Barrett 2010; Potts 2010), operationalisation in the organisational context is not straightforward, and gains can be difficult to sustain.

The remainder of this chapter explores the rights-based approach to service development (referred to as 'the initiative') in a Melbourne NGO. Its emphasis is on identifying factors that can support the sustainability of the approach, ensuring that organisations embed this into future work. There are four sections. The first gives an overview of the approach used for inclusive service development. The second discusses the four mechanisms that were found to be effective in fostering inclusion. The third discusses the barriers and limits to inclusive practice, and the final section offers a framework for organisations who wish to pursue an inclusive approach to service development.

Overview of the inclusive approach to service development

The initiative sets out to involve service users and their families in organisational decision-making processes for service development and future service delivery, as equal partners alongside others from within the organisation and in the government departments responsible for funding the services. It was hoped that the voices of experts by profession would not dominate service development, nor exclude the people that the organisation intended to serve (Potts 2010). The initiative was designed with intentional vigilance on the operation of power in the local service development context, to counter the tendency to silence some voices and ways of knowing, whilst privileging others (Taket 2012). Finally it set out to increase people's agency in relation to organisational decisions that impacted them, in particular, service users and the frontline staff who worked with them.

The initiative comprised a participatory approach to service evaluation trialled in three settings (referred to as 'the project/s'): Wesley Aged Care Housing Service, a residential aged care service for elders with long-term histories of homelessness associated with mental ill health and/or drug and alcohol misuse (WACHS); a planning service for people with disability with individualised packages (ISP); and Resilient Kids, a short-term therapeutic intervention for children whose families had experienced homelessness (RK). It had support within the NGO from senior management and the Board and willing engagement from the relevant government departments that funded and administered the three selected services, and it took place in the context of an organisation-wide policy on social inclusion and belonging. Everyone involved in the service in each setting was invited to take part, including service users and their families, frontline service delivery staff, middle and senior managers, and government officials. In each location, diverse groups of people were engaged in each stage of the project, and there were multiple ways to take part. People worked within an interlinked governance structure that comprised community and management reference groups, embedded within the organisation's existing governance and line-management arrangements. The projects used a programme logic process as the basis for evaluating the outcomes the service was currently achieving and to ask questions about what could or should be done differently. Participants then worked together to plan for improvement, locally and in the immediate system context. In each setting, groups worked separately and together to make sense of what they learned as the evaluations proceeded and to plan future action. Each of the three projects had a dedicated researcher/facilitator from within the organisation but not involved in the delivery of any service.

In each setting, the projects delivered a range of outcomes that were useful to each group of participants (Pollock 2016). Service users and family members reported health and well-being benefits and a greater sense of agency. Staff, managers, and government officials gained insights into their service delivery that were not available to them through other channels and were able to make practical changes to service delivery on the basis of the new knowledge. However, despite these gains, it was difficult to sustain the transformative potential that the participatory process offered or extend beyond the local setting to achieve organisational or systemic change.

Fostering inclusive practice

This section outlines what worked to foster inclusive practice. It examines the discursive context that made inclusion possible, at the same time as it made it difficult to sustain temporarily or extend beyond the local context. At the completion of the initiative, all participants were invited to take part in an interview that formed part of the author's PhD study (Pollock 2016). The theoretical approach undertaken in this analysis is described elsewhere (Pollock and Taket 2014a), as is a more detailed description of the initiative and the strategies employed to facilitate effective participation (Pollock and Taket 2014b). The study found that there were four mechanisms that were effective in fostering social inclusion in the NGO setting: authentic voice; inclusive dialogue; critical facilitation; and valuing alternate ways of knowing. These are considered in turn as follows.

Authentic voice

The participatory processes employed in each project provided opportunities for service users and family members to talk about what mattered to them and to describe themselves and the world as they saw it in their own voices. This self-description stood out as materially different to the experience of being described in ways that were oppressive, through the language and practices of the service delivery system. Creating the conditions for authentic voice applied in both separate and together spaces during the projects. When service users and family members can talk authentically about difficulties, the help they need and what is and is not working for them interactions potentially become safer and service delivery more efficient. This was most obvious in the homelessness service, where all the mothers were also subject to child protection orders. Compliance with these was a source of great stress for the mothers, who felt as though not only were they trying to deal with being a parent whilst homeless but were at constant risk of losing their children to the authorities. This circumstance typically created a tense and hostile environment for interactions between the mothers and service system actors. In the projects, this environment changed significantly to one of mutual cooperation and respect, noted and appreciated by all participants alike.

> I think that the important thing for me was that I was listened to and I was asked. I hadn't really drawn a connection [. . . but] I'm at a point where I'm saying I want support that's supportive and this isn't helping. I will actually attend a meeting with my respite carer and say these things to her face, and not only will I do that but I will also follow through.
>
> (Brady, service user, RK)

Being able to describe one's experience in one's own words and having these interpretations valued and validated by professional participants was instrumental in shifting from oppressive to inclusive relations.

It has been noted elsewhere that benefits accrue when service users and family members are able to speak in an authentic voice, unencumbered by the dialogic requirements of institutional practices that constitute 'client', 'staff', and 'official' identities (Hodge 2005; Martin 2012). Importantly, it was not the content of dialogue that changed, but control over what the information meant and how it could be used, as the following quote from one of the mothers in the RK project illustrates,

> Yep, and [child protection case workers] really dig into your background and your previous history and everything, and at the end of it they write

up a report based on the bad things, not the good things. Whereas with [the researcher], I got the good things, in the sense that talking about domestic violence, the homelessness, financial difficulties and everything. It was a safe place to do it in. Whereas, like I say, Department or anyone else, they out to nitpick the gritty bits out for their own purpose.

(Dora, service user, RK)

At play is control over identity and over what constitutes a legitimate description of what it means to be a mother, parenting in extreme circumstances. What is counted as a legitimate description of a social problem (e.g. homelessness whilst being a mother) becomes the basis of institutional practices (e.g. the surveillance of the child protection system) and the services and supports that are made available. For the mothers in the RK project, being able to self-describe and to have their version of themselves legitimated was transformational. Rather than a story told through official records created by professionals for an organisational purpose about her and from which she is excluded, in the earlier example, Dora is able to take part in a dialogue about the same events where she remains in control of what she shares and how meaning is ascribed to her experiences. The transformation occurs because legitimated self-description counters the oppressive and deficit identity of 'risky mother' made available in the dominant discourses that circulate in the service delivery environment (Gillies 2005). Most importantly, these shifts in subject position occurred regardless of whether there were practical changes in the service delivery arrangements, supporting the argument that it is the opportunity to speak in an authentic voice that fosters inclusion.

Inclusive dialogue

The second mechanism was the establishment of spaces for inclusive dialogue within and between groups. This gave service users and family members a role as equal and legitimate participants in a process of knowledge production rather than as the objects of others' knowledge about them. In inclusive dialogue, the flow of control over meaning is multidirectional as all groups of participants work together to understand the shared situation in new ways. No longer is the dialogue and dialogic form dominated by one way or knowing and speaking, but becomes a process of negotiation, learning, and reimagining. As the participants engaged with others in the projects, whether they were from the same group or not, the ways in which they saw themselves and each other shifted. This shift occurred in multiple directions. For instance, service users shifted from seeing other service users as competitors for scarce resources to seeing them as people experiencing hardship with whom they shared an identity that could be valued in a process of social change.

I guess you just see other people as just a block to what you want, which is a house. So you don't actually perceive, oh ok, well other people are struggling, Maybe you don't have enough energy to take it on. You can't. It's like, I'm struggling. [. . .] And they're not obstacles. You realise that they're people that have had [similar experiences], even though they might have completely different lives to you.

(Brady, service user, RK)

Similarly, professional participants saw service users differently.

I think I've got a little bit more respect for the service users now, just because of the involvement with the project. And it's not just the people who have been involved. I've kinda taken a minute to reflect and consider the way I'm working with people. I realised service users have a much greater understanding of what we do than I gave them credit for, and that I need to give people a bit more credit.

(Gabrielle, staff, ISP)

As well as the material benefits of inclusive dialogue (i.e. feedback on current service delivery), these shifts were humanising for all participants, as the following exchange between a service user and a senior manager from the relevant government department in the ISP setting illustrates.

Ursula (service user):   This is good because we meet each other, and [government department] is not the big bad wolf.
David (gov official):   We are just people too.

Staff talked about the emotional impact of their work to each other and with service users and families, revealing their vulnerability and humanity. This had the effect of making available constructions of service delivery that did not rely on the unidirectional provision of 'help' from a relatively empowered staff member to a relatively disempowered service user. By drawing on a more personal language that legitimated staff's emotional experiences and value, professional participants positioned themselves alongside service users and families within the service system. This had the effect of exposing the impacts of the managerial and technical practices of the dominant discursive paradigms of service delivery on service users, families, and staff alike. Accordingly, it was possible to counter the dominant narratives with others that were situated in a shared humanity and desire to reduce suffering.

As was noted with authentic voice, inclusive dialogue was effective in making available new, more empowered subject positions, regardless of whether practical change was achieved in the local service setting. A clear example of this came from the WACHS project, where very little changed in the service delivery context as a result of the evaluation.

I mean, we ask for things, and they used to say, yes we'll do it, we'll do it, and we never heard any more. Whereas [in this process] we've got somewhere with those two things.

(Nellie, resident, WACHS)

Materially, nothing had changed. Nellie's comment that they were getting somewhere can be read as a reference to her sense of being engaged in an ongoing struggle for change, where she was able to represent her own and other residents' needs and report back to them on progress rather than the achievement of a material outcome. Throughout the projects, service user and family participants were realistic about what could be achieved and the difficulties involved. It was being part of the struggle and having a direct, equal voice that counted in terms of inclusive practice. The multidirectional shifts in how people saw each other generated a greater sense of 'we', a collective voice with a shared interest in countering the oppressive effects of ascribed expert knowledge, and that could offer new insights into the present and generate new ideas for future action. The development of the collective voice also helped to create a sustainable process whereby the stakeholders in the service could examine the impacts of changes and improvement as they occurred.

Facilitated critical reflection

The third mechanism was facilitated critical reflection on the structures and practices that needed to be transformed in order to counter the oppressive tendencies of service delivery systems. In each project, a researcher/facilitator worked with groups of participants separately and together to facilitate their reflection on the situation as they variously described it. Tensions in descriptions were noted and discussed, with the researchers ensuring that no specific description or way of knowing was given greater privilege than any other. Disagreements in ways of knowing and seeing were critically examined to try to understand why there might be differing views and what each way of knowing might mean for particular groups of participants (who benefited, who suffered, and how). The combination of separate/together spaces for dialogue, facilitated by someone who was from outside of the service setting but inside the organisation, was important for creating the necessary safety for authentic critical reflection. Extending the argument for the use of external facilitators (Martin 2012; Romm and Gregory 2001), the internal/external status of the facilitator was materially important in creating a sense of safety for all participants and led to the creation of alliances within and between groups, particularly service users and families, that were the basis for future action. The insider/outside location of the facilitator was also useful to understand and analyse the ways in which participants constructed power relations in each local context whilst the projects were underway. This capacity for real-time analysis thus rendered the power relations in each local context more readily available for reflection in group processes.

Facilitated critical reflection worked to shift the meaning of individual experiences in ways that were empowering for individuals. In the homelessness service context, the mothers shared their experiences with each other and reflected together on these with the researcher-facilitator and then later with the professional participants. Through collectively reflecting on their experiences of the service system, the mothers were able to challenge the deficit client identity made available to them by the dominant paradigm and negotiate a new narrative that explained homelessness as a systemic rather than an individual failure.

> It made me feel a bit differently about myself. It made me feel that this is a circumstance. This isn't me. This isn't who I am.
>
> (Adele, service user, RK)

The shifts in meaning and explanatory narrative extended across group boundaries and had an impact on action planning. Celia, a government official involved in the RK project, remarked that when she first saw the list of recommendations that the service users had drawn up, starting with wanting a house, her initial response had been to dismiss out of hand what she regarded as a naïve suggestion. However, as she reflected on her own position, relative to that of the service users, her view changed.

> [The service users] just want somewhere to live. At its bare bones, life and death, hand to mouth, day to day cliché cliché, I know, from their point of view. Whereas we're comfortable, well-fed bureaucrats who live in a well-paid world [. . .] without having the real visceral understanding of what it's like to be homeless. We haven't got a clue, to be perfectly frank.
>
> (Celia, government official, RK)

The importance of shifts such as this is that they extend to what is counted as legitimate knowledge or a legitimate position as the basis for future action. Celia's comment illustrates the limitations of relying only on a limited range of meanings about what constitutes high-quality care and the potential inefficiency of doing this as a means of making service-related decisions. It is her reflection on her own position in the service delivery system that enables her to see the limitations of her regular way of working and the liberating benefits, if these ways of working are changed, that flow to her and to the people using the service she administers.

Whilst power relations shifted and new subject positions were made available, power itself was not an overt topic in discussions within or across groups. It was discussion on the local arrangements for delivering services that was effective, by revealing the way power worked to legitimate some meanings whilst silencing others. All participants benefited from seeing how their position in the dominant discursive formations of service delivery gave them particular ways of seeing the world and made others unavailable to them. They were also able to see that the material benefits of the shifts in discursive position were greater the more marginalised the participant was. Like other participatory endeavours that achieved transformational outcomes for participants locally, it was possible to maintain these shifts during the projects, but difficult to extend them temporally and beyond the local setting (Newman et al. 2004). Maintenance of the shift in subject positions required constant and ongoing work to reflect on what was happening in each setting as the relationships between participants changed and developed and vigilance on which ways of knowing were centred or excluded.

Alternate ways of knowing

The final mechanism was making available and valuing alternate ways of knowing about social problems and social care that each participant brought with them, including ways of knowing generally silenced in mainstream dialogue. The importance and benefits of including the voices of those from marginalised communities, in particular service users and families, have been widely remarked in the current vogue on co-design and coproduction in health service delivery settings. However, the need to ensure the inclusion of *all* participants' authentic voices and to treat these as being equally important is less frequently remarked. Service user accounts were able to highlight aspects of service delivery that they experienced as being unhelpful and were consequently inefficient, unsafe, or both. Staff accounts made visible their emotional and personal experience of service delivery, generally silenced in mainstream conversations about service development despite the centrality of service users' emotional and personal experiences in dominant discursive formations on social care service delivery. The inclusive and equal treatment of alternate ways of knowing had the effect of positioning service users alongside staff, making them equally, although differently, vulnerable in the context of the service delivery system in the same way. It also made available local meanings for service delivery that developed around staff's shared values and practices that are generally unavailable for consideration or are dismissed as being outside legitimate process in relation to service development.

These alternate narratives centred the question of what it means to give and receive care. An example of this comes from the WACHS project where Evelyn, a staff member, had experienced the death of her son from a protracted illness in his early twenties. She talked about her loss as a human experience that linked her to the elders she gave care to and located herself as care worker in the same discursive space as elder-cared-for.

> Coming back to work, I was able to focus on their needs and they helped me, the residents here, even though not many of them knew what happened. I'd come here and for that six, seven hours that I was here, I concentrated on them and I knew they all had issues, so it wasn't just about me and my loss. They've lost a lot too.
>
> (Evelyn, staff, aged housing service)

As with the issue of power, it was not necessary for Evelyn to share her experiences with the elders to shift what it meant to provide care from a transactional exchange to a relationship constructed around the common human experience of suffering. This conceptualisation of the care relationship is more humanising because it is based on an equal positioning of giver and receiver and on the individuality of the actors. It is a view that brings all parties together into a common human experience of caring that is also democratic and hopeful.

Barriers to sustaining inclusive practice

In a service delivery system that relies on privileged knowledge about social problems and social care, a rights-based approach that effectively included silenced voices will inevitably and intentionally be disruptive. Facilitated critical reflection enables all participants to see how they and each other are positioned in the relations of power and affords them the chance to rebalance those relations through listening, empathy, and collective action. Where these actions threaten to overturn sedimented arrangements, then there is likely to be push back of one sort or another from those immediately outside of the locale of inclusive practice. The application of a critical lens to what is regarded as 'mainstream' makes visible the ways in which mainstream meanings and values placed on particular forms of activity or identity exclude certain individuals and ways of life, even when these are meaningful to those individuals and their communities (Steinart and Pilgram 2007). Consequently, a process that seeks to surface and validate alternate ways of knowing will initiate various forms of counteractivity as the destabilised system tries to reassert its former shape. In each of the projects, despite the gains and benefits to individuals, the services, and the organisation, there were various barriers to sustaining a more inclusive way of working.

Australian social care NGOs operate in an everyday environment that is time-poor, fraught with uncertainty and ambiguity, and changing ceaselessly. Being busy, not having enough time, working within restrictive service delivery guidelines, and needing to meet compliance requirements all impacted on the projects. Managers and government officials were clear that the approach taken in the service development initiative delivered unique value but found that their time was taken up with other priorities, such as meeting compliance requirements or responding to ministerial requests. Staff felt disempowered and unable to make changes to their services in response to what they learned in the projects, without the say-so from whomever they deemed to have authority (their senior managers, the researchers, the case managers, or senior managers in government departments). Government officials did not know how to respond to a much richer picture of their programme landscape and its inhabitants. Staff turnover and poor leadership compounded these problems so that whilst the projects were completed successfully and the approach was demonstrably effective, sustaining these gains proved impossible beyond the duration and locale of each project (Pollock 2016).

A brief example from the ISP project serves to illustrate this situation. In the ISP project, the programme logic workshop had been a particularly powerful and successful event, where all participants spoke with authenticity and honesty about matters that were usually silenced or discussed only within groups. As an outcome of this, the participants, through their joint steering committee, agreed to work together to advocate to trial a process of approving people's funding plans locally, cutting out the invisible authority within the regional government department office. All parties, including the government officials, were excited about pursuing the possibility and began the work to advocate for this change. Also during this workshop, the frontline staff had learned about more the appeals process for plans that were rejected by the invisible authority. In the weeks that followed, staff began to use the process to appeal plans that they felt had been unreasonably rejected. After a few weeks, despite direct involvement in the decision-making, the regional office of the government department rejected out of hand the possibility of local plan approval and, moreover, censured staff and the organisation for inappropriate use of the appeals process. One interpretation is to see this is a form of bureaucratic resistance and a means of rebalancing unsettled power relations to return them to their former state. It is noteworthy that the push-back occurred at a time when the ISP service staff had no manager, nor senior manager, to support them to continue their actions.

Rights-informed inclusive practice unsettles prevailing power in service delivery systems (Yates et al. 2008). When ways of knowing that derive from people's lived experiences are centred, a tension point is created where individual's experiences collide with the meanings or prevailing discursive frameworks, causing those meanings to become unstable. Once a system is unstable, it is vulnerable to reinscription (Ney et al. 2013). As the examples in this chapter illustrate, inclusive practice makes it possible to see how possibilities in dominant discursive practices are delimiting for service users and providers alike, albeit in different ways and with more or less oppressive impact. However, when a process opens up a multidirectional vulnerability, it brings with it new opportunities for shared action that can be of benefit to all. The principles of rights-based approaches to service delivery, combined with strong leadership, offer one possibility for sustained inclusive practice and democratic hope. The next section offers a framework for organisations that wish to pursue a sustainable approach to inclusive practice.

An organisational framework for sustaining inclusive practice

The following builds on earlier work, affirming and extending and organisational framework for inclusive practice by focusing on elements that aim to counter the tendency to reinscription and return to previous system dynamics (Pollock and Taket 2014b). The elements presented here have taken account of the barriers, strengthening what is required to sustain inclusive practice in service development.

Ensure knowing commitment at the whole-organisation level

The approach intentionally sought to surface and unsettle prevailing power relations by centreing and legitimating the silenced voices of all participants. Strong, committed leadership was required to counter the tendencies to reinscription that emerged in each project setting. Organisations wanting to undertake inclusive practice must be prepared for the resistance they will encounter, regardless of the impact this may have on their business and brand. Commitment to a clear and stated purpose, in relation to both the democratic and disruptive intents, is required at all levels of and functions within the organisation. Senior staff in particular need to understand the disruptive nature of the inclusive endeavour and be trained and supported in how to facilitate and sustain inclusive practice.

Value and utilise diverse ways of knowing

It was possible to build opportunities for groups of participants to explore their experiences and ideas together and separately into routine service delivery. Bringing together diverse ways of knowing gave rise to opportunities for service innovation and made available more empowered subject positions for service users, families, and staff in particular. Facilitated critical reflection was central to exploring how the local arrangements of service delivery impacted on different groups and to challenge oppressive meanings and practices with immediate practical and well-being benefits to participants. Sustaining inclusive practice requires giving due consideration to how to maintain a critical exploration of current arrangements that can be sustained within routine service delivery, so that as systems develop and change, they remain subject to review from within and across different ways of knowing.

Build systems to support organisational capability

What emerged from the projects was a potential role for frontline staff and managers in encouraging and supporting participation in local decision-making and action planning. As local service delivery teams grew clearer and more confident about the value of inclusive practice, they began to implement changes in the immediate environment that had clear benefits for all. Organisations wanting to sustain and extend the benefits of inclusive practice need to consider the systems that will continue to build organisational capability. These include training for staff in engagement and participation; inclusion of individual capabilities in position descriptions; systems for collecting, collating, and analysing outputs of participatory activities in order to identify patterns, trends, and themes; and ways of responding to new knowledge that can support actions for change beyond the local context.

Hold the organisation accountable for its practice

The intractability of institutional practices lies, in part, in their circular processes of implementation, measurement, and reporting. By ensuring that performance indicators for participation are built into individual-, service-, and organisation-level plans, an organisation can establish its own system of implementation and reporting that reflects the value it places on participation as a central practice. A strong and stated link between commitment to participation and what needs to be measured will ensure accountability back to community and to funders, who will be left in no doubt about the organisation's democratic intentions. The initiative in this Melbourne NGO demonstrated that all this can be achieved within routine arrangements for service delivery and, as a consequence, should be nothing to fear but rather to offer hope for a more humanised, shared future for all.

In concluding, this chapter has presented a rights-based organisational practice for service development that is practical and sustainable. At a time when the rhetoric on consumer participation, coproduction, and co-design is strong, there is less evidence of change in practice in organisations that make up health and social welfare service systems (Byrne et al. 2014; Slay and Stephens 2013). The framework offers one way for organisations to reshape their practices so service users, providers, and government officials can work together as equal partners to develop service responses that are efficient and safe and offer hope to all who come in contact with them.

References

Byrne, L., Wilson, M., Burke, K.J., Gaskin, C.J. and Happell, B. (2014) 'Mental health service delivery: a profile of mental health non-government organisations in south-east Queensland, Australia' *Australian Health Review*, 38: 202–7.

Cousins, J.B. and Whitmore, E. (1998) 'Framing participatory evaluation', *New Directions for Evaluation*, 80: 87–105.

Gaventa, J. and Barrett, G. (2010) *So What Difference Does it Make? Mapping the Outcomes of Citizen Engagement*, Brighton: Institute of Development Studies, IDS Working Paper 347. Online. Available at www.ids.ac.uk/files/dmfile/Wp347.pdf (accessed 11 April 2019).

Gillies, V. (2005) 'Meeting parents' needs? Discourses of 'support' and inclusion in family policy', *Critical Social Policy*, 25: 70–90.

Gruskin, S., Bogecho, D. and Ferguson, L. (2010) ' "Rights-based approaches" to health policies and programs: articulations, ambiguities, and assessment', *Journal of Public Health Policy*, 31: 129–45.

Gustafsson, U. and Driver, S. (2005) 'Parents, power and public participation: sure start, an experiment in new labour governance', *Social Policy and Administration*, 39: 528–43.

Hodge, S. (2005) 'Participation, discourse and power: a case study in service user involvement', *Critical Social Policy*, 25: 164–79.

Martin, G.P. (2012) 'Public deliberation in action: emotion, inclusion and exclusion in participatory decision making', *Critical Social Policy*, 32: 163–83.

Newman, J., Barnes, M., Sullivan, H. and Knops, A. (2004) 'Public participation and collaborative governance', *Journal of Social Policy*, 33: 203–23.

Ney, T., Stoltz, J-A. and Maloney, M. (2013) 'Voice, power and discourse: experiences of participants in family group conferences in the context of child protection', *Journal of Social Work*, 13: 184–202.

Ottmann, G.F., Laragy, C. and Damonze, G. (2009) 'Consumer participation in designing community based consumer-directed disability care: lessons from a participatory action research-inspired project', *Systemic Practice and Action Research*, 22: 31–44.

Pollock, S. (2016) 'Power and participation: enhancing service user agency in social care', unpublished PhD thesis, Deakin University.

Pollock, S. and Taket, A. (2014a) 'Achieving socially inclusive practice: analysing power dynamics in a participatory approach to service development', *International Journal of Interdisciplinary Organizational Studies*, 8(2): 1–11.

Pollock, S. and Taket, A. (2014b) 'Inclusive service development: exploring a whole-of-organisation approach in the community services sector', in A. Taket, B.R. Crisp, M. Graham, L. Hanna, S. Goldingay and L. Wilson (eds) *Practising Social Inclusion*, London: Routledge.

Potts, H. (2010) *Participation and the Right to the Highest Attainable Standard of Health*, Colchester: Human Rights Centre, University of Essex. Online. Available at http://repository.essex.ac.uk/9714/1/participation-right-highest-attainable-standard-health.pdf (accessed 11 April 2019).

Romm, N. and Gregory, W. (2001) 'Critical facilitation: learning through intervention in group processes', *Management Learning*, 32: 453–67.

Rorty, R. (1989) *Contingency, Irony and Solidarity*, Cambridge: Cambridge University Press.

Rose, D., Fleischmann, P., Tonkiss, F., Campbell, P. and Wykes, T. (2003) *User and Carer Involvement in Change Management in a Mental Health Context: Review of the Literature*, London: National Co-ordinating Centre for NHS Service Delivery and Organisation Research and Development. Online. Available at www.netscc.ac.uk/hsdr/files/project/SDO_FR_08-1201-017_V01.pdf (accessed 11 April 2019).

Slay, J. and Stephens, L. (2013) *Co-production in Mental Health: A Literature Review. Commissioned by Mind*, London: New Economics Foundation. Online. Available at https://b.3cdn.net/nefoundation/ca0975b7cd88125c3e_ywm6bp3ll.pdf (accessed 11 April 2019).

Singh, A. (2010) 'Commentary rights-based approaches to health policies and programmes: why are they important to use', *Journal of Public Health Policy*, 31: 146–9.

Steinart, H. and Pilgram, A. (2007) *Welfare Policy from Below: Struggles Against Social Exclusion in Europe*, Aldershot: Ashgate.

Taket, A. (2012) *Health Equity, Social Justice, and Human Rights*, London: Routledge.

Triggs, G. (2013) 'Social inclusion and human rights in Australia'. Online. Available at www.humanrights.gov.au/news/speeches/social-inclusion-and-human-rights-australia (accessed 11 April 2019).

Wilson, M.G., Lavis, J.N. and Guta, A. (2012) 'Community-based organizations in the health sector: a scoping review', *Health Research Policy and Systems*, 10: 36.

Yates, S., Dyson, S. and Hiles, D. (2008) 'Beyond normalization and impairment: theorizing subjectivity in learning difficulties—theory and practice', *Disability and Society*, 23: 247–58.

12 The space to think critically

How supervision can support sustainable practice in social service organisations

Matt Rankine and Liz Beddoe

Introduction

Creating and maintaining sustainable organisations that are inclusive and adaptable for service users remain a challenge to health and social welfare professionals in the current neoliberal environment. Sustainability is multifaceted, with points of tension at systemic, organisational, and environmental levels that require professionals to consider the impact of organisations on the broad social and physical environment and how resources are developed and renewed (Clegg et al. 2008). Moreover, sustainability requires the preservation of core values and principles. In Canada, Barter (2012: 241) argued that, 'given contemporary social and political climates, and knowing the challenges being expressed about and within the profession, there is reason for concern for professional sustainability', linking the concept of professional sustainability to the preservation of values of inclusion and social justice for individuals and communities in social work. Thus, sustainable services are those which address consumers' complex social needs and concerns with those values in the foreground, requiring critical thinking and an integrated response in practice (Schmitz et al. 2012).

In addition, at organisational levels, social service organisations need to nurture staff to ensure retention and continuing commitment. Employers and managers must foster commitment to innovation and inclusionary practice in the workplace as part of a workforce sustainability strategy. A study conducted in Australia, Aotearoa New Zealand, and Canada found that commitment to the agency 'mission', along with support from supervisors, remained 'centrally important to workers' identity and willingness to remain employed in social care' (Baines et al. 2014: 433). The ability to reflect critically holds an important place in challenging contradictory systems that oppress people in society, to support disadvantaged groups and promote human rights and social justice. In this chapter, we argue that critical reflection in supervision can support sustainable practice for workers in social services. Concepts drawn from Bourdieu's social theory support a critical examination of the supervision space and the impact of wider, structural issues. We explore how to align supervision to current demands on the workforce. By way of illustration, we draw on a small qualitative study regarding the supervision of social workers in community-based child welfare organisations in Aotearoa New Zealand.

Supervision in the organisational context of human services

Essentially, supervision is a professional working relationship between the supervisee, supervisor, and the organisation (Davys and Beddoe 2010). The practice of supervision has, over 100 years, developed across a range of helping professions including counselling, social work, nursing, midwifery, and psychology, often reflecting the underpinning theoretical orientations of those professions (Beddoe and Davys 2016). Developmental models used in counselling and psychology have described the process of supervisors and supervisees moving through organic stages of professional development (Hawkins and Shohet 2012). Experiential learning has become central in self-evaluation and improvement of practice in supervision. Underpinning experiential learning has been the application of cyclical reflective structures in supervision practice, such as the reflective learning model (Davys and Beddoe 2010). Momentum has gathered regarding the importance of critical reflection in ensuring social justice is addressed in professional practice (Asakura and Maurer 2018; Fook and Gardner 2007). Critical reflection in supervision provides the space to explore diverse perspectives and encompasses the professional, organisational, administrative, and cultural contexts of the work undertaken with service users (Beddoe and Egan 2009). The exploration of broader and contextual perspectives in supervision then provides a strategic and action focus as a foundation to support critical practice (Noble et al. 2016). As a space for critical reflection to occur, supervision needs to be transformational so that changes in thinking and behaviour occur in practice (Davys and Beddoe 2010).

The quality of critical discussions in supervision has been increasingly influenced by the local and global context of where practice takes place. Neoliberal preoccupations with maintaining efficiency, fiscal restraint, and scrutiny of practice have shifted the focus of supervision toward risk management, meeting pre-arranged targets with service users and support for organisational agendas (Beddoe 2010). Baines et al. (2014: 438) note that critical management perspectives suggest that supervisors can make a significant contribution to mediating the impact of management for both consumers of services and for human services staff by employing 'organisational and discretionary power to challenge and destabilise the overarching dominance of New Public Management (NPM). . . . This critical management literature views these practices as forms of resistance'. Together, supervisors and supervisees need to proactively explore how supervision can be improved and be part of developing an environment within organisations that ensures worker well-being, ongoing learning, and sustainability.

To promote professional sustainability, critical conversations related to oppression and social justice require ongoing scrutiny in supervision alongside individual practice, relationships with others, the organisation, and the political environment (Noble et al. 2016; Rankine et al. 2018). The challenge for supervision practice is to develop a wider systemic approach (Lambley 2018), explore diversity and co-construction of knowledge (Hair and O'Donoghue 2009), and critical practice (Noble et al. 2016).

The current human services environment requires practitioners in different disciplines to think more critically and creatively about the present use of supervision. An examination of supervision has led to the development of alternative supervision approaches to promote anti-oppressive practice, such as strengths-based approaches (Engelbrecht 2010), cross-cultural supervision (Tsui et al. 2014), and indigenous models of supervision (Eruera 2012). Utilising alternative methods including arts and creative approaches in supervision has supported deeper understanding of the emotions associated with the practice experience (Hafford-Letchfield and Huss 2018; Markos et al. 2008).

Enriching the supervision experience in new and creative ways provides practitioners with the opportunity to understand the wider macro areas influencing their practice, repositioning associated challenges and the feelings of working in what can be a corrosive environment. Understanding that environment and its impacts on the sustainability of social service practice is enhanced by drawing on the work of Bourdieu, whose conceptual framework provides perspective and clarity to an examination of where supervision 'sits' in the contemporary social services environment.

Bourdieu's concepts and understanding the social services environment

Bourdieu's conceptual framework of field, capital, and habitus, often referred to as his 'conceptual arsenal' (Garrett 2007a; Houston 2002), has been noted as particularly pertinent to understanding practice across a range of health and social welfare disciplines through analysis of societal structures and power relations (Garrett 2007a; Gill et al. 2014; Houston 2002; Taket et al. 2009). Bourdieu has described how dominant structures reproduce and maintain inequality but also provide potential opportunities for change. We briefly define Bourdieu's terms here.

Habitus refers to the identity of individuals and encompasses the day-to-day habitual practices and meaning of the social world around them (Bourdieu 1989). Habitus is seen by some as a *product* of the social world but as a *reproducer* of the social world for others (Houston 2002). The structures within an individual's habitus provide socialisation that leads to either privileges or disadvantages. In addition, Houston (2002) has stated that there is also margin for innovation and improvisation with such structures, which is an important consideration in exploring sustainability in social services work.

Field is the structured social space occupied by the individual or institution in society (Bourdieu 1999). The occupants of a field are defined by the dominance and subordination that exists between their positions. Fields are dependent on sets of rules and discourses that govern relationships with others (Garrett 2007a). This discourse can change and evolve with an individual's position over time. Fields can also be used to define broader, unequal, social constructs where there is competition for knowledge, skills, and resources.

Capital is Bourdieu's third interrelated concept and can take different forms: economic, social, cultural, and symbolic capital (Garrett 2013). Beddoe (2013) has also employed the construct of 'professional capital' to represent the qualifications and attributes related to the status of professions in complex social fields. The different forms of capital create hierarchies within society which 'makes it possible to keep undesirable persons and things at a distance' (Bourdieu 1999: 127).

Bourdieu refers to *doxa*, which are the taken-for-granted assumptions, hidden agendas, and traditions that operate within society, culture, and education (Garrett 2007a). Doxa, when identified and unpacked, help explain how oppression by a ruling class or dominant force such as patriarchy or colonisation is maintained within society. This unequal distribution of capital, Bourdieu argues, can be confronted through the process of practitioners scrutinising their personal and social environments (Bourdieu 2001). This scrutiny provides the basis for challenging oppression and developing inclusion and sustainability. Bourdieu has referred to public services such as social work and education as 'agents of the state' under neoliberalism (Bourdieu 1999). The oppression that marginalised groups experience requires social welfare professionals to critically consider their position. Bourdieu highlighted the contradiction that social services workers are simultaneously part of administering welfare for the state while paradoxically opposing systems that oppress marginalised groups. In this chapter, Bourdieu's concepts are used to assist with redefining critical reflection within supervision. This process supports sustainability in the workforce through the development of critical reflection of practice in supervision.

Supervision in community child welfare: an Aotearoa New Zealand, case study

A critical realist epistemology (Baines 2017) influenced the qualitative study drawn upon here, where diverse participant perspectives were captured highlighting the impact of oppressive structures as well as the development of social justice strategies in practice (Rankine 2017). In this approach, we understand that participants construct their understandings of the social world of human services practice within the realities of societies and driven by measurable injustice and inequality.

The study explored supervisory dyads' use of supervision within the current context of different community-based, nongovernment child welfare organisations across Auckland, the largest multicultural city in Aotearoa New Zealand (Rankine 2017; Rankine et al. 2018). Social workers were chosen as study participants, as their profession is associated with supporting and promoting the wellbeing of diverse populations in an environment dominated by organisational and government agendas (Gray and Webb 2013). A thinking-aloud process of recording supervision sessions, transcribing, and examining transcribed material was developed to aid the critical reflection, analysis, and review of supervision practice by supervisors and supervisees (Maidment and Cooper 2002; Rankine and Thompson 2015).

Participant data were gathered from two separate, audio-recorded, and transcribed sessions, including a supervision session between each supervisor and supervisee and a follow-up session with the researcher several weeks later. To assist with anonymity in the study, participants chose pseudonyms to use. Rankine completed an initial content analysis of the supervision session where content was grouped into themes to assist the facilitation of the follow-up session. Both members of each dyad participated in the follow-up meeting and had copies of the transcript. The findings from the dyads' follow-up session revealed the current themes that occupied the supervisory space for both parties. This included self-awareness, navigating professional relationships, organisational pressures to meet targets, and uncertainties within the current professional environment (Rankine 2017). The application of Bourdieusian concepts to these themes presents the realities and further possibilities for developing sustainable and inclusive practice for the practitioners involved. Examples from the data follow.

The application of Bourdieu's concepts to supervision practice

The application of the concepts, habitus, field, and capital to the themes identified in the study signals a sustainable approach for practitioners within community-based child welfare organisations and their use of supervision. Supervision can contribute to enabling practitioners to sustain their core values and deepen insight into their day-to-day practice; appreciate the complexity of professional relationships within and outside the organisation; and strengthen professional identity weakened in managerialised workplaces while highlighting opportunities to create change and inclusion.

Habitus

How individuals identify who they are and make sense of their daily practices are central to habitus (Bourdieu 1999). Safe, supportive supervision provides the necessary container to regulate and assess well-being, make connections, and critically reflect. Participants, such as Susan, commented on supervision being the place to discuss personal experiences and the impact this may have on professional work:

> I've had a pretty tough year with my mum passing away . . . so I need to talk about [in supervision] those things and not just think that it's separate from my work . . . it's important for my safety and my client's safety. . . . You'd be silly to think that your personal life doesn't impinge on your work life.
>
> (Susan)

Houston (2002) reminds us that habitus provides a framework to adapt, innovate, and improvise. Supervision enables the practitioner to adapt and adjust to the social services environment while holding firm to the values that first attracted them to this sector (Baines et al. 2014). Jessica acknowledged how the supervision habitus was a continually emerging process (supervision is seen as lifelong in social work practice rather than as a professional development tool as in education and internships) and an integration of professional and personal values for her supervisee over time:

> What I've noticed with Grace, that you [are using] supervision for . . . the personal journey [and] the professional journey. So it's about that integration . . . of ideas and values and life philosophy with the work. You carry your consciousness . . . this is a steep learning time for you.
>
> (Jessica)

Habitus provides understanding of an individual's 'place' and the positioning of 'others' (Bourdieu 1989). In complex environments where various practitioners operate, a clear understanding of professional roles, boundaries, and values is essential. Supervision provides clarity of roles, guidelines, and associated codes of practice conduct for the supervisee operating in an organisation. Analysis of the participant data concurred—through critical discussions in supervision, the supervisee was able to examine perspectives and develop professional confidence.

> I'm really clear about where I stand on this and where it needs to go. . . . To express without being judged around what I'm thinking.
>
> (Jackie)

> It just gave me the opportunity to put the whole thing in perspective, see myself as a person in the middle of something complex with many interactions. And that I did not have to hold it all, it could be put into [perspective].
>
> (Grace)

Through a Bourdieusian lens, an exploration of habitus involves specific rituals and practices in order to perform appropriately in an environment. The supervisor's enquiry into the supervisee's emotions in supervision allows for nonjudgemental ownership of feelings and resolution in complicated and emotionally draining work (Davys and Beddoe 2010). Jock highlighted the purpose of supervision to 'park' emotions, critically examine situations, and 'rejuvenate'.

> It's a human thing that we get . . . emotionally attached to people we're trying to help and support, and for me, supervision is the vehicle to actually help us contain, cope and park our emotions when we get attached. We do want the best for the families [in community child welfare]. . . . I think [supervision] is a really good vehicle to think things through in a positive, safe way . . . that's where you can rejuvenate yourself and get a fresh start.
>
> (Jock)

Supervision that fosters critical reflection enables the supervisee to address the mission and values of the agency, illuminate strengths, build resilience, and come up with their own solutions.

[I]t was like trying to find a way of helping Grace to think about what other strengths and resources she's got . . . to get in touch with those. And that needed to be something that she came up with—not me telling her how I thought she could've handled it.

(Jessica)

Field

Bourdieu's concept of field enables the practitioner to understand the structured space of relationships in social services practice within potentially corrosive and damaging workplaces. Within the supervisory space, the influences of organisational and professional forces permeate the discourses and agendas and structure how knowledge is produced in the session. The interaction and relationship the practitioner has with others, such as their supervisor, consumers of services, colleagues, and other professionals, are all important areas that require critical consideration for effective and sustainable practice.

In order for practitioners to feel rejuvenated in their work, the supervision session itself needs to contribute as a positive socialising process that supports professional well-being and development. Analysis of the supervisory dyads' data highlighted key skills required by the supervisor to assist with an effective relationship.

I believe that my relationship with Debbie is sufficiently honest enough—if Debbie thought there's a complete lack of connection here she would ask a question that would lead into a conversation about that. Trust in a relationship [and] certainly a connection [are important].

(Jane)

I think we have a good, open, honest relationship . . . if I have something I'm concerned about I can talk to Jock about it. . . . I always feel that I've been listened to and that's really important that I'm supported.

(Susan)

The organisational and professional 'fields of forces' (Bourdieu 1999) demonstrate opposing tensions in the supervisory relationship. In the study, this relationship was highlighted by the commitment to external supervision (supervisor external to the organisation) by some community child welfare agencies for social workers to maintain professional obligations.

The fact that Jessica [external supervisor] is outside the organisation, I take this time—it's all about me. Whereas in the organisation, it's about the cases and how the cases are moving. . . . So there's a different focus.

(Grace)

Internal supervision relationships tend to focus on administration, completion of tasks, tight time frames, and external targets that do not necessarily reflect service users' needs and with little focus on critical reflection on practice (Beddoe 2011). In such arrangements, the supervisee has learnt to feedback information as a mechanism to measure compliance. In this way, dominant neoliberal discourses are maintained, reproduced, and unchallenged within organisations (Garrett 2007b). The lack of opportunity for critical exploration and a sense of powerlessness within internal supervision left Yvonne considering with her supervisee what could change.

> Quite often I find . . . that supervisees want the answer from me. 'Tell me' . . . then I just continue to enable them to be powerless. How can I give you the feeling that you actually do have power in that organisation?
>
> (Yvonne)

An important aspect of Bourdieu's work is the importance of amplifying discourses of disadvantaged groups (Bourdieu 1999)—a core value of professional disciplines in social services. Critical supervision, exploring the 'field of forces' that Bourdieu would argue are present in this sector, provides the practitioner the opportunity to analyse their relationships with service users within an understanding of power and structure. The participants in the study, for example, emphasised the importance of supervision being child focused when other dominant agendas prevailed.

> It's really . . . what's going to benefit that child . . . I really felt that [the family] are focusing on the adult issue rather than the child and that was one of my goals—to discuss this with my supervisor [and] find a way to bring the focus back on the child rather than themselves.
>
> (Jackie)

When community-based organisations are dominated by managerial targets, practitioners struggle to explore creative solutions to issues experienced by service users (Connolly and Cashmore 2009). The space to critically reflect in supervision offers the supervisee a chance to view different perspectives and find alternatives, as this dyad's commentary attests.

> Jock [supervisor] has given me different ideas . . . when I'm talking about the grandmother that I'm working with and the problems that she's having. Jock's looking at it from a different perspective [and] angle.
>
> (Susan)

> [Supervision] allows us to think about the skills that Susan has employed and it's a really positive piece of work . . . a task-centred, cooperative working partnership . . . you are standing alongside her and helping her come to informed choices.
>
> (Jock)

Actors in the field of social services are rendered unequal by dimensions of power and dominant beliefs (Bourdieu 1989). A Bourdieusian analysis of differing professional fields highlights the power imbalances internal and external to the organisation. Critical examination of the internal relationships within the organisation includes staff operating within teams where hierarchies and power dynamics may privilege some and disadvantage others. Analysis of the supervisory dyads' data stressed the prominence of power struggles within community-based child welfare services.

> I think it's a challenge to work with a big team of different professions. There's decisions that are made at a hierarchical level, higher up, and they're making the decisions without talking to you. . . . I think our communication could be stronger . . . but they've already made up their mind in leadership so they do what they want . . . nothing changes.
>
> (Tracey)

Similarly, professional interactions outside the organisation can create conflict and miscommunication. The child welfare system, from a Bourdieusian perspective, exemplifies a complex system comprising a number of agencies and professionals where there is a dominant discourse controlled by a risk-averse state (Featherstone et al. 2018). Within supervision, conversations reflecting disillusionment are common, as illustrated by Alice who described some working relationships with professionals in statutory child protection as 'banging my head up against a wall'.

> My concerns were how it was managed from the external agencies. I . . . spoke to [name of agency] and . . . when it comes to dealing with suicidal comments I expect a response that makes you feel like the concerns are being heard and that you are putting everything in place that you possibly can.
>
> (Alice)

When working within complex and competing fields, Bourdieu's theorisations encourage the practitioner to 'correspond to the multiplicity of co-existing, and sometimes directly competing points of view' (Bourdieu 1999: 3). The supervisor has a key role in enhancing this unique position and the potential for working alongside others. Supervision becomes an essential process for critical reflection of the supervisee's navigation of multiple, complex systems so that practice remains effective and sustainable within community organisations.

> I do come back to relationship being one of the things that is the very foundation of the work. So if I don't have that relationship then the work cannot be done . . . I see that [supervision] is one of the unique places where I can be allowed to [critically reflect on relationships] completely safely. My understanding of supervision is there has to be that trust that this is the place to do that.
>
> (Grace)

Capital

Bourdieu has described capital as the influence an individual or group has over others and how this can be measured over time relative to economic, cultural, social, and professional influence (Garrett 2013). Beddoe (2013) has previously described signs of weak professional capital as including invisibility in the public discourse of professionalism; a lack of recognition for its contributions to the public institutions; a weak or disputed knowledge claim; and a passive role in institutions rather than taking leadership. Demonstrating features of weak professional capital threatens the sustainability of practice in community service organisations that aim to support disadvantaged groups.

In this study, struggles for greater professional capital were intensified by managerial discourses on professional practice (Rankine 2017). Constant changes to service delivery in community-based child welfare work, restructuring of personnel and reduced funding by the state were central to the challenges raised in supervision.

> We have a really high turnover of staff. How can you build a solid team when your team's always changing? . . . that's just something that I have to consider if I want to stay here or not.
>
> (Tracey)

> It is a theme that runs through a lot of supervision work at the moment because of the broader context [in] which we are operating . . . and the fact that . . . the goalposts have been changed. . . [resulting in] negative deficit talk about resourcing, not enough staff . . . and downsizing.
>
> (Debbie)

An unequal distribution of capital, according to Bourdieu, maintains doxa (taken-for-granted assumptions) and disadvantages individuals and groups within society (Bourdieu 1999). The levels of oppression are also apparent in how professionals operate with inadequate resources, skill bases, and social connections. For many social workers in the study, operating in community-based child welfare led to a persistent mind-set of disempowerment. This was an important topic in Debbie and Jane's supervision.

> [Some staff's] thinking is poisonous and we've got these young, energetic grads that are coming through with enthusiasm, lots of wonderful vibrant ideas . . . and then they catch on to that train of. . . 'We don't have enough' deficit type . . . negativity.
>
> (Jane)

> That is the external impact it's having on the cultures of teams generally. . . . I think that you work very hard to establish an organisational culture [that is positive]. But the challenge is how you get those staff holding the hope and . . . vision.
>
> (Debbie)

The concept of capital assists with a closer inspection of existing structures and colonising processes that impact on professional practises and supervision. Moreover, choices can be explored that enhance professional capital, identity, and work undertaken with others. Bourdieu's theorisations align with principles of critical reflection in that an exploration of the wider environment of society provides the opportunity to strategise and critically examine the impact of capital-influencing institutions (Bourdieu 2001). Supervision provides the space for the practitioner to critically explore alternatives to practice within institutions.

The study found an overall lack of critical analysis within supervision of connections between organisational functioning and external forces. However, the importance of having reflective time in supervision to discuss wider factors impacting on work, other than administrative matters alone, created a shift in thinking for some participants. Kath acknowledged the busyness of her job prevented her from examining her practice, and the value of participating in the study and its process had made her evaluate practice in more detail.

> I think having the opportunity to talk about [the use of critical reflection in supervision] is really great. To even think about all that is really different to last time . . . in my work, it is so crisis driven, it is really difficult to step out of that and reflect in a really healthy way.
>
> (Kath)

Bourdieu reminds professionals of the importance of multiple voices often concealed by dominant discourses in practice (Bourdieu 2001). The unpacking of culture, connection, and narratives in the supervisory relationship allows for the recognition of different ways of inclusive working. From an Aotearoa New Zealand, perspective, Ohaki and Rangi, as one supervisory dyad in the study, provided an example of this.

> It's the sense of being able to connect with my ahua [character], my wairua [spirit] and Ohaki has that strong sense. She's happy to let me finish just whatever that looks like. I don't feel I've just got to cut off. . . . It really affirms for me that there is a place for Māori doing supervision together because I have a Pākehā [European] internal supervisor and . . . it's a very different feel . . . a whole lot of stuff gets unsaid.
>
> (Rangi)

Implications for sustainable practice

For organisations to be sustainable now and in the future, health and social care professionals require stronger opportunities for critical reflection on the wider environment and its impact both on service consumers and social services work itself (Baines et al. 2014). Commonly not recognised within texts related to helping professions (Garrett 2013), is the significance of Bourdieu's critical theorising of contemporary sociocultural and sociopolitical issues. Good supervision and effective interprofessional and inter-agency relationships can foster greater connection between individuals, groups, and their environment and ultimately stronger social services. These organisations, in turn, can enhance their contribution to social inclusion within communities (Gill et al. 2014).

Supervision provides the ideal space for professionals within health and social care settings to critically reflect on the context of the work, to become strategic, purposeful, and transformative in their practice whilst resisting the tendency to devalue and remove professional knowledge and practice wisdom from services (Noble et al. 2016). Applying Bourdieu's critical concepts to the study of supervisory dyads working in community child welfare settings in Auckland, New Zealand, illustrated how sustainable and more effective forms of practice can evolve and be operationalised within a reflective supervisory space. *Habitus* provides greater self-examination and insight of thoughts, feelings, and communication. This includes a closer inspection of a practitioner's taken-for-granted assumptions and beliefs and how these are challenged when working in a particular organisation with different norms and rules. *Field* permits the practitioner to develop a more comprehensive appreciation of systemic relationships. In doing so, a professional can view power imbalances within and outside of organisations and how dominant discourses are inadvertently played out within professional relationships. *Capital* allows the practitioner to see the tenuous political nature of professional work, the ongoing power struggles to promote professionalism within a managerial climate, as well as the opportunities to promote inclusive and alternative practices. Furthermore, the themes from the study also illuminated a need for the ongoing development of critical reflection by the supervisee and supervisor of their habitus, interrelationship with other fields, and the impact of dominant discourses on professional practice.

To develop sustainability in practice, practitioners and organisations need to continually make visible and strengthen social justice strategies. Supervision can often be influenced by a neoliberal discourse and requires ongoing examination over how existing supervision frameworks inculcate social justice principles and cultural identity (Beddoe 2015). In a Bourdieusian sense, supervisors and supervisees who can reflexively scrutinise their own habitus have the potential to challenge existing doxa and practices (Garrett 2013). Strategies for critical practice have become more prevalent within the supervision literature emphasising the need to examine the wider sociopolitical, sociocultural, and structural factors influencing practice (Noble et al. 2016; Rankine 2017). However, practitioners, supervisees, supervisors, and managers operating in organisations have much to do in promoting interdisciplinary and coordinated conversations around sustainability and critical reflection in practice (Schmitz et al. 2012). Practitioners need to be proactive within organisations in developing critical reflection and more sustainable practice. Supervisors can hone their skills in facilitating critical reflection within supervision while supervisees need to have a willingness to explore the value of critical reflection in sessions. Managers need to understand these organisational practices and support the significance of critical conversations held in supervision toward sustainability, social inclusion, and learning for the organisation in policy and service design. Each has a connected and distributed role to ensure the development of supervision models that are context-responsive, to critically examine the wider environment, and to ultimately promote social justice and the human rights of consumers of services in practice.

Conclusion

Crucial to sustainable, renewable, and socially inclusive services is the practitioner's ability to develop critical reflection and social justice strategies in health and social care organisations. To do so, practitioners require spaces such as supervision to reinvigorate their passion and integrate and reshape professional practice within organisations. The hope for a sustainable future necessitates a collaborative and more informed approach in organisations where the impact of sociocultural and sociopolitical factors on practice and people can be critically examined and alternatives implemented.

References

Asakura, K. and Maurer, K. (2018) 'Attending to social justice in clinical social work: supervision as a pedagogical space', *Clinical Social Work Journal*, 46: 289–97.

Baines, D. (2017) *Doing Anti-oppressive Practice: Social Justice Social Work*, Halifax: Fernwood.

Baines, D., Charlesworth, S., Turner, D. and O'Neill, L. (2014) 'Lean social care and worker identity: the role of outcomes, supervision and mission', *Critical Social Policy*, 34: 433–53.

Barter, K. (2012) 'Competency-based standards and regulating social work practice: liabilities to professional sustainability', *Canadian Social Work Review/Revue Canadienne de Service Social*, 29: 229–46.

Beddoe, L. (2010) 'Surveillance or reflection: professional supervision in "the risk society"', *British Journal of Social Work*, 40: 1279–96.

Beddoe, L. (2011) 'External supervision in social work: power, space, risk, and the search for safety', *Australian Social Work*, 65: 197–213.

Beddoe, L. (2013) 'A "profession of faith" or a profession: social work, knowledge and professional capital', *New Zealand Sociology*, 28: 44–63.

Beddoe, L. (2015) 'Supervision and developing the profession: one supervision or many?' *China Journal of Social Work*, 8: 150–63.

Beddoe, L. and Davys, A. (2016) *Challenges in Professional Supervision: Current Themes and Models for Practice*, London: Jessica Kingsley.

Beddoe, L. and Egan, R. (2009) 'Social work supervision', in M. Connolly and L. Harms (eds) *Social Work: Contexts and Practice*, 2nd edn, South Melbourne: Oxford University Press.

Bourdieu, P. (1989) 'Social space and symbolic power', *Sociological Theory*, 7: 14–25.

Bourdieu, P. (1999) 'An impossible mission', in P. Bourdieu and P. Parkhurst Ferguson (eds) *The Weight of the World: Social Suffering in Contemporary Society*, Stanford: Stanford University Press.

Bourdieu, P. (2001) *Acts of Resistance: Against the New Myths of Our Time*, 2nd reprint, Cambridge: Polity Press.

Clegg, S., Kornberger, M. and Pitsis, T. (2008) *Managing and Organizations: An Introduction to Theory and Practice*, London: Sage.

Connolly, M. and Cashmore, J. (2009) 'Child welfare practice', in M. Connolly and L. Harms (eds) *Social Work: Contexts and Practice*, Melbourne: Oxford University Press.

Davys, A. and Beddoe, L. (2010) *Best Practice in Professional Supervision: A Guide for the Helping Professions*, London: Jessica Kingsley.

Engelbrecht, L.K. (2010) 'A strengths perspective on supervision of social workers: an alternative management paradigm within a social development context', *Social Work and Social Sciences Review*, 14: 47–58.

Eruera, M. (2012) 'He korari, he kete, he korero', *Aotearoa New Zealand Social Work*, 24(3/4): 12–19.

Featherstone, B., Gupta, A., Morris, K. and Warner, J. (2018) 'Let's stop feeding the risk monster: towards a social model of "child protection"', *Families, Relationships and Societies*, 7: 7–22.

Fook, J. and Gardner, F. (2007) *Practising Critical Reflection: A Resource Handbook*, Maidenhead: Open University Press.

Garrett, P. (2007a) 'The relevance of Bourdieu for social work: a reflection on obstacles and omissions', *Journal of Social Work*, 7: 355–79.

Garrett, P. (2007b) 'Making social work more Bourdieusian: why the social professions should critically engage with the work of Pierre Bourdieu', *European Journal of Social Work*, 10: 225–43.

Garrett, P. (2013) 'Pierre Bourdieu', in M. Gray and S. Webb (eds) *Social Work Theories and Methods*, 2nd edn, London: Sage.

Gill, J., Liamputtong, P. and Hoban, E. (2014) 'Practicing social inclusion: comfort zone— a social support group for teenagers with high-functioning autism', in A. Taket, B.R. Crisp, M. Graham, L. Hanna, S. Goldingay and L. Wilson (eds) *Practising Social Inclusion*, London: Routledge.

Gray, M. and Webb, S. (eds) (2013) *Social Work Theories and Methods*, 2nd edn, London: Sage.

Hafford-Letchfield, T. and Huss, E. (2018) 'Putting you in the picture: the use of visual imagery in social work supervision', *European Journal of Social Work*, 21: 441–53.

Hair, H. and O'Donoghue, K. (2009) 'Culturally relevant, socially just social work supervision: becoming visible through a social constructionist lens', *Journal of Ethnic and Cultural Diversity in Social Work*, 18: 70–88.

Hawkins, P. and Shohet, R. (2012) *Supervision in the Helping Professions*, 4th edn, Maidenhead: Open University Press.

Houston, S. (2002) 'Reflecting on habitus, field and capital: towards a culturally sensitive social work', *Journal of Social Work*, 2: 149–67.

Lambley, S. (2018) 'A semi-open supervision systems model for evaluating staff supervision in adult care settings: a conceptual framework', *European Journal of Social Work*, 21: 389–99.

Maidment, J. and Cooper, L. (2002) 'Acknowledgement of client diversity and oppression in social work student supervision', *Social Work Education*, 21: 399–407.

Markos, P., Coker, K. and Jones, P. (2008) 'Play in supervision', *Journal of Creativity in Mental Health*, 2(3): 3–15.

Noble, C., Gray, M. and Johnston, L. (2016) *Critical Supervision for the Human Services: A Social Model to Promote Learning and Value-based Practice*, London: Jessica Kingsley.

Rankine, M. (2017) 'What are we thinking? Supervision as the vehicle for reflective practice in community-based child welfare services', unpublished thesis, University of Auckland, NZ.

Rankine, M., Beddoe, L., O'Brien, M. and Fouché, C. (2018) 'What's your agenda? reflective supervision in community-based child welfare services', *European Journal of Social Work*, 21: 428–40.

Rankine, M. and Thompson, A. (2015) ' "Swimming to shore": co-constructing supervision with a thinking-aloud process', *Reflective Practice*, 16: 508–21.

Schmitz, C.L., Matyók, T., Sloan, L.M. and James, C. (2012) 'The relationship between social work and environmental sustainability: implications for interdisciplinary practice', *International Journal of Social Welfare*, 21: 278–86.

Taket, A., Crisp, B., Nevill, A., Lamaro, G., Graham, M. and Barter-Godfrey, S. (eds) (2009) *Theorising Social Exclusion*, London: Routledge.

Tsui, M-S., O'Donoghue, K. and Ng, A.K.T. (2014) 'Culturally competent and diversity-sensitive clinical supervision', in C.E. Watkins Jr and D.L. Milne (eds) *The Wiley International Handbook of Clinical Supervision*, Chichester: John Wiley and Sons.

Part 5

Sustainable social inclusion outcomes

13 Embedding change

Designing short-term projects for sustainable effects

Elena Jenkin, Erin Wilson, Robert Campain,
Kevin Murfitt and Matthew Clarke

Introduction

Projects or interventions, whether of a service delivery, community development, or research focus, are frequently established with finite time and resource
parameters. While often funders/donors propose that projects that offer strategies
for ongoing 'sustainability' are preferred (where 'sustainability' infers the ability
to continue project activity without the current funding source), in most cases,
both funders/donors and grant recipients (usually nongovernment organisations
[NGOs]) are complicit in the knowledge that this may not be possible. This poses
a significant problem for the sustainability of the change intended through the
project activity, as the project has a necessarily limited window of time in which
to both create and embed change in an ongoing way. Given that continuation of
funding or resources is not guaranteed in most programs or organisations, we
need to find ways to embed change at a range of levels that have likelihood of
longevity, including at the level of individual and community attitudes as well as
within organisational practice and within social structures such as policy. Such an
approach can be considered as a means to achieve sustainable outcomes for social
inclusion. It is this aspect of 'sustainability', that is, sustainability as embedding
change beyond the life of a project or intervention, that is the focus of this chapter,
drawing on the strategy used by the 'Voices of Pacific Children with Disability'
project to do this.

Project context

Globally, we know that children with disability experience high levels of social
exclusion and are frequently denied their human rights (McCallum and Martin
2013), despite the mandate of the *Convention on the Rights of Persons with Disabilities* [CRPD] (United Nations 2006) and the *Convention on the Rights of the
Child* (United Nations 1989). Such denial of social inclusion and human rights
is even more evident in certain regions, such as the Pacific, where there are low
levels of development (Clarke et al. 2014). In addition, children with disabilities
appear to be largely excluded from child research in general, and human rights
reports openly declare the absence of data pertaining to the human rights situation

for Pacific children with disability (Office of the United Nations High Commissioner for Human Rights Regional Office for the Pacific 2012).

In Vanuatu and Papua New Guinea (PNG) specifically, available data suggests that children with disability experience poverty, lack basic services such as health care and education, and face ongoing discrimination and abuse (Department of Community Development 2005; Robinson et al. 2013; United Nations 2003; Walji and Palmer 2012), but the level of data available is limited with very little engaging with the views of children with disability themselves. This means that, in addition to the ongoing barriers to human rights attainment for children with disability, their self-identified needs and priorities are not adequately addressed in service delivery and policy design, with the potential to further perpetuate experiences of exclusion and oppression. Liebel and Invernizzi note of children more broadly that

> when programmes and policies are devised without children themselves, significant aspects of their problems are ignored and dismissed. . . . Badly thought out policies and programmes might even be detrimental to children when they undermine their survival strategies and scarce resources they are confronted with in a difficult environment or when they specifically violate other rights.
>
> (Liebel and Invernizzi 2016: 2)

Underpinning this complex set of circumstances that contribute to the ongoing exclusion of children with disability, especially those in the Global South, are views held about children and disability that construct them as 'underdeveloped, deficient, and incompetent' (Jenkin et al. 2018). These views permeate individual and community attitudes, services, research, and policies.

The Voices of Pacific Children with Disability project

In this context, the 'Voices of Pacific Children with Disability' research project was a two-year project conducted in Vanuatu and PNG between 2013 and 2015, led by Deakin University with Save the Children Vanuatu, PNG, and Australia and the Disabled Persons Organisation (DPO) in each country, specifically Vanuatu Disability Promotion and Advocacy Association (DPA) and Papua New Guinea Assembly of Disabled Persons (PNG ADP), as the industry partners. The project aimed to address the research question, 'What are the human rights needs and priorities of children with disability in Vanuatu and Papua New Guinea?', through an inclusive research design that focused on enabling the self-report of children with diverse disabilities. Data were collected from 89 children with disability (aged 5 to 18) across both countries.

While the data collection method developed for the project (further discussed in Jenkin et al. 2017) was designed to be inclusive through offering a range of aural, visual, oral, and tactile modes to support the self-report of children, a particular focus of the wider research design was on mechanisms for fostering and embedding changes to support social inclusion.

Design of method for change

The project was constructed within a paradigm of social change or social justice research (Ife 2013; Tuck and Yang 2014). Social change fundamentally encompasses 'transformational processes related to the (re)distribution of power' (Guijt 2008: vi). These processes address power inequalities and require numerous actions across different levels of society in order to pursue attitudinal, structural, or systemic change (Guijt 2008). Such research involves intentional consideration of the methodology and method to ensure that both the research process as well as the outcome are anti-oppressive and challenge existing power inequalities toward enacting social change (Grieshaber 2010).

The first consideration in this method was the role of children with disability themselves in the research project. Literature related to child participation in research identifies central elements by which to involve children and affect change. First, 'it is essential to understand and respect children not only as executing actors but also as independently-acting subjects with their own rights' (Liebel 2012: 25). Our response to this was primarily to focus our resources on offering methods to children to support their engagement and communication in diverse ways, to enable them to report their own views and experiences. However, as described by several researchers, there is a risk that this becomes the means and the ends of child research (Lundy 2007). Merely listening to children restricts the political right and power of children to influence the political sphere (Liebel 2012) and can lead to 'unintended negative impacts on their lives' (Johnson 2017: 3), with little room for children's voices to contribute toward change (Kraftl 2013). Harcourt and Sargeant (2009: 175) have argued that there is little evidence of change occurring as a result of child participatory research and recommend an increased 'emphasis on the process of translating research findings into positive changes in children's lives'. With this critique in mind, we sought ways to enable children to engage with roles in dissemination and influencing activities through their involvement in films (funded through the project) and in public film screenings and dissemination events (discussed later).

A social justice research approach propels a focus beyond the immediate and requires an engagement with both the local and global contexts that together construct the child's world and their experiences of exclusion. Hart (2008) argued that failure to identify larger systemic issues limits the ability for change resulting from child research. Undertaking this broader analysis of the context in which children reside assists in positioning children's priorities within this broader schema of influences in order to support lasting change (Ife 2010). This understanding of change led us to a focus on considering change at both local and global levels, along with consideration of how our research activity, including both the process and the 'products' of the research project, could be developed to maximise and sustain change at all levels (Muirhead et al. 2017) targeting local and global audiences.

In this project, change can be thought of in terms of both capacity building and awareness raising with regards to understanding and supporting the rights and capabilities of children with disabilities. Change was targeted at different audiences as Muirhead et al. (2017) argue that targeting various stakeholders from the beginning of the research enables researchers to develop different products to achieve change across all levels of society. In this context, we defined our 'change' audience as

1   Child participants, their family, and communities;
2   Partners—DPOs and a child rights nongovernment organisation;
3   Governments of PNG and Vanuatu, donors;
4   Researchers, international development practitioners, and organisations; and
5   United Nations members, donors, and global audience (see Table 13.1).

In designing our change method, we targeted a number of underlying barriers to social inclusion for children with disability. As stated previously, negative

Table 13.1 Change audience, products, and change focus

Target audience	Change strategies (process and products of research)	Change focus
Child participants, their family and communities	Research method of engagement and self-report Films	Attitudinal change: Increased experience of children's capacity to express views and engage in activities Attitudinal change: Increased understanding that children with disability have human rights equal to others Attitudinal change: Increased understanding of the life aspirations of children with disability
Partners—DPOs and Save the Children	Employment of people with disability as co-researchers Training and resources for inclusive method of consulting/research children with disability Human rights findings	Practice expansion: Increased organisational capacity to employ people with disability Practice expansion: Increased organisational capacity to consult children with disability to inform design and delivery of relevant services Practice expansion: Increased organisational understanding of children's human rights needs, used to inform advocacy and service delivery

Target audience	Change strategies (process and products of research)	Change focus
Governments of PNG and Vanuatu, donors	Policy recommendations Human rights findings Policy brief Films	Policy change: Increased understanding of children's human rights needs and actions to address them linked to policy and programme change Attitudinal change: Increased understanding of the capacities and aspirations of children with disability
Researchers, international development practitioners, and organisations	Training and resources for inclusive method of consulting/research with children with disability Films	Attitudinal change: Increased understanding of the capacities and aspirations of children with disability Practice expansion: Increased skills and knowledge to consult/ research with children with disability Practice expansion: Increased research activity to document the human rights needs of children with disability in the Global South
United Nations members, donors, and global audience	Human rights findings Films	Attitudinal change: Increased understanding of the capacities and aspirations of children with disability Policy change: Increased understanding of children's human rights needs, used to inform programme and policy

attitudes about disability prevail at both the local and global level, with assumptions of deficit and incapacity. We aimed to tackle this in two main ways. First, the data collection methods enabled children to participate and communicate their views: children took photos, drew pictures, listened to audio recordings, worked with tactile objects, guided researchers around their communities, and told stories of their lives. Such engagement showcased both their inherent capacity (with appropriate supports) as well as affirming the value of their views (see Jenkin et al. 2015). Secondly, a subset of children participated in films, commissioned by the project, of children engaging in the research.

Two fourteen-minute films of the research in each country and one three-minute short film of one child participant in Vanuatu were developed in accessible formats (audio described or closed captions), with children speaking or signing their views in local languages. Film screenings were held in multiple locations in both countries at international events and widely viewed on YouTube and other websites (see www.voicesofchildrenwithdisability.com/films/). Both the data collection methods with children and the development of films to report their views provided evidence that children were capable of self-report, of engaging in a range of activities, and of sharing life aspirations in common with their non-disabled peers and community members (such as gaining employment, attending school, caring for family and community). These change methods had considerable reach, both in a local and global context, and we considered them to be a sustainable method of disseminating findings and of continuing the attitude change process (see Jenkin et al. 2016).

Our second change method targeted our research partners, particularly NGOs and local communities. A key aspect of our method was the employment of local adults with disability as co-researchers to undertake the bulk of data collection with children in each country. This was a deliberate strategy, not only to capitalise on the significant lived experience and local insight that each brought, but also to model the employment of people with disability to children, their communities, and also our partner organisations. Recruiting adults with a disability as researchers was a new experience for our partner child-rights organisation and changes to traditional recruitment processes were required to ensure these were accessible. This included advertising through disability networks and word of mouth rather than via formal advertisement, valuing lived experience of disability and relationship skills, rather than résumés and academic qualifications, to ensure that people with disabilities who may have had no previous employment experience were able to apply. Whilst the recruitment of people with disabilities for the research role was actively encouraged, it was ultimately the partner organisations' choice as to whom they employed, resulting in four out of the six researchers having a disability. Through this change strategy, we hoped to embed inclusive employment practice in participating organisations and model this to others, also contributing to attitude change about the capabilities and aspirations of people with disability.

A main concern of the project was how to extend its reach, so we focused significant attention on our change strategy to enable inclusive practice replication. The inclusive research method used offers a way of working to collect data from children with disability and/or consult them in the development and delivery of services and policies. We used a variety of approaches. The main strategy was the development and dissemination of a practice guide, *Inclusive Practice for Research with Children with Disability: A Guide* (Jenkin et al. 2015). Including a clear framework of ethics and principles for inclusive practice, the *Guide* also includes step-by-step prompts for communicating with children with disabilities and developing aural, oral, visual, and tactile data collection tools or communication supports to suit each context. The *Guide* was made available both at training workshops for DPO, NGO, and government personnel in both countries at the end of the project, at other training events and conference presentations in Australia, and via the project website (www.voicesofchildrenwithdisability.com/).

To accompany this, additionally at the local level, throughout the project several training workshops were held with co-researchers, DPO members, and other interested stakeholders. (For example, personnel from the government data collection agency in Vanuatu attended.) This change strategy aimed to enable the inclusive research approach to be replicated widely and build a community of practitioners able to positively engage children with disability in developing countries in issues of relevance to them in order to use this information to improve policy and programs.

Finally, we considered that structural change needed to target policies of relevant governments in each country as well as those of donor countries (providing international development funding). Achieving policies that are relevant to and inclusive of children with disability at a country level is a clear way to achieve change at scale. To this end, we summarised research findings into short reports for the governments of Vanuatu and PNG, identifying human rights needs and priorities of children with disability in each country, aligned to the *Convention on the Rights of Persons with Disabilities* (United Nations 2006), and the implications for policy. A similar approach was taken in attempting to influence the project donor, the Australian Department of Foreign Affairs and Trade (DFAT), via providing a policy brief outlining key policy implications.

Overall, our change activities aimed to extend the reach of the project through changing attitudes locally and globally, fostering practice replication, and informing policy change with the potential to scale-up inclusion initiatives for children with disability.

Results of project

Reporting upon and measuring change throughout a two-year research process is challenging as many changes are subtle, not always visible and usually incremental (Guijt 2008). Change is not always evident in short-term work, and Guijt (2008: 12) reports that 'focusing entirely on a tangible change as evidence of impact ignores what is often slow shifts in norms, institutions, [and] political reform over the longer term'. Furthermore, any such change is hard to attribute solely to a single cause as there are always a range of forces at play.

However, given we had an explicit change strategy, we attempted to note change and collect 'evidence' through a variety of mechanisms. Child participants and their families shared their reflections of the research process at the end of each data collection period. Co-researchers were also encouraged to journal their own reflections and sometimes shared thoughts and feelings with us, and at the end of the research, the primary author met with co-researchers over several sessions to discuss observed changes, no matter how small. Changes observed or that were reported to the research team, for example, by the co-researchers, partner organisations, government representatives, and other organisations, were documented throughout the project and for three years after its end. The changes captured are likely to reflect individual events/outcomes, and there is no way of knowing if these are representative of the experience of the cohorts or within a domain more broadly. A summary of embedded changes is reported as follows.

Changes as a result of the research process: change for children and families

Children generally provided very positive evaluations of their involvement in the research. For many, it was reported as a unique and empowering experience, as explained by this child participant in the project,

> I am so happy to be part of this big research project because there's never been a group of people coming around and talking to me and asking me about my problems. I really liked that you wanted to hear straight from me.

Families' attitudes about the level to which their children could contribute to the research process were reported as challenged during the data collection period. They were often surprised by the level and depth at which their children could participate in the research. Change was recorded in detail from one family. The family had lost trust in 'others' (disability service providers) who kept telling them what to do and had never listened to what they had to say. By contrast, the inclusive process used in this project (across four visits) emphasised building trust over time and the value of listening and respecting the expertise of the child and family. As captured by co-researchers:

> Timu (Agnes's father) is so pleased we included Agnes in the research because no-one has ever asked her what she thinks or what she needs or what might help her improve her life. He is very committed to improving Agnes's lifestyle and providing what she needs. He tells us that it is important to him that we listened to him tell the story of his family, their struggles—the heartbreak of losing their son (who died of what appears to be the same condition that Agnes is experiencing), and their achievements. He is so proud of Agnes but he worries about her future.

Some parents who participated in the research appeared to take up new or increased roles in advocacy and public speaking, either through films, presentations at film screenings, or via the development of a family advocacy group that was established in PNG with the assistance of PNG ADP. As was noted by co-researchers:

> Timu has become an important advocate for children with disabilities in his community. He said that being involved in the research gave him more confidence to understand that all children deserve to be heard and he was encouraging all the families with children with disabilities in his community to either send their children to school or teach them at home. He acted as messenger to all parents and children who do not have phone contact. His support to the research and to the co-researchers in this role was invaluable.

Attitude change through the films

The films appear to have had a significant emotional impact on viewers fostering an awareness of children with disabilities—that they exist, they can speak for themselves, they have desires and dreams, and just like other children, they ought to be able to realise them. The gentle respect of the co-researchers and their willingness to listen to and learn from children with disabilities is powerfully presented, along with the parents who speak of their children, their acceptance of disability, and their love for their children. The films appeared to have both local and global resonance. Locally, all child participants and their families were invited to film screenings that were organised by partner organisations and held in urban and remote locations. Transport assistance and meals made these events accessible. These events were reported to be valued by the children, families, and village chiefs. In addition, each child participant and their family were provided with a DVD of the films.

The accessibility features of the films were a new concept in both Vanuatu and PNG, and this aspect brought about awareness amongst viewers. Viewers with vision impairments in PNG enjoyed hearing the audio description that, for many of them, was a first-time experience. It has been reported to us that films have been drawn on for disability awareness in multiple countries, particularly Vanuatu, PNG, and Timor-Leste. It is hard to quantify this as, due to poor internet connections, DPOs in Pacific Island countries utilised both internet versions as well as DVD copies of films that were shared with DPOs.

The films have had significant global reach. Between 5 June 2017 and 9 March 2019, there have been 4,951 views combined of the films on YouTube and Tedx platforms, and they have been shared via social media by various organisations such as Enabling Education Network (EENET). The films have been shortlisted and screened by the United Nations in New York as part of their Enable film competition by DFAT during the International Day of People with Disabilities in 2015 and at TEDx Sydney in 2015. The PNG film was selected as the opening film in 2015 for the sixth PNG Human Rights Film Festival, which toured regionally. The festival director Alithia Barampataz explained in a radio interview that the films shown have a valuable role in supporting social change and will 'preserve a moment in time that can really tell its story for years and generations to come' (Walsh 2015). Alithia described that there are entire districts in PNG of people who are unable to pass a high school certificate, yet films in their language are accessible. She explained that everyone can understand them, and it promotes talking points in viewers' conversations with others for years (Walsh 2015).

Organisational change through employment of people with disability

Providing employment to people with disabilities as researchers was an opportunity to practice and demonstrate disability inclusion throughout the research. After the research, each of the four co-researchers with disability was able to gain employment or enter study, even where they previously had been unable to. While there have been positive employment outcomes for co-researchers with disabilities, it is harder to evidence ongoing change in organisational recruitment and inclusive employment practices. The partner DPOs already had a history of employing people with disability and have continued to do so, whereas this was a new experience for the child rights organisation. For this organisation in Vanuatu, continuation of employment of staff with disability was evident for a time follow-ing the completion of the project. Upon the completion of the research, the organi-sation also established a disability specific role to ensure that disability became a cross-cutting issue across all of their humanitarian and development work though this role has since been discontinued due to funding limitations.

Replicating practice

As discussed, the method and tools developed in this research offer a relevant and inclusive method for consultation with children, needs analysis for service devel-opment and planning, monitoring and evaluation, research, and in any other situa-tion that requires aids for the self-report of children with disability. The *Inclusive Practice for Research with Children with Disability: A Guide* (Jenkin et al. 2015) was intentionally developed as a user-friendly guide to promote inclusive prac-tice. As reported by researchers and development workers, the inclusive method promoted in the *Guide* has already assisted researchers and development workers to listen more intentionally to children with disabilities in different contexts and generate knowledge as reported by them. In turn, this has led to direct policy recommendations, meetings with government leaders, and the development of further resources (such as toolkits, discussed further later on) for the sector.

To date, this methodology and method have been drawn upon in a number of ways across the globe. Furthermore, the research methodology and methods have led to increased knowledge about children with disabilities in two developing countries. The methodology and method have now been used in Ethiopia by the Women's Refugee Commission (WRC) with refugee children with and without disabilities in participatory research regarding gender-based violence and have heavily informed the WRC's toolkit *Building Capacity for Disability Inclusion in Gender-Based Violence Programming in Humanitarian Settings* (Pearce 2015). Similarly, PLAN International, a global nongovernment organisation with a focus on children, has heavily drawn upon the *Guide* to develop a manual for the inter-national development sector titled *Guidelines for Consulting with Children and Young People with Disabilities* (Kuper et al. 2017). It is hoped that these guide-lines will further assist to generate practitioners' knowledge and commitment to inclusive practice in programming and research.

The methods have also been adapted for use with children with disabilities living in Cambodia. Funded by the United Nations International Children's Emer-gency Fund (UNICEF) and facilitated by the Nossal Institute for Global Health, research was conducted with 63 children living both with their families in urban and rural locations as well as in out of home care, in this case, institutions. Feed-back provided to the authors from the lead researcher found that the tools were adaptable and useful in gathering the data from children with disabilities. Quali-tative and quantitative data from children with disabilities have been interpreted thematically along with corresponding policy recommendations that have been directly communicated by UNICEF and research partner organisations to the Cambodian government. In addition, the method was recently drawn upon for an entirely different research focus, a multi-country evaluation of child sponsorship within international development. Various methods were used to evaluate this programme, and this method and tools were used when engaging with children in Ethiopia, Georgia, Senegal, Peru, and Sri Lanka, though findings from this study have not yet been released.

As the *Guide* is freely accessible on the website, it is unknown where else and in what form the method has been drawn upon. However, the knowledge that is gleaned from what we know of this rapid uptake of research methods is significant. The fact that there is now self-reported evidence about the situation and preferences of children with disabilities in not just Vanuatu and PNG, but in Ethiopia and Cambodia in very different contexts is a substantial addition to knowledge about children with disabilities' lives. As Craig et al. (2000) and Ife (2013) propose, this strategy appears to validate the use of new technologies, such as film, electronic publications, and the internet, to intentionally build alliances for change and share information and strategies across a global audience.

Scaling change through policy

The strategy to influence policy through policy briefs, reports, and various engagement activities with government personnel is, at this point, the least embedded of change strategies. During the project life cycle, government personnel in both countries engaged with the project, including attending training in inclusive research/consultation methods. The disability desk officer for the government of Vanuatu became an advocate of the research approach and, while in New York for the United Nations Conference of State Parties in 2015, met with the ambassador of Vanuatu (to USA) to advocate for the rights of children with disabilities in Vanuatu. Both DPOs continue to utilise project resources to advocate to government. For example, since the findings have been released, DPA has made key policy recommendations to the national government that it is hoped will progress the child participants' priorities. This is a work in progress that will be interesting to observe over time.

One priority identified by children was communication support, particularly access to sign language communication. DPA has reported that DFAT has since funded a further consultancy to co-investigate with DPA how sign language can be further supported in Vanuatu. DPA are now implementing recommendations to further facilitate sign language development in Vanuatu amongst the deaf population. DPA have also reported that they incorporated the research human rights findings and policy recommendations into their first Alternative Report to the CRPD. A draft of this report has been sent to Geneva in May 2018. It is hoped that these findings will form part of the CRPD committee's recommendations to the government of Vanuatu.

Conclusion

Claiming changes as a result of the research must be done with caution. Change is difficult to measure and even more challenging to attribute. Social change relies on a range of mediums over time by which to affect change, and changes are likely to be incremental (Campbell et al. 2012). Thinking strategically about how changes can be brought about is the responsibility of researchers and project developers if we are to achieve sustainability of change beyond the life span of a project or intervention. This requires us to think beyond specific programs and the immediate worlds of our participants and to support change to happen across various layers of society, targeting both local and global levels in order to achieve lasting or sustainable change (Ife 2013). However, fundamental to the change brought about in this project was the connection to and collaboration with local people and organisations, as well as with global actors. Craig et al. (2000: 331) identify the building of 'alliances for change' as a core activity of social change, but these alliances must commence at the level of the local in order to maintain relevance to local situations and cultures.

References

Campbell, C., Mayo, M. and Taylor, M. (2012) ' "Dissemination as intervention": building local HIV competence through the report back of research findings to a South Africal rural community', *Antipode*, 44: 702–24.

Clarke, M., Feeny, S. and McDonald, L. (2014) 'Vulnerability to what? Multidimensional poverty in Melanesia', in S. Feeny (ed) *Household Vulnerability and Resilience to Economic Shocks: Findings from Melanesia*, Farnham: Ashgate.

Craig, G., Mayo, M. and Taylor, M. (2000) 'Globalization from below: implications for the community', *Community Development Journal*, 35: 323–35.

Department of Community Development (2005) *Papua New Guinea National Policy on Disability*, Port Moresby: Department of Community Development.

Grieshaber, S. (2010) 'Equity and research design', in G. Mac Naughton, S. Rolfe and I. Siraj-Blatchford (eds) *Doing Early Childhood Research: International Perspectives on Theory and Practice*, 2nd edn, Sydney: Allen and Unwin.

Guijt, I. (2008) *Assessing and Learning for Social Change: A Discussion Paper*, Brighton: Institute of Development Studies. Online. Available at www.ids.ac.uk/files/dmfile/ASClowresfinalversion.pdf (accessed 1 November 2019).

Harcourt, D. and Sargeant, J. (2009) 'Major themes and considerations', in *Involving Children and Young People in Research: Compendium of Papers and Reflections from a Think Tank*, Canberra: Australian Research Alliance for Children and Youth and Sydney: New South Wales Commission for Children and Young People. Online. Available at www.aracy.org.au/publications-resources/command/download_file/id/108/filename/Involving_children_and_young_people_in_research.pdf (accessed 1 November 2019).

Hart, J. (2008) 'Children's participation and international development: attending to the political', *The International Journal of Children's Rights*, 16: 407–18.

Ife, J. (2010) *Human Rights from Below: Achieving Rights Through Community Development*, Port Melbourne: Cambridge University Press.

Ife, J. (2013) *Community Development in an Uncertain World*, Port Melbourne: Cambridge University Press.

Jenkin, E., Wilson, E., Campain, R. and Clarke, M. (2018) 'Beyond childhood, disability and postcolonial theory: young children with disability in developing countries can tell their own story', in M. Twomey and C. Carroll, C. (eds) *Seen and Heard: Exploring Participation, Engagement, and Voice of Children with Disabilities*, London: Peter Lang Publishers.

Jenkin, E., Wilson, E., Clarke, M., Campain, R. and Murfitt, K. (2016) 'Spreading the word: using accessible film to share research findings and knowledge', *Knowledge Management for Development Journal*, 12(1): 69–84. Online. Available at www.km4djour nal.org/index.php/km4dj/article/view/306/386 (accessed 1 November 2019).

Jenkin, E., Wilson, E., Clarke, M., Murfitt, K. and Campain, R. (2017) 'Children with disability: human rights case study', in S. Kenny, B. McGrath and R. Phillips (eds) *The Routledge Handbook of Community Development*, New York: Routledge.

Jenkin, E., Wilson, E., Murfitt, K., Clarke, M., Campain, R. and Stockman, L. (2015) *Inclusive Practice for Research with Children with Disability: A Guide*, Melbourne: Deakin University. Online: Available at www.voicesofchildrenwithdisability.com/wp-content/uploads/2015/03/DEA-Inclusive-Practice-Research_ACCESSIBLE.pdf (accessed 1 November 2019).

Johnson, V. (2017) 'Moving beyond voice in children and young people's participation', *Action Research*, 15: 104–24.

Kraftl, P. (2013) 'Beyond "voice", beyond "agency", beyond "politics"? Hybrid childhoods and some critical reflections on children's emotional geographies', *Emotion, Space and Society*, 9: 13–23.

Kuper, H., Banks, M., Velthuizen, F. and Duffy, G. (2017) *Guidelines for Consulting with Children and Young People with Disabilities*, Plan International. Online. Available at file:///C:/Users/bethc/Downloads/guidelines_for_consulting_with_children_and_young_people_with_disabilities_0.pdf (accessed 1 November 2019).

Liebel, M. (2012) 'Framing the issue: rethinking children's rights', in M. Liebel (ed) *Children's Rights from Below*, Basingstoke: Palgrave Macmillan.

Liebel, M. and Invernizzi, A. (2016) 'Introduction', in A. Invernizzi, M. Liebel, B. Milne and R. Budde (eds) *Children Out of Place' and Human Rights*, Cham: Springer International Publishing.

Lundy, L. (2007) ' "Voice" is not enough: conceptualising Article 12 of the United Nations convention on the rights of the child', *British Educational Research Journal*, 33: 927–42.

McCallum, R. and Martin, H. (2013) 'Comment: the CRPD and children with disabilities', *Australian International Law Journal*, 20: 17.

Muirhead, D., Willetts, J., Crawford, J., Hutchison, J. and Smales, P. (2017) *From Evidence to Impact: Development Contribution of Australian Aid Funded Research. A Study Based on Research Undertaken Through the Australian Development Research Awards Scheme 2007–2016*, Research for Development Impact Network. Online. Available at https://acfid.asn.au/sites/site.acfid/files/resource_document/From%20Evidence%20to%20Impact%20Full%20Report.pdf (accessed 1 November 2019).

Office of the United Nations High Commissioner for Human Rights (OHCHR) Regional Office for the Pacific (2012) *Human Rights in the Pacific: Country Outlines 2012*, Suva: Office of the High Commissioner for Human Rights Regional Office for the Pacific. Online. Available at https://pacific.ohchr.org/docs/HR_Pacific_v7_July_25.pdf (accessed 1 November 2019).

Pearce, E. (2015) *I see That It Is Possible: Building Capacity for Disability Inclusion in Gender-Based Violence (GBV) Programming in Humanitarian Settings*, New York: Women's Refugee Commission. Online. Available at file:///C:/Users/bethc/Downloads/Disability-Inclusion-in-GBV-English.pdf (accessed 1 November 2019).

Robinson, G., Baker, S. and Goulding, M. (2013) *Factors Which Facilitate and Limit Inclusion of Children with Disability in Kindergarten in Vanuatu: Sample Study, Shefa Province*, Save the Children Australia. Online. Available at https://mjcs.gov.vu/images/research_database/Disability_Sample_Study_Vanuatu_2013_FINAL.pdf (accessed 1 November 2019).

Tuck, E. and Yang, K.W. (2014) 'R-words: refusing research', in D. Paris and M.T. Winn (eds) *Humanizing Research: Decolonizing Qualitative Inquiry with Youth and Communities*, Thousand Oaks, CA: Sage.

United Nations (1989) 'Convention on the rights of the child'. Online. Available at www. ohchr.org/EN/ProfessionalInterest/Pages/CRC.aspx (accessed 1 November 2019).

United Nations (2003) 'UN committee on the rights of the child: state party report: Papua New Guinea'. Online. Available at www.refworld.org/docid/3f8d18e74.html (accessed 1 November 2019).

United Nations (2006) 'Convention on the rights of persons with disabilities'. Online. Available at www.un.org/development/desa/disabilities/convention-on-the-rights-of-persons-with-disabilities.html (accessed 16 October 2018).

Walji, F. and Palmer, M. (2012) *Improving Access to and Provision of Disability Services and Facilities for People with Disabilities in the Pacific: Disability Service and Human Resource Mapping*, Melbourne: CBM Australia—Nossal Institute Partnership for Disability Inclusive Development.

Walsh, M. (2015) 'Local issues a focus of 6th Papua New Guinea Human Rights Film Festival'. Online. Available at www.abc.net.au/radio-australia/programs/pacificbeat/localissues-a-focus-of-6th-papua-new-guinea-human/6664128 (accessed 1 November 2019).

14 Philosophy and ethics

Sustaining social inclusion in the disability sector

Emma Rush, Monica Short, Giselle Burningham and Joan Cartledge

Introduction

The concept of personhood is the central philosophical underpinning for social inclusion policies and practice, which strive to enable all individuals and communities to fully participate across all areas of life. Our purpose in this paper is to strengthen the practice of professionals working to sustain social inclusion, through empowering them to better respond to the challenges faced in this field. We pursue two interrelated questions:

- How are the three major Western ethical frameworks that operate throughout the field of social inclusion policy, professional ethics, and practice related to the concept of personhood?
- How can a sharper awareness of these ethical frameworks help to inform and sustain responses to the challenges faced by socially inclusive policies in the disability sector?

Our approach is theoretical, supported by relevant literature review and illustrated through two auto-ethnographic case studies in the disability sector.

We begin by defining social inclusion and then demonstrate the practical importance of three major Western ethical frameworks—utilitarianism, deontology, and virtue ethics—through a brief analysis of international codes of ethics relevant to professionals working in social inclusion. Our analysis suggests that deontology and virtue ethics are primary for professionals in their interactions with individuals, whereas later in the chapter we demonstrate that utilitarianism is more prominent at a policy level. We then discuss key strengths and weaknesses of each framework and conclude this part of the chapter with an answer to our first research question: an explanation of how these three major Western ethical frameworks are related to the concept of personhood.

We then turn to our case studies' area, the disability sector, and introduce the marketisation of care as a form of social inclusion implemented by governments around the world over the last two decades. The challenges faced by these socially inclusive policies can be clearly seen in the impact on participants of specific systems' implementation of marketisation of care, illustrated through the lived experiences of two authors, Giselle and Joan. Finally we conclude with an answer to our second research question: showing how a sharper awareness of the ethical frameworks underlying these systems can help inform successful and sustainable policy and practice responses to such challenges.

Social inclusion

The United Nations' 2030 Agenda advocates for social inclusion 'as the process of improving the terms of participation in society for people who are disadvantaged on the basis of age, sex, disability, race, ethnicity, and economic and migration status' (United Nations 2016: 1). Taket et al. (2014: 3) refine this further by stating that social inclusion 'occurs when the participation or involvement achieved in any particular case can be demonstrated to be real rather than tokenistic or manipulative', specifying that such real participation involves 'citizen control, delegated power and partnership'.

Hargreaves argues that an inclusive society is characterised by 'a striving for reduced inequality, a balance between an individual's rights and duties and increased social cohesion' (Centre for Economic and Social Inclusion 2002 in Hargreaves 2005: 6). A socially inclusive society is made up of communities that are attractive and attentive and understand what it means to remember all people (Short 2018). Their atmosphere, actions, and language encompass everyone where all are nurtured and can participate (Short 2015, 2018). Each member of the community's personhood is respected.

Ethical frameworks, personhood, and social inclusion

Professional codes of ethics

Each profession working in the area of social inclusion is committed to its own code of ethics, but all of these *specific* contemporary codes are based on insights from more *general* ethical frameworks: utilitarianism, deontology and virtue ethics (see Table 14.1). As discussed in the following sections, utilitarianism focuses on acting to create the best consequences (often expressed in terms of the 'most happiness') overall; deontology focuses on people's rights and the ethical rules and obligations that seek to protect those rights; virtue ethics focuses on personal character traits and their contribution to a good life for the community and the individual.

The codes in Table 14.1 cover many professionals working within the area of social inclusion. Our review of these codes revealed that they focus on practitioner/client interaction and are primarily based on deontology and virtue ethics. Deontology and virtue ethics result in similar practical prescriptions within codes of ethics because many ethical rules can be reframed as character traits; for example, in Table 14.1, the rule 'Respect all people' (Social Work, example of deontology) can be reframed as the good character trait of 'respectfulness' (Nursing, example of virtue ethics). Utilitarianism is difficult to find in these codes,

Table 14.1 Examples of ethical frameworks from Codes of Ethics for professionals who work in social inclusion contexts

Professional code	Example of Utilitarianism	Example of Deontology	Example of Virtue Ethics
International Association of Schools of Social Work (2018)	[E]ncourage social workers across the world to reflect on the challenges and dilemmas that face them [including]: • The conflicts between the duty of social workers to protect the interests of the people with whom they work and societal demands for efficiency and utility. • The fact that resources in society are limited. (1)	Social work is based on respect for the inherent worth and dignity of all people, and the rights that follow from this. Social workers should uphold and defend each person's physical, psychological, emotional and spiritual integrity and well-being. (4.1)	Social workers should act with integrity. (5.3)
World Medical Association (2018)	A physician shall strive to use health care resources in the best way to benefit patients and their community. (Duties of physicians in general–Number 10)	A physician shall give emergency care as a humanitarian duty unless he/she is assured that others are willing and able to give such care. (Duties of physicians to patients–Number 5)	A physician shall deal honestly with patients and colleagues. (Duties of physicians in general–Number 4)
World Confederation for Physical Therapy (2017)	*Utilitarianism not clearly evident anywhere in code.*	Respect the rights and dignity of all individuals (Point 2)	Provide honest, competent and accountable professional services (Point 4)
International Council of Nurses (2012)	*Utilitarianism not clearly evident anywhere in code.*	The nurse ensures that the individual receives accurate, sufficient and timely information in a culturally appropriate manner on which to base consent for care and related treatment. (p. 2)	The nurse demonstrates professional values such as respectfulness, responsiveness, compassion, trustworthiness and integrity. (p. 2)

(Continued)

Table 14.1 (Continued)

Professional code	Example of Utilitarianism	Example of Deontology	Example of Virtue Ethics
International Union of Psychological Science and International Association of Applied Psychology (2008)	Competent caring for the well-being of persons and peoples involves working for their benefit and, above all, doing no harm. It includes maximizing benefits, minimizing potential harm, and offsetting or correcting harm. (Principle II)	[P]sychologists accept as fundamental the Principle of Competent Caring for the Well-Being of Persons and Peoples. (Principle II)	Integrity is vital to the advancement of scientific knowledge and to the maintenance of public confidence in the discipline of psychology. (Principle III)

and in some codes, it is not clearly present at all, as indicated in Table 14.1. We suggest an interpretation of this based upon our own experience of working in social inclusion. First, in practitioner/client relationships, utilitarianism is most likely to be used as a secondary guide to action when circumstances are such that the standard course of action suggested by ethical rules or character traits is not applicable. Secondly, utilitarianism is more commonly present at a policy level than at a practitioner/client level, and as such, it can lead to 'challenges and dilemmas' for professionals who are primarily committed to clients, as indicated in Table 14.1 (Social Work, example of utilitarianism). Nonetheless, we see these three frameworks as complementary approaches to ethics: each has a characteristic range of strengths and weaknesses. Later, we focus on how relevant strengths and weaknesses are mobilised in inter-professional discourse; awareness of this is powerful for sustaining social inclusion, as will be illustrated in the case studies in the following sections.

Utilitarianism

Utilitarianism extends our own intuitive individual search for happiness to a rational search for the greatest overall collective happiness (Weston 2011). Theoretically, the utilitarian method of 'rational calculus' identifies all costs and benefits for everyone affected by two (or more) different courses of action and then aggregates and compares these costs and benefits in order to choose what utilitarianism sees as the best ethical action: that which results in the greatest net benefit (Shafer-Landau 2012). First clearly articulated in England during the nineteenth century by Jeremy Bentham and further refined by John Stuart Mill, modern variants of utilitarianism remain a powerful force in contemporary ethics (Preston 2014).

Utilitarianism provides a modern, quasi-scientific perspective from which to reevaluate conventional ethics and thus has a history of supporting progressive social movements, for example, women's rights (Mill 1869) and animal welfare (Singer 1975). It also offers a neat theoretical solution for the comparison of policy options affecting large numbers of people in a range of ways, promising to translate such complexity into a single metric enabling simple comparison of the overall net benefit of different scenarios (Preston 2014).

Useful as a utilitarian approach can be, its method of 'rational calculus' has serious limitations, in particular, negative consequences for social inclusion. In reality, it often proves impossible to agree on how to measure different kinds of benefit and cost for different people and then combine them into an overall measure for comparison purposes (Shafer-Landau 2012). Since utilitarianism lacks a principle of justice, creating the greatest net benefit suffices to justify the sacrifice of the interests (perhaps even the lives) of some or even many people (Shafer-Landau 2012). Moreover, it is always the same groups of people who are excluded: those whose happiness is 'costly' to achieve. For example, Preston (2014) notes that decisions to exclude children with disabilities from mainstream education are usually defended on utilitarian grounds.

Deontology

Ethical rules and obligations, which are the focus of deontology, are present in all human cultures (Rachels and Rachels 2010). Many of these rules and obligations uphold principles of social inclusion. A deontological approach remains central to contemporary theoretical ethics (Preston 2014), and the most philosophically influential form of deontology, developed by seminal thinker Immanuel Kant in the eighteenth century, is still prominent (Preston 2014).

Strengths of Kantian deontology include its focus on the importance of universal rules and its insistence on respect for persons (Dell'Olio and Simon 2010). Both of these Kantian characteristics can be seen in the *Universal Declaration of Human Rights* (United Nations 1948) and the legally binding instrument created to reaffirm it, the *Convention on the Rights of Persons with Disabilities* [CRPD] (United Nations 2006). This Convention currently has 160 signatories and 175 parties, including Australia, Canada, United Kingdom of Great Britain and Northern Ireland, and the United States of America (United Nations 2017a). One of the Convention principles is 'respect for inherent dignity, individual autonomy including the freedom to make one's own choices, and independence of persons' (United Nations 2006: Article 3.1).

Rights are a modern counterpart to ancient ethical rules and obligations: a rule or obligation for one person frequently protects another person's right to something. For example, many professions have an *obligation* to promote the autonomy of a person with a disability and to protect that person's *right* to self-determination. Nations have obligations to people living with disabilities through insurance and similar schemes, such as the National Disability Insurance Scheme [NDIS] in Australia (Australian Department of Human Services 2017: Section 4.4.1 para 2).

Whilst in America, under the *Affordable Care Act*, the federal government, state governments, insurers, employers, and individuals are given shared responsibility to reform and improve the availability, quality, and affordability of Health Insurance Coverage in the United States for employees (ObamaCare Facts 2017). Insurance companies are obliged to ensure that people with prior health conditions, such as experienced by people living with disabilities, cannot be denied a health policy or be offered a higher costing policy with the prior condition not recognised (National Council of Independent Living 2017).

One major weakness of Kantian deontology was its focus on rationality, which unfortunately facilitated later philosophers (including those from other theoretical traditions such as utilitarianism) downgrading or dismissing respect for persons who are less than fully rational (see for example, Singer 2011), with profoundly negative consequences for social inclusion.

Virtue ethics

While the promotion of good character traits can be found across cultures and religions, the most philosophically influential proponent of virtue ethics was Aristotle (379 BC/ 1976), who wrote at length about the relationship between the virtues and human flourishing. For Aristotle (379 BC/ 1976), good character traits (for example, courage and generosity) could be valued both extrinsically because they were important for achieving social cohesion and intrinsically because they represented individual fulfilment of human moral potential.

Although good character traits can typically be redescribed as ethical rules (for example, generosity can be described as behaviour following the rule 'be generous'), virtue ethics goes substantially further than deontology in that it 'builds in' motivation for ethical behaviour—the truly virtuous person *wants* to be generous (Shafer-Landau 2012). Hence, the social cultivation of the right disposition, including emotional responses, through training, habit, and reference to moral exemplars, is a fundamental part of virtue ethics (Preston 2014): rationality remains crucially important to virtue ethics (Dell'Olio and Simon 2010), but an ethical approach is grounded in the whole person, not just the rational mind. This social cultivation process has clear echoes in the more specific process of professional formation both before and after graduation (Moorhead et al. 2016).

Virtue ethics in its original Aristotelian form, however, did not recognise universal personhood (Stevenson 2013). Its focus on the full development of human intellectual and moral potential as part of the good life is an essential foundation for social inclusion, but this must also be handled with care: the potential of individual persons is highly variable, and any 'metric' for interpersonal comparison of potential may undermine universal personhood (Short et al. 2018).

As demonstrated earlier, indicated in Table 14.1 and in the discussion of case studies, all three ethical frameworks—utilitarianism, deontology, and virtue ethics—have a role to play in promoting social inclusion, so it will be useful for professionals practising in social inclusion contexts to recognise the operation of all three in professional and political discourses. But, as we discuss later, not all three ethical frameworks are equally compatible with the recognition of universal personhood, which is the crucial philosophical underpinning for social inclusion.

Personhood and social inclusion

As the legal framework surrounding social inclusion indicates, the importance of social inclusion is justified on the basis of universal human rights (for example, United Nations 2017a). But universal human rights are themselves based on a prior recognition of the fundamental importance of the human person. As one member of the drafting sub-Committee for the *Universal Declaration of Human Rights*, Hernán Santa Cruz of Chile, wrote about the adoption of the *Declaration*,

> a consensus had been reached as to the supreme value of the human person, a value that did not originate in the decision of a worldly power, but rather in the fact of existing—which gave rise to the inalienable right to live free from want and oppression and to fully develop one's personality.
>
> (United Nations 2017b)

Later, we discuss the relationship between recognition of the fundamental importance of personhood (and consequent promotion of social inclusion) and the three ethical frameworks.

As discussed earlier, utilitarianism, while useful for assessing collective cost-benefit scenarios, lacks the principle of justice which is essential for ensuring that rights are not overridden. Moreover, the very calculation procedures of utilitarianism—isolate, aggregate, and maximise—mean that both individual persons and their existence in relation to other persons tend to disappear from view. These weaknesses with respect to recognition of the fundamental importance of the person mean that while utilitarian frameworks remain useful, they should be handled with care in social inclusion contexts.

Kantian deontology addresses the lack of a principle of justice in utilitarianism by protecting rights—as discussed earlier, recognition of personhood is central to Kantian deontology, and deontological frameworks (rules, obligations, and rights) are therefore very important to social inclusion contexts. But deontology is similar to utilitarianism in its lack of attention to the social formation of persons, and neither considers the importance of virtuous activity in a good life. Recognition of the social formation of persons—which is so fundamental for professionals promoting social inclusion—is central to virtue ethics. Moreover, virtue ethics' understanding of the importance of virtuous activity to a good *individual* life fosters personal resilience for professionals, and understanding the importance of virtuous activity for a good *collective* life underlines a broader dimension to the importance of social inclusion: it is best for everyone.

As noted earlier, classical Aristotelian virtue ethics itself lacked insight about universal personhood; however, so such insight must be explicitly included in what we call a personhood-informed virtue ethics approach. Insight about universal personhood is available from a secular (human rights) perspective, as illustrated by the quotation from Cruz, or from some traditional religious perspectives, such as illustrated by the idea of everyone made in the image of God (Genesis 1:26–27): either provides the basis for professionals to better sustain social inclusion. We have argued that although all three ethical frameworks have a role to play in promoting social inclusion, a personhood-informed virtue ethics approach will best promote positive sustainable social inclusion. With this in mind, we now turn to our second, related, research question: How can a sharper awareness of these ethical frameworks help to inform and sustain responses to the challenges faced by socially inclusive policies in the disability sector?

Marketisation and personhood

Marketisation of care as a form of social inclusion

The marketisation of care for people living with disabilities through cash-for-care schemes such as insurances and plans and their association with social inclusion is a worldwide trend. Australia implemented the NDIS in 2013 (NDIS 2017). If it is determined that someone living with disabilities requires 'reasonable and necessary supports' then through a market-based system with a lifetime approach, participants are involved in the decision-making about their funds and how they are spent (NDIS 2017: 12). Social inclusion is one of the indicators of success of the Scheme (NDIS 2017).

The Australian NDIS was partly inspired by the Canadian Registered Disability Savings Plan (RDSP), which was established in 2008 and is a ten-year long-term savings plan to help Canadians with disabilities and their families save for the future (Etmanski 2018; Government of Canada 2016; RDSP 2018). This Plan is a partnership between the Canadian government through bonds and grants and individuals through personal contributions (Government of Canada 2016). Canada recognises that social inclusion is affected by income amongst other determinants (Senate Canada 2013) and that the RDSP provides long-term financial security for people and children living with disabilities (Government of Canada 2016).

Since 1997, people living with disabilities in the UK have been able to opt for direct payments, that is, cash in lieu of directly provided services (Dickinson and Glasby 2010). Currently in the UK, people living with disabilities develop a care plan, often with a social worker or care manager, which determines the value of their personalised (individualised) budget (NHS 2018). Each individual can be in charge of their budget and informed how the money is allocated, where it is directed, and how it is spent (NHS 2018). If included in the process, the social workers and others as part of their role promote social inclusion for each person (SCIE 2010).

Next we analyse cash-for-care schemes through the lived experience in Australia, the UK, and Canada. As the case studies show, specific features of the implementation of these schemes pose challenges for social inclusion. Discussion during and after the case studies reveals the operation of the different ethical frameworks—utilitarianism, deontology, and virtue ethics—within scheme implementation.

Giselle's story (Australia): the lived experience

I have a condition called 'neurological non-specific', which results in chronic pain and tetraplegia, which has stabilised. The ability to walk to the park and breathe in the smells of fresh eucalyptus leaves is such a simple act that I never truly appreciated it. Mobility provides stimulation of the senses; it provides access to community and freedom! A wheelchair is my mobility, but after 20 years my secondhand electric wheelchair would suddenly slow to a crawl. This happened a few times whilst crossing the road, and understandably I no longer felt safe. Without mobility, during the day, my only human interaction was the cleaner; once a fortnight, occasionally friends popped round at the weekend. My partner came home each night, and I would listen eagerly to the mundane gossip of office life, but in reality, I was alone. I was 54, too young for day groups, but not disabled enough to join disability groups. With limited mobility, my world became smaller and smaller.

Thankfully, National Disability Insurance Scheme (NDIS) arrived, and I was finally able to get my chair serviced. The results came back: sad to say my 20-year-old electric wheelchair's 'brain' was dying, and I needed a new chair urgently. The National Disability Insurance Agency (NDIA) was new, and this was my first experience of asking for help. I am a social worker and had worked in government for years, so I thought I had realistic expectations of a bureaucratic system. Sadly I found a massive disconnect between the NDIS governance statement on the individual and the NDIA's focus on a utilitarian model based on 'insurance principles'. Somehow in this gap, the intent of the NDIS has been lost. I am a self-funded participant, and I am grateful that at least I have some control. Horror stories abound with others being lost in the system.

Initially I was part of the roll-out under the Australian Capital Territory (State) control of the NDIA, which allowed me a case manager via the Multiple Sclerosis (MS) Society. We worked out my plan and submitted it. Despite being prompted to ask for more assistance, my sole focus was a new chair so I could maintain my independence. I met my NDIA state plan coordinator, and she was wonderful. She realised that I was isolated and insisted that I expand my world by supporting my endeavours with my art work and church through paid support workers. Moreover, she understood and supported my request for a new chair. Plans under this system were flexible to the needs of the participant and could be changed as many times as needed throughout the year. But to me the most important part of my plan was approval to sort out a replacement chair. I thought that I could just pop out to the shops. Unfortunately, that is not how the system works.

In the midst of this process, the NDIA system changed over to federal control, and so did the philosophical position. The Australian Capital Territory model was person-focused (virtue ethics and deontological-based); the federal system was utilitarian. Suddenly I was a number and not a person. Everything became focused on clinical reports and not my direct experience or needs. Moreover, my personal plan now could only be changed once a year! I had to accept the plan I was given (not necessarily agreed to by all parties). You can only ask for a change to the plan through the review process, but this takes a minimum of three months and is not flexible to any changing needs that often occur for clients. By now my wheelchair had died, and I was trapped at home. Under the new system, I no longer had a caseworker—I faced navigating this new system all through a call centre. Typically I felt that NDIA staff did not understand my needs: I felt they saw all disabled people as the same. The most insulting process I had to endure was phone calls checking my need for a wheelchair(!) despite NDIA having full medical records and occupational therapist (OT) reports.

I notified NDIA that my current wheelchair had died, and they logged the urgency for a replacement wheelchair on my record. I was told I could use any OT I wanted, but this proved to be very difficult because the system was not set up. I finally found a specialist OT, and after my initial assessment, she agreed I needed a wheelchair. But she only offered me a choice of two chairs from one Canadian company, and I felt neither chair was suitable for me to use on uneven ground. At this point, I took control! I am lucky that I am able to. I went online and found an Australian wheelchair company that met ALL my needs at nearly half the cost. However I needed another OT report to approve it.

Unfortunately, the saga did not stop there. Despite being logged as a critical need and having an OT report for the wheelchair, the bureaucracy would not approve the purchase of the wheelchair as it was four months before the end of my NDIA-approved plan. NDIA stated that I needed to wait until my next plan to ask for the money for the wheelchair! This process took 18 months in total from the first request!

During this process, nowhere was my voice heard. My disability needs were questioned, and my choices were ignored. The system made me feel disempowered. The NDIS core values focus on the individual; however, the managing body, NDIA, has focused on the financial cost over the individual by following a utilitarian model. The focus on a utilitarian model and following associated 'insurance principles' took away my voice, and I felt I had no rights. I felt so passionately about my loss of rights that I told my story at the NDIS Senate hearings in Canberra. Sadly, my story was not unique. The NDIA's response to the Senate hearing was a two-page letter of incomprehensible government jargon that even I (with years of government training) could not understand! It was clear they did not understand the participants' issues.

In reflecting upon Giselle's story, although the NDIS offered an outcome that promised ongoing social inclusion—for Giselle, achieved through a new wheelchair—creating sustainable social inclusion requires the philosophy of the service to determine the operational mode. Giselle's experience and the experience of many other people with disability has been that the socially inclusive philosophy of the NDIS was undermined by an operational mode incompatible with the stated philosophy (Parliament of Australia 2017).

Joan's story (UK and USA): the lived experience

Twenty-five years ago, I was working as a community development worker in the UK when I was diagnosed with MS. As a professional, I had worked supporting people who lived with disabilities in communities known for experiencing disadvantage. But I had no personal understanding of how it felt to be 'characterised' as disabled or socially excluded. I was a new mum when I was first diagnosed, when it became clear that I could not sustain a job as well as looking after a young child. I was required to 'prove' to the Benefits Agency that I was unable to contribute to the working community due to my incapacity. I received financial support, but little emotional or professional support was offered to me that would help me adapt to living with disability and make adjustments in order to continue my career. My experience is not uncommon because a person who is diagnosed with a condition such as MS is often viewed as a recipient of social care rather than someone who has a contribution to make. I was provided with information about support groups, but when I attended one, I found the emphasis was on accepting my incapacity. At that time, I was not ready to give up the possibility of having a career.

For me, one of the most difficult things about receiving disability support was the reassessment of my condition every three years, requiring me to explain each time the details of my inability to perform basic daily tasks. Whilst I recognise that assessment is necessary, the process was emotionally damaging in terms of my sense of well-being. I believe in the philosophy of universal healthcare provided by the National Health Service (NHS) and the provision of support for those living with disability. I do, however, believe that the implementation of this support sees recipients as noncontributing members of society and is focused more on economics (utilitarianism) than on social inclusion (deontology or virtue ethics).

Four years ago, I moved to the United States of America with my husband. I am fortunate to have excellent health insurance through my husband's work, for which we pay an insurance premium, and we also pay a fee for each treatment I receive. In contrast to my own experience, I volunteer in a community, where many have no insurance and so receive only emergency care. Social exclusion for those who live with disability in the USA can be a consequence of poverty. The implementation of the *Patient Protection and Affordable Care Act* has enabled many who live with disability to have fairer access to treatment, but the process of accessing disability benefits is complex and difficult to navigate, and it can take years to make a successful application. *The Patient Protection and Affordable Care Act* is also administered by states, with states able to opt out of implementation of the programme.

My experience of living with disability in the UK and the USA has enabled me to appreciate the strengths and weaknesses of cash-for-care provision in each country. The welfare system in the USA requires recipients to be active in seeking services and necessitates both medical and legal support to succeed in being awarded disability payments. My observation is that the system generally disadvantages those who do not have capacity or resources. In the UK, services and financial support for people with disabilities is more easily accessible, although I acknowledge that I have seen the system abused by people who have manipulated the rules for financial gain. My personal preference is for a system that provides universal health care as it protects those who have limited capacity, whether it is physical, mental, or educational.

In reviewing Joan's story, as her experience with universal health care in the UK in the 1990s showed, universal provision of care should also actively promote social inclusion—otherwise disability support will continue to be suboptimal.

Conclusion

The utilitarian model appeals through its promise of optimal overall outcomes: in principle, resources are efficiently allocated where they can achieve most happiness. However, in practice, as illustrated by Giselle and Joan's stories, if the fundamental importance of the person is not kept at the centre of social inclusion policies and processes, then the experience for participants is frequently one of having to 'fight' the system. Although marketisation of care aims to promote personal agency, attention to the lived experience suggests that particular systems may either promote or undermine this aim.

Sustainable social inclusion would be best promoted through a whole-of-government policy approach that recognised the theoretical limitations of utilitarianism. Genuine recognition of universal personhood requires that the deontological and virtue ethical requirement of social justice be met *before* utilitarian attempts to maximise overall social benefits are applied—and this philosophical priority must also be reflected in the operational modes used to deliver services. Under such an integrated policy and practice approach, service recipients would experience true social inclusion—and social inclusion professionals would be well supported by systems that facilitate the provision of services.

In the meantime, it is essential that professionals working within social inclusion contexts continue to recognise, speak out against, and resist depersonalising actions that frequently occur in the name of efficiency—for example, call centres, unnecessary assessments, and unduly protracted application processes—in favour of actions that support the person, such as a dedicated case manager who promotes personal agency and social inclusion. The 'economic' arguments that drive depersonalising actions have a utilitarian underpinning: the assumption is that 'it's worth saving money here so that it can be better spent elsewhere'. We argue for an authentic commitment to social inclusion, one that sets a limit to what kinds of savings can be acceptable—it is nonsensical to undermine social inclusion while supposedly promoting it. Professionals can articulate this contradiction and suggest the need for a systemic solution to it by calling attention to the fundamental importance of the person and using concepts of rights (deontological) and virtues to differentiate the kinds of savings that are acceptable from the kinds of savings that are not.

As demonstrated earlier, all three major Western ethical frameworks are operative in social inclusion policy, professional ethics, and practice. We have argued that sustainable social inclusion will be best promoted through giving priority to deontological and virtue ethics, thus ensuring social justice before applying utilitarian frameworks. In particular, in both policy and practice, a personhood-informed virtue ethics not only promotes attention to the particularity of each person in their circumstances but also recognises that genuine social inclusion leads to a better life for everyone, giving everyone in society more diverse opportunities to develop and flourish.

References

Aristotle (379 BC/1976) *Ethics*, London: Penguin Books.

Australian Department of Human Services (2017) 'Overview of the NDIS'. Online. Available at www.ndis.gov.au/operational-guideline/overview (accessed 16 October 2018).

Dell'Olio, A.J. and Simon, C.J. (2010) *Introduction to Ethics: A Reader*, Lanham, MD: Rowman and Littlefield.

Dickinson, H. and Glasby, J. (2010) *The Personalisation Agenda: Implications for the Third Sector*, Third Sector Research Centre, Working Paper 30. Online. Available at www.birmingham.ac.uk/generic/tsrc/documents/tsrc/working-papers/working-paper-30.pdf (accessed 16 October 2018).

Etmanski, A. (2018) 'Thanks to Jim Flaherty, disabled Canadians can fulfill their dreams'. Online. Available at www.theglobeandmail.com/opinion/thanks-to-jim-flaherty-disabled-canadians-can-fulfill-their-dreams/article18037166/ (accessed 16 October 2018).

Government of Canada (2016) 'Registered disability savings plan (RDSP)'. Online. Available at www.canada.ca/en/revenue-agency/services/tax/individuals/topics/registered-disability-savings-plan-rdsp.html (accessed 16 October 2018).

Hargreaves, D. (2005) 'Social inclusion and participation: what does this mean for the social work service?' in M. Pawar (ed) *Capacity Building for Participation: Social Workers' Thoughts and Reflections*, Wagga Wagga, NSW: Centre for Rural Social Research, Charles Sturt University.

International Association of Schools of Social Work (IASSW) (2018) 'Global social work statement on ethical principles'. Online. Available at www.ifsw.org/wp-content/uploads/2018/07/Global-Social-Work-Statement-of-Ethical-Principles-IASSW-27-April-2018-1.pdf (accessed 11 January 2019).

International Council of Nurses (2012) 'The ICN code of ethics for nurses'. Online. Available at www.icn.ch/sites/default/files/inline-files/2012_ICN_Codeofethicsfornurses_%20eng.pdf (accessed 21 December 2018).

International Union of Psychological Science and International Association of Applied Psychology (2008) 'Universal declaration of ethical principles for psychologists'. Online. Available at https://iaapsy.org/site/assets/files/1057/ethical_principles_for_psychologists.pdf (accessed 16 October 2018).

Mill, J.S. (1869) *The Subjection of Women*, London: Longmans, Green, Reader and Dyer.

Moorhead, B., Bell, K. and Bowles, W. (2016) 'Exploring the development of professional identity with newly qualified social workers', *Australian Social Work*, 69: 456–67.

National Council of Independent Living (2017) 'Fact sheet: the affordable care act and the disability community'. Online. Available at www.advocacymonitor.com/fact-sheet-the-affordable-care-act-and-the-disability-community/ (accessed 16 October 2018).

National Disability Insurance Scheme (NDIS) (2017) *Annual Report*. Online. Available at www.ndis.gov.au/medias/documents/h28/h9e/8805113626654/1617-AnnualReport-lock.pdf (accessed 16 October 2018).

National Health Service (NHS) (2018) 'Personal budgets'. Online. Available at www.nhs.uk/conditions/social-care-and-support/personalisation/#how-does-personalised-care-work (accessed 16 October 2018).

ObamaCare Facts (2017) 'ObamaCare employer mandate'. Online. Available at https://obamacarefacts.com/obamacare-employer-mandate/ (accessed 16 October 2018).

Parliament of Australia (2017) Joint standing committee on the national disability insurance scheme: services for people with psychosocial disabilities related to a mental health condition, 12 May. Online. Available at http://parlinfo.aph.gov.au/parlInfo/search/display/display.w3p;query=Id%3A%22committees%2Fcommjnt%2F9b3b9f5f-8397-402e-a518-478f6bb74dbe%2F0006%22;src1=sm1 (accessed 11 January 2019).

Preston, N. (2014) *Understanding Ethics*, 2nd edn, Sydney: The Federation Press.

Rachels, J. and Rachels, S. (2010) *The Elements of Moral Philosophy*, 6th edn, Boston: McGraw-Hill.

Registered Disability Savings Plan (RDSP) (2018) 'A bit of history'. Online. Available at www.rdsp.com/tutorial/a-bit-of-history/ (accessed 16 October 2018).

Senate Canada (2013) *In From the Margins, Part II: Reducing Barriers to Social Inclusion and Social Cohesion*. Online. Available at https://sencanada.ca/content/sen/Committee/411/soci/rep/rep26jun13ExecSummary-e.pdf (accessed 16 October 2018).

Shafer-Landau, R. (2012) *The Fundamentals of Ethics*, 2nd edn, New York: Oxford University Press.

Short, M. (2015) *Three Anglican Churches Engaging with People from Culturally and Linguistically Diverse Backgrounds*, Sydney: The Bush Church Aid Society of Australia.

Short, M. (2018) *Anglican Churches Engaging with People Living with Disabilities*, Sydney: The Bush Church Aid Society of Australia and CBM Australia's Luke 14 Program.

Short, M., Dempsey, K., Ackland, J., Rush, E., Heller, E. and Dwyer, H. (2018) 'What is a person? Deepening students' and colleagues' understanding of person-centeredness', *Advances in Social Work and Welfare Education*, 20(1): 139–56.

Singer, P. (1975) *Animal Liberation: A New Ethic for Our Treatment of Animals*, New York: Random House.

Singer, P. (2011) *Practical Ethics*, 3rd edn, New York: Cambridge University Press.

Social Care Institute for Excellence (SCIE) (2010) 'Personalisation for social workers in adults' services'. Online. Available at www.scie.org.uk/personalisation/practice/social-workers (accessed 16 October 2018).

Stevenson, L. (2013) 'Aristotle: the ideal of human fulfilment', in L. Stevenson, D.L. Haberman and P. Matthews Wright (eds) *Twelve Theories of Human Nature*, 6th edn, New York: Oxford University Press.

Taket, A., Crisp, B.R., Graham, M., Hanna, L. and Goldingay, S. (2014) 'Scoping social inclusion practice', in A. Taket, B.R. Crisp, M. Graham, L. Hanna, S. Goldingay and L. Wilson (eds) *Practising Social Inclusion*, London: Routledge.

United Nations (1948) 'The universal declaration of human rights'. Online. Available at www.un.org/en/documents/udhr/index.shtml (accessed 16 October 2018).

United Nations (2006) 'Convention on the rights of persons with disabilities'. Online. Available at www.un.org/development/desa/disabilities/convention-on-the-rights-of-persons-with-disabilities.html (accessed 16 October 2018).

United Nations (2016) *Leaving No One Behind: The Imperative of Inclusive Development. Report on the World Social Situation 2016*. Online. Available at www.un.org/esa/socdev/rwss/2016/full-report.pdf (accessed 16 October 2018).

United Nations (2017a) 'Convention on the rights of persons with disabilities: signatories and parties'. Online. Available at https://treaties.un.org/Pages/ViewDetails.aspx?src=TREATY&mtdsg_no=IV-15&chapter=4&clang=_en (accessed 16 October 2018).

United Nations (2017b) 'Universal declaration of human rights: history of the document'. Online. Available at www.un.org/en/sections/universal-declaration/history-document/index.html (accessed 16 October 2018).

Weston, A. (2011) *A Practical Companion to Ethics*, 4th edn, New York: Oxford University Press.

World Confederation for Physical Therapy (2017) 'WCPT ethical principles'. Online. Available at www.wcpt.org/ethical-principles (accessed 16 October 2018).

World Medical Association (2018) 'WMA international code of medical ethics'. Online. Available at www.wma.net/policies-post/wma-international-code-of-medical-ethics/ (accessed 16 October 2018).

15 Spirituality and religion

Sustaining individuals and communities or replicating colonisation?

Beth R. Crisp

Introduction

Had the principles enshrined in the United Nations (2007) *Declaration on the Rights of Indigenous Peoples* been those of the European powers which colonised the rest of the world for centuries, history might have been very different. Perhaps we might live in a world in which we would not need to be

> Concerned that indigenous peoples have suffered from historical injustices as a result of, inter alia, their colonization and dispossession of their lands, territories and resources, thus preventing them from exercising, in particular, their right to development in accordance with their own needs and interests.
>
> (United Nations 2007: 2)

Instead we live in a world where the violence, abuse, and disrespect of Indigenous peoples in many countries form not just catalogues of historical events (Brett 2016) but lives on in the disadvantage experienced by Indigenous peoples compared to non-Indigenous settlers in countries such as Australia (Sherwood 2013), Canada (Shackleton 2007), New Zealand (Fraser 2014; Walsh-Tapiata 2008), and the United States (Weaver 2008). The religious beliefs of the colonisers and the ways in which they were manifested are increasingly being recognised as contributors to the disadvantage experienced by Indigenous peoples (Dallaire 2014).

In secular societies in which the prevailing modernity of the nineteenth and twentieth centuries promoted the idea that the place of religion was in the private sphere, the role of religion in colonisation could flourish and not be subject to public debate (Dinham et al. 2018). While there are many who would 'characterize the West as a colonial overlord' (Modood 2013: 124), particularly in respect of religion, such simplification is problematic and denies the possibility that religion and spirituality can also be part of the process of sustaining individuals and communities rather than replicating colonisation.

Positioning

There are at least three distinct discourses on the impacts of colonialism for Indigenous populations. The first of these is by European writers where the postcolonial experience is about coming to terms with influxes of migrants from former colonies and the impact of migration on both individual immigrants and the societies where they have moved (Murphy 2007).

A second strand of postcolonial writing has emerged from many African, Asian, and Pacific countries where European powers saw it as their right to do whatever they considered warranted to tap the wealth and resources of their distant colonies and withdraw when the benefits of remaining were too diminished or they had outstayed their welcome. Either way, for many of the colonists, their lives away from Europe was often time-limited rather than embarking on permanent migration to a new 'home', and during their time in the colonies, they were part of a minority white population. Although they may be long gone, the impacts, positive and negative, of the colonists remain as a legacy of earlier eras.

It is a third strand of postcolonial experience in which I am positioned, as a member of Australia's white settler community (see also Stephens and Monro 2018). As with other settler communities in countries such as Canada, United States, and New Zealand, generations of migrants have sought to make permanent homes here, and the typically white, European settlers and their descendants are now the majority of the population (Coombes 2006). In some cases, this is relatively recent, and although my father's family arrived from England in the nineteenth century, my mother's family migrated from England less than five years before my birth, making me the first Australian-born member of their family.

As a primary school child, I learnt early the colonialist disregard of Indigenous Australians, when in response to the question 'Who discovered Australia?' I suggested the Aboriginal people had been here long before Captain Cook's travels in 1770. It was much later that I learnt that the promotion of the view that Cook 'discovered Australia' also represented a British Imperialism, given that the Dutch had mapped much of the northern and western coastline decades before Cook (Williams 2018). Others who had come prior to the British included French and Spanish sailors from Europe as well as those from within the region, including the area now known as Indonesia (Russell 2018).

Writing about the role of religion in colonisation requires me as a practising Christian to understand that some religious organisations I have been involved with historically may have treated Indigenous Australians atrociously (Brett 2016). As a child, I also had distant relations who worked as missionaries with Indigenous peoples and observed how missionaries were considered to be so virtuous by some members of the Christian community. While I have no doubt there were many missionaries who did excellent work, a much more sceptical understanding of missionary work is now rightly justified.

In addition to being part of a settler family and a Christian, I am also a social worker. Welfare provision in settler countries has a long history of reinforcing the worst aspects of colonialism, often under the aegis of religious organisations (Gray et al. 2008). Therefore engaging with issues of religion and colonialism forces me to deal with a history of abuse perpetrated by my profession. Although it may be more comfortable to avoid,

> For non-Indigenous Peoples, an exploration of their own beliefs, assumptions and knowledge, and how they have benefitted from and been complicit in, the colonizing, dehumanizing and othering of Indigenous Peoples is imperative.
>
> (Coates 2016: 73)

Nevertheless, on doing so, I acknowledge that as a non-Indigenous Australian, I do not have the right to speak on behalf of Indigenous peoples, which would be a further form of colonisation (Briskman 2008). However, the responsibility for change cannot be left solely to Indigenous peoples. Those of us who are members of the settler majority communities need to rethink how we work with Indigenous peoples and not assume our ways of thinking and doing are necessarily the only or best approaches (Briskman 2008; Gair 2008).

Disrespect for humanity

Although Australia has been a home to peoples for over 65,000 years and at the time of European settlement was already home to more than 600 tribes and more than 250 language groups (Russell 2018), the settlers treated the land as '*terra nullius*' or land not belonging to anyone which they were free to claim (Brittan 2007).While this could perhaps be understood had European explorers and early settlers arrived in places not inhabited by Indigenous Australians, this was not the case. Rather as occurred elsewhere, colonial representations of non-Europeans were typically as primitive and inferior (Singh and Cowden 2011). In his diary, Captain Cook referred to the Indigenous people of Australia he encountered in 1770 as 'animals' (Brittan 2007: 73) due to their lack of interest in engaging in trade with the incomers.

By failing to acknowledge Indigenous peoples as human, vast areas of land could be taken from them and given to settlers who lacked the 'sophisticated ecological, environmental and faunal knowledge' (Russell 2018: 29) to effectively farm in landscapes very different from what they were used to in Europe (Gammage 2011). Indeed, in the period 1810–1821, more than half a million acres of Aboriginal lands was granted to European settlers by the colonial powers in Australia as part of a comprehensive approach to establishing the European dominance (Leahy et al. 2018). While acknowledging there were exceptions,

> Generally, Aborigines were treated by pastoralists as chattels and kept in a position of virtual slavery where their wives and daughters were often sexually exploited; again they were subject to spasmodic massacres and arbitrary detention, while their children were often removed "for their own good". "Genocide" is not a word which should be used lightly but this pattern of

cruel repression resulted in the near extinction of many Aboriginal groups and the disappearance of their languages, kinship systems, and above all their rich and complex religions.

(Charlesworth 1998: xxiv)

The sentiments underpinning colonisation in Australia were not dissimilar from European colonisation in many other parts of the globe (Charlesworth 1998; McLeod 2007). Although dispossession is difficult in any circumstances, for Indigenous peoples for whom their relationship with the land is central to their spirituality (Gray et al. 2008) such difficulties are compounded. It was not until 1992 when the notion of *terra nullius* was overturned in Australia (Brett 2016) and the impact of the early settlers in Australia is still felt by Indigenous Australians today.

At the time of the invasion we were unaware that this encounter would impact on the lives of generations, dispossess us of our country and destroy our right to practice our culture and ceremony. The ongoing impact of this on the First Peoples, in this land now known as Australia, has been denied, accepted and normalised.

(rea 2018: 196)

Religion and colonisation

There is a long history of Christian teachings being (mis)used to support the ambitions of rulers and nations (Pace 2011). Hence, readings of biblical texts which focussed on conquest supported the quest for colonisation and suppressed questioning of this, much to the horror of some contemporary biblical scholars (e.g. Brett 2016). Such unshakeable belief that it was their religious right, if not duty, to claim foreign lands on behalf of Christian nations was often coupled with the 'belief that they were benefitting the local Indigenous Peoples with the technologies, systems, values and the Christian religion of the industrialized world' (Faith 2008: 245). In other words, it was about imposing a view of a so-called superior European civilisation. Indigenous peoples were required by the missionaries to adopt Western clothing and speak English and were forcibly not only exposed to but expected to adopt the teachings and practices of Christianity (Gray et al. 2008). Rather than an improvement, Indigenous peoples experienced this as cultural destruction. In the words of John Packham, an Indigenous Australian:

Christianity played a big part in the death of our culture by turning our people from our god to a white god, thus destroying the ways of our people. Then farmers took the land, put up fences and built churches. With the clearing of the land and killing of our native animals came the loss of our hunting skills, thus driving a stake through the very soul of our culture.

(Packham 2018: 40)

The possibility that Indigenous peoples may have their own forms of religion was not considered by the colonialists. Emile Durkheim, in the early years of the twentieth century, summed up the view of centuries of European thinking when he wrote,

> If then we wish to discover the true nature of religion, we must observe it at the zenith of its evolution; it is in the most refined forms of Christianity and not in the puerile magic of the Australian aborigine or the Iroquois that we must expect to find the elements of the definition we are seeking.
>
> (in Pickering 1975: 75–6)

Indeed it is only in the latter part of the twentieth century have scholars of religion come to the position that the religions and belief systems of Indigenous peoples can be compared with religions such as Christianity, Islam, Judaism, or Buddhism (Charlesworth 1998) and is still questioned today by some (Boisvert 2015). As religion is essentially a European concept, other belief systems do not necessarily fit the Christian framework around which functionalist models of religion are based (Bruce 2011).

While some ways of defining religion include the possibility of 'New Religious Movements' (Dobbelaere 2011: 196) when considering religious traditions outside a Christian framework, such designation is inappropriate when discussing much older traditions such as those of Indigenous peoples. When asked to nominate their religion in Australia's 2016 Census of Population and Housing, approximately 2 per cent of Indigenous Australians reported adherence to 'Australian Aboriginal Traditional religions or beliefs' as their primary religion (ABS 2017).

But not only were Indigenous peoples assumed not to have a religion, at least one conforming to Western concepts, Indigenous Australians were not perceived as having the mental capacity to engage in religious thinking by some colonists. Such thinking may, however, have been based on the misapprehension that there not being a tradition of reading and writing reflected an inability for complex and abstract thinking (Stanner 1998).

If 'the catalogue of complaints than can be brought against colonial Christianity is so impressive one might wonder why it is still the majority religion in many countries of Africa, Latin America, and Oceania' (Brett 2016: 3). This is true for Australia also. More than half (54 per cent) of the Aboriginal and Torres Strait Islander population reported a Christian affiliation in the 2016 Census, almost the same proportion as the non-Indigenous population (55 per cent) (ABS 2017). In this context, it is important that non-Indigenous peoples do not unwittingly engage in a further form of colonial behaviour by asking Indigenous Christians why they persist with a religion that has caused so many difficulties for their communities (Brett 2016). It is also necessary to recognise that not all missionary groups conformed to the stereotypes of showing a lack of respect for the Indigenous Peoples they encountered.

> Others, with a wider vision, sought to learn the heart languages of the people among whom they lived, sought to grow the love in families and

communities. They sought to graft the body and blood of Christ into cultural customs.

(Sherman and Mattingley 2017: 17)

In adopting Christianity, many Indigenous peoples have blended Western forms of religious expression with elements of their own traditions in community rituals and in the decoration of religious buildings (Brett 2016; Fraser 2014).

Indigenous spirituality

Despite the lack of consensus as to whether the beliefs and practices of many Indigenous communities constitute a religion, there is widespread agreement as to the centrality of spirituality in the lives of Indigenous peoples (Hart 2008). Although customs and beliefs vary, a reverence for the earth and the natural environment it supports is a common point for Indigenous peoples both in Australia (Charlesworth 1998) and elsewhere (Coates 2016). While there are some forms of Christian spirituality which also place a strong importance on the sacredness of the natural environment (Tacey 2009), a spirituality centred on the land was regarded as pagan by many colonialists (Dallaire 2014). Nor was there any understanding as to why an emphasis on collective rather than individual self-determination in respect of the land is critical (Walsh-Tapiata 2008).

> The Aborigines, found abhorrent, for example and plainly incomprehensible the idea that land could be treated as private property, to be bought and sold, or even to be owned in the first imaginative and spiritual life, no more of a commodity for sale than a parent or child. In the immensely complex and variable web of beliefs and customs that shaped Aboriginal relationships to land there was no place for the central and unquestioned premise of British colonists: that land was merchandise to be traded for money for goods, claimed with words written on paper, or simply taken by force.
>
> (Brittan 2007: 74)

In other words, for many Indigenous peoples, there is no distinction between spirituality and the rest of human experience (Fraser 2014) or notions of sacred versus profane. As such, spirituality is part of everyday living and hence not readily apparent to outsiders. Furthermore, because outsiders are often excluded from the ceremonial rituals of many Indigenous communities (Berndt 1998), the spiritualities of Indigenous peoples could readily go unrecognised by the early colonists as they set up social structures, such as schools and welfare services, based on the norms of their European homelands (Jones 2014).

Sustaining social inclusion

In Australia, the 'Closing the Gap Strategy' (Holland 2018) came about after an agreement in 2008 by heads of government at federal and state levels for a long-term strategy to tackle the social determinants of health, including housing, education, and community infrastructure, with the aim of improving not just life expectancy but also levels of health and well-being of Indigenous Australians. Such problems cannot be tackled overnight, and it was envisaged that Closing the Gap would require 25 years of effort and investment. However, after five years, changes in priority have led some to claim that the Closing the Gap Strategy continues to exist in name only. Consequently, a decade after being launched, the achievements have been limited the prospect of health equality for Indigenous Australians within a generation is unlikely (Holland 2018).

The rhetoric of the 'Closing the Gap Strategy' is that it represented a partnership of government with Indigenous Australians, but in fact was 'without any significant Aboriginal and Torres Strait Islander engagement, let alone partnership' (Holland 2018: 17). As such, it was not unlike the efforts of the colonists of previous generations in imposing a White European way of doing things (Modood 2012).

Moving toward, let alone sustaining, social inclusion with Indigenous peoples arguably requires a different approach than those involving the imposition, however well-meaning, of programmes on individuals and communities. To begin with, this requires recognition of the expertise in many Indigenous communities which has enabled them to survive for generations in environments which non-Indigenous Peoples often regard as completely inhospitable (Gray et al. 2008). As such,

> Indigenous Peoples have exhibited remarkable resilience in resisting colonial incursions and attempts to eliminate them completely have failed. Indigenous people have and will continue to survive and resist further incursions into their territories, natural resources, sacred sites, languages, beliefs, values, networks and systems of governance, intellectual property rights and sovereignty.
>
> (Yellow Bird 2016: xxii)

It has been argued that it is a Western fallacy to think that social inclusion for Indigenous peoples can be sustained with strategies which take no account of spirituality (Hart 2008). Yet for Western health and welfare workers whose professional socialisation may well have included the message that there was no place for religion (Crisp 2011) or spirituality (Crisp 2010) in their professional practice, incorporating religion and spirituality into their practice with Indigenous peoples may require a fundamental change in thought and action. However, there is now a growing acceptance that spirituality has a place to play in addressing issues of social exclusion (de Souza and Halahoff 2018). This can start with deep listening and taking the time to really listen to Indigenous peoples who have difficult stories which need to be able to be told and heard (Buttigieg 2018).

> Deep, inner listening is a spiritual experience. It invites you to be fully present. When we are fully present our attention is focused and our whole being begins to slow down. The ability to connect is nurtured through cultivating the spiritual characteristic of presence.
>
> (Buttigieg 2018: 167)

In the Ngan'gikurunggurr and Ngen'giwumirri languages of the Indigenous peoples of the Daly River Region of the Northern Territory in Australia, this deep listening is known as 'Dadirri'.

> In our Aboriginal way, we learnt to listen from our earliest days. We could not live good and useful lives unless we listened. This was the normal way for us to learn—not by asking questions. We learnt by watching and listening, waiting and then acting. Our people have passed on this way of listening for over 40,000 years.
>
> There is no need to reflect too much and to do a lot of thinking. It is just being aware.
>
> (Ungunmerr 1998: 1–2)

Opportunities to meet and learn from Indigenous peoples about their spirituality and sacred stories are often difficult for non-Indigenous peoples as they may be confronted with their own prejudices and ignorance. Nevertheless, such meeting can be openings not just to reconciliation (Buttigieg 2018) but a step in building sustained social inclusion. Deep listening requires an openness to different ways of communicating and a realisation that Eurocentric methods of question and answering may lead to superficial discussions. Rather for Indigenous peoples in many countries, storytelling is an important means of communication. For Indigenous peoples in Australia, this is known as 'yarning' (Bessarab and Ng'andu 2010). This is a dynamic process in which stories are told and reinterpreted through the contributions of different members and over time and, in doing so, become part of the oral tradition of the community:

> Yarning almost always contains the threads of Aboriginal and Torres Strait Island history as it moves into the present tense, its parameters within present time is filtered through the memories of the past as the two move simultaneously and at points collide and reveals fragments of the future. This type of Aboriginal storytelling or yarning enables Aboriginal and Torres Strait Island people to reconstruct their lives in new ways while at the same time keeping their cultural integrity intact.
>
> (Geia et al. 2013: 15)

While the protocols and processes of yarning vary between communities (Bessarab and Ng'andu 2010), there is nevertheless widespread agreement that yarning is an appropriate method for engaging either individuals or groups in health and social care (Dudgeon et al. 2014; Nagel et al. 2012) and research/community consultations (Bessarab and Ng'andu 2010; Geia et al. 2013). As relationships develop, the depth of stories may increase (Bessarab and Ng'andu 2010; Geia et al. 2013), but it can be months or years, if ever, for non-Indigenous individuals or groups to be accepted to the point at which some yarns can be shared with them (McCoy 2008).

The importance of relationality underpins the notion of 'kanyirninpa', a word in the Kukatja language used by four communities in the Kimberley region in the far north of Western Australia. Sometimes translated as 'holding',

> Kanyirninpa is expressed in a number of interconnected ways. It includes nurturance but it also involves older people taking responsibility for those they hold. This relationship between generations is named as "respect". Kanyirninpa is also expressed in relationships that involve teaching and learning where older people will help young people "grow up the right way". While some aspects of kanyirninpa remain constant over one's lifetime, others assume different cultural expressions as those who are held grow older and in turn hold others.
>
> (McCoy 2008: 22)

While kanyirninpa includes taking responsibility for ensuring those in one's care have adequate food, clothing, housing, and are protected from harm, it is not about control or possession but about nurturing relationships. Kanyirninpa is something everyone can play a role in, such as the parents who 'see holding as a reciprocal relationship where they have experienced their children supporting and encouraging them as parents' (McCoy 2008: 27). However, kanyirninpa is not confined to family relationships and can also occur in time-limited contexts such as prisons, health, and education settings, where non-Indigenous peoples may not even realise at the time how significant some of their efforts in holding were to those in their care (McCoy 2008).

Notwithstanding their mistreatment by many missionary groups, some have recognised the importance of supporting Indigenous peoples to retain their language and culture by playing a major role in documenting Australian Indigenous languages and keeping them alive for future generations. For Indigenous peoples, having one's language recognised promotes a sense of identity and worth (Sherman and Mattingley 2017). This sense of worth and identity intrinsic to understandings of spirituality (Crisp 2010) as well as implicit in understandings of social inclusion which are not limited by a focus on economic well-being (Taket et al. 2009). Yet endeavours by non-Indigenous peoples to create social inclusion with Indigenous peoples 'are unlikely to address either the spiritual goals or use the culturally appropriate pedagogy that would be required to meet the . . . needs' (Zoellner et al. 2017: 57) of participants.

One example of a training organisation which takes seriously the spiritual needs of Indigenous Australians is Wontulp-Bi-Buya-College, originally founded as a Bible college run by Indigenous Australians for Indigenous Australians but which now also teaches a range of vocational courses in community development, addictions, Indigenous mental health, and suicide prevention. In particular,

> The training foregrounds contemporary social contexts to post-European Indigenous perspectives of Australian history to build a narrative of hope, cultural enrichment and fulfilment through the vehicle of training. . . . Proud

graduates receive . . . above all, a collective understanding of intergenerational and postcolonial trauma and its connectedness to family and community violence

(Stephens and Monro 2018: 2)

This approach has resulted in much higher completion rates than generally achieved by vocational training programmes for Indigenous Australians (Stephens and Monro 2018). However, such achievements are not cheap, and in addition to government funding, Wontulp-Bi-Buya-College has relied on funding from various church organisations and philanthropy (Zoellner et al. 2017).

Conclusion

This chapter has demonstrated that while European understandings of religion and spirituality have been used to condone the unjust treatment of Indigenous peoples both in Australia and elsewhere, religion and spirituality can also contribute to the building and sustaining of social inclusion for those marginalised by colonisation. The examples provided in the previous section will not necessarily be applicable in every Indigenous community, but are provided as examples of what is possible and to encourage readers to enter into a process of 'decolonisation' which requires 'deconstructing old myths and practices used to problematize Australian Indigenous peoples in the past and currently' (Sherwood 2013: 29).

It is now increasingly common in Australia for public events to have an acknowledgement to the traditional owners of the land on which one is meeting. Such acknowledgements typically recognise the place of land as central to the spirituality of Indigenous Australians. For meetings held at Deakin University's Geelong campuses, the following wording is used:

I wish to begin by acknowledging we are gathered here today on the traditional lands of the Waddawurrung people. And pay our respects to Elders past and present.

(Deakin University 2018)

While far more is needed to ensure than verbal acknowledgements, it is perhaps an early step in the decolonisation process, in that there are many more Australians who know the names of the lands on which they live and work than was the case only 20 years ago. On the other hand, it would be a pity is Acknowledgements of Country allowed non-Indigenous peoples to become complacent (Brennan 1998) rather than encourage us to do our part in working with the aim of ensuring a society which is equally inclusive of Indigenous and non-Indigenous Australians (Brett 2016). Hopefully, in time this will result in a situation in which Article 12 of the *Declaration on the Rights of Indigenous Peoples*, which calls for 'Indigenous peoples [to] have the right to manifest, practise, develop and teach their spiritual and religious traditions, customs and ceremonies.' (United Nations 2007: 6) will be a reality rather than aspiration.

References

Australian Bureau of Statistics [ABS] (2017) 'Religion in Australia, 2016'. Online. Available at www.abs.gov.au/ausstats/abs@.nsf/Lookup/by%20Subject/2071.0~2016~Main%20Features~Religion%20Article~80 (accessed 4 March 2018).

Berndt, R.M. (1998) 'The profile of good and bad in Australian Aboriginal religion', in M. Charlesworth (ed) *Religious Business: Essays on Australian Aboriginal Spirituality*, Cambridge: Cambridge University Press.

Bessarab, D. and Ng'andu, B. (2010) 'Yarning about yarning as a legitimate method in indigenous research', *International Journal of Critical Religious Studies*, 3: 37–50.

Boisvert, D. (2015) 'Quebec's ethics and religious culture school curriculum: a critical perspective', *Journal of Intercultural Studies*, 36: 380–93.

Brennan, F. (1998) 'Land rights: the religious factor', in M. Charlesworth (ed) *Religious Business: Essays on Australian Aboriginal Spirituality*, Cambridge: Cambridge University Press.

Brett, M.G. (2016) *Political Trauma and Healing: Biblical Ethics for a Postcolonial World*, Grand Rapids, MI: William B. Eerdmans Publishing Company.

Briskman, L. (2008) 'Decolonizing social work in Australia: prospect or illusion', in M. Gray, J. Coates and M. Yellow Bird (eds) *Indigenous Social Work Around the World: Towards Culturally Relevant Education and Practice*, Farnham: Ashgate.

Brittan, A. (2007) 'Australasia', in J. McLeod (ed) *The Routledge Companion to Postcolonial Studies*, London: Routledge.

Bruce, S. (2011) 'Defining religion: a practical response', *International Review of Sociology*, 21: 107–20.

Buttigieg, O. (2018) 'Yingadi Aboriginal immersion: a program to nurture spirituality', in M. de Souza and A. Halahoff (eds) *Re-Enchanting Education and Spiritual Well-being: Fostering Belonging and Meaning-making for Global Citizens*, London: Routledge.

Charlesworth, M. (1998) 'Introduction', in M. Charlesworth (ed) *Religious Business: Essays on Australian Aboriginal Spirituality*, Cambridge: Cambridge University Press.

Coates, J. (2016) 'Ecospiritual approaches: a path to decolonizing social work', in M. Gray, J. Coates, M. Yellow Bird and T. Hetherington (eds) *Decolonizing Social Work*, London: Routledge.

Coombes, A.E. (ed) (2006) *Rethinking Settler Colonialism: History and Memory in Australia, Canada, Aotearoa New Zealand and South Africa*, Manchester: Manchester University Press.

Crisp, B.R. (2010) *Spirituality and Social Work*, Farnham: Ashgate.

Crisp, B.R. (2011) 'If a holistic approach to social work requires acknowledgement of religion, what does this mean for social work education?' *Social Work Education*, 30: 657–68.

Dallaire, M. (2014) 'Spirituality in Canadian education', in J. Watson, M. de Souza and A. Trousdale (eds) *Global Perspectives on Spirituality and Education*, New York: Routledge.

Deakin University (2018) 'Welcome to country'. Online. Available at www.deakin.edu.au/courses/ike/welcome-to-country (accessed 1 January 2019).

De Souza, M. and Halahoff, A. (2018) 'Introduction', in M. de Souza and A. Halahoff (eds) *Re-Enchanting Education and Spiritual Well-being: Fostering Belonging and Meaning-making for Global Citizens*, London: Routledge.

Dinham, A., Baker, C. and Crisp, B.R. (2018) 'The need to re-imagine religion and belief', in C. Baker, B.R. Crisp and A. Dinham (eds) *Re-imagining Religion and Belief: 21st Century Policy and Practice*, Bristol: Policy Press.

Dobbelaere, K. (2011) 'The contextualization of definitions of religion', *International Review of Sociology*, 21: 191–204.

Dudgeon, P., Milroy, H. and Walker, R. (2014) (eds) *Working Together: Aboriginal and Torres Strait Islander Mental Health and Wellbeing Principles and Practice*, 2nd edn, Perth: Telethon Institute for Child Health.

Faith, E. (2008) 'Indigenous social work education: a project for all of us?' in M. Gray, J. Coates and M. Yellow Bird (eds) *Indigenous Social Work Around the World: Towards Culturally Relevant Education and Practice*, Farnham: Ashgate.

Fraser, D. (2014) 'Taha Wairua: the spiritual in state education in New Zealand', in J. Watson, M. de Souza and A. Trousdale (eds) *Global Perspectives on Spirituality and Education*, New York: Routledge.

Gair, S. (2008) 'Missing the "Flight from responsibility": tales from a non-indigenous educator pursuing spaces for social work education relevant to Indigenous Australians', in M. Gray, J. Coates and M. Yellow Bird (eds) *Indigenous Social Work Around the World: Towards Culturally Relevant Education and Practice*, Farnham: Ashgate.

Gammage, B. (2011) *The Biggest Estate on Earth: How Aborigines Made Australia*, Sydney: Allen and Unwin.

Geia, L.K., Hayes, B. and Usher, K. (2013) 'Yarning/Aboriginal storytelling: towards an understanding of an Indigenous perspective and its implications for research practice', *Contemporary Nurse*, 46: 13–17.

Gray, M., Yellow Bird, M. and Coates, J. (2008) 'Towards an understanding of Indigenous social work', in M. Gray, J. Coates and M. Yellow Bird (eds) *Indigenous Social Work Around the World: Towards Culturally Relevant Education and Practice*, Farnham: Ashgate.

Hart, M.A. (2008) 'Critical reflections on an Aboriginal approach to helping', in M. Gray, J. Coates and M. Yellow Bird (eds) *Indigenous Social Work Around the World: Towards Culturally Relevant Education and Practice*, Farnham: Ashgate.

Holland, C. (2018) *A Ten-Year Review: The Closing the Gap Strategy and Recommendations for Reset*. Online. Available at www.humanrights.gov.au/sites/default/files/document/publication/CTG%202018_FINAL-WEB.pdf (accessed 7 May 2018).

Jones, N. (2014) 'Buddhism in Bhutanese education', in J. Watson, M. de Souza and A. Trousdale (eds) *Global Perspectives on Spirituality and Education*, New York: Routledge.

Leahy, C., Ryan, J. and van Wyk, S. (2018) 'Colony', in C. Leahy and J. Ryan (eds) *Colony: Australia 1770–1861/ Frontier Wars*, Melbourne: National Gallery of Victoria.

McCoy, B. (2008) *Holding Men: Kanyirninpa and the Health of Aboriginal Men*, Canberra, ACT: Aboriginal Studies Press.

McLeod, J. (2007) 'Introduction', in J. McLeod (ed) *The Routledge Companion to Postcolonial Studies*, London: Routledge.

Modood, T. (2012) '2011 Paul Hanly Furfey lecture. Is there a crisis of secularism in Western Europe?' *Sociology of Religion*, 73: 130–49.

Modood, T. (2013) 'Multiculturalism and religion: a three part debate. Part one Accommodating religions: multiculturalism's new fault line', *Critical Social Policy*, 24: 121–7.

Murphy, D. (2007) 'Africa: North and Sub-Saharan', in J. McLeod (ed) *The Routledge Companion to Postcolonial Studies*, London: Routledge.

Nagel, T., Hinton, R. and Griffin, C. (2012) 'Yarning about Indigenous mental health: translation of a recovery paradigm to practice', *Advances in Mental Health*, 10: 216–23.

Pace, E. (2011) 'Religion as communication', *International Review of Sociology*, 21: 205–29.

Packham, J. (2018) 'John Packham on Petin: to abduct, to steal', in C. Leahy and J. Ryan (eds) *Colony: Australia 1770–1861/ Frontier Wars*, Melbourne: National Gallery of Victoria.

Pickering, W.S.F. (1975) *Durkheim on Religion: A Selection of Readings with Bibliographies*, London: Routledge and Kegan Paul.

rea (2018) 'rea on Poles Apart', in C. Leahy and J. Ryan (eds) *Colony: Australia 1770–1861/ Frontier Wars*, Melbourne: National Gallery of Victoria.

Russell, L. (2018) 'Worlds collide and contested histories', in C. Leahy and J. Ryan (eds) *Colony: Australia 1770–1861/ Frontier Wars*, Melbourne: National Gallery of Victoria.

Shackleton, M. (2007) 'Canada', in J. McLeod (ed) *The Routledge Companion to Postcolonial Studies*, London: Routledge.

Sherman, L. and Mattingley, C. (eds) (2017) *Our Mob, God's Story: Aboriginal and Torres Strait Islander Artists Share Their Faith*, Sydney: Bible Society Australia.

Sherwood, J. (2013) 'Colonisation—It's bad for your health: the context of Aboriginal health', *Contemporary Nurse*, 46: 28–40.

Singh, G. and Cowden, S. (2011) 'Multiculturalism's new fault lines: religious fundamentalisms and public policy', *Critical Social Policy*, 31: 343–64.

Stanner, W.E.H. (1998) 'Some aspects of aboriginal religion', in M. Charlesworth (ed) *Religious Business: Essays on Australian Aboriginal Spirituality*, Cambridge: Cambridge University Press.

Stephens, A. and Monro, D. (2018) 'Training for life and healing: the systemic empowerment of Aboriginal and Torres Strait Islander men and women through vocational education and training', *The Australian Journal of Indigenous Education*, DOI: 10.1017/jie.2018.5.

Tacey, D. (2009) 'Environmental spirituality', *International Journal of New Perspectives in Christianity*, 1(1): Article 3. Online. Available at https://research.avondale.edu.au/npc/vol1/iss1/3 (accessed 1 January 2019).

Taket, A., Crisp, B.R., Nevill, A., Lamaro, G., Graham, M. and Barter-Godfrey (2009) 'Introducing theories of social exclusion and social connectedness', in A. Taket, B.R. Crisp, A. Nevill, G. Lamaro, M. Graham and S. Barter-Godfrey (eds) *Theorising Social Exclusion*, London: Routledge.

Ungunmerr, M.R. (1998) 'Dadirri: inner deep listening and quiet still awareness'. Online. Available at www.miriamrosefoundation.org.au/about-dadirri (accessed 29 April 2018).

United Nations (2007) *Declaration on the Rights of Indigenous Peoples*. Online. Available at www.un.org/esa/socdev/unpfii/documents/DRIPS_en.pdf (accessed 10 May 2018).

Walsh-Tapiata, W. (2008) 'The past, the present and the future: the New Zealand indigenous experience of social work', in M. Gray, J. Coates and M. Yellow Bird (eds) *Indigenous Social Work Around the World: Towards Culturally Relevant Education and Practice*, Farnham: Ashgate.

Weaver, H.N. (2008) 'Indigenous social work in the United States: reflections on Indian tacos, Trojan horses and canoes filled with indigenous revolutionaries', in M. Gray, J. Coates and M. Yellow Bird (eds) *Indigenous Social Work Around the World: Towards Culturally Relevant Education and Practice*, Farnham: Ashgate.

Williams, N. (2018) 'Unfinished business: Australia as palimpsest', in C. Leahy and J. Ryan (eds) *Colony: Australia 1770–1861/ Frontier Wars*, Melbourne: National Gallery of Victoria.

Yellow Bird, M. (2016) 'Preface', in M. Gray, J. Coates, M. Yellow Bird and T. Hetherington (eds) *Decolonizing Social Work*, London: Routledge.

Zoellner, D., Stephens, A., Joseph, V. and Monro, D. (2017) 'Mission-driven adaptability in a changing national training system', *The Australian Journal of Indigenous Education*, 46: 54–63.

16 A 'good news' story of social inclusion

Refugee resettlement in Australia

Kim Robinson

Introduction

The response of the developed world to forced migration is both a politically fraught and challenging area of public policy at national and international levels. Humanitarian migrants face increasing barriers to settlement that are rooted in what Crock et al. (2017: 2) refer to as 'economic uncertainty, rising xenophobia and increased economic migration'. The United Nations High Commissioner for Refugees (UNHCR 2018a) notes that there are 68.5 million forcibly displaced people worldwide, with 85 per cent of them living in developing countries. Of the 25.4 million refugees, 3.1 million are claiming protection as asylum seekers, and only 102,800 refugees are resettled (UNHCR 2018a). Australia, as a country of resettlement, claims adherence to its international human rights obligations and a long-standing successful humanitarian settlement programme (Australian Government 2016). However, currently Australian politicians are engaging in the politics of race and what has been described as 'race-baiting' to revise and question the role of assimilation and integration of newly arrived refugees (Seccombe 2018). The treatment of asylum seekers in Australia and in offshore detention, while not the focus of this chapter, also contributes to an unsettled and contentious public discourse about immigration (Silove and Mares 2018).

The Australian government has a commitment to providing support to refugees via its Humanitarian Settlement Programme (HSP), which establishes an annual quota for entry, based on assessments provided by UNCHR in its refugee camps. Services considered key to settlement are funded by both federal and state government and consist of housing, employment programmes, health care, education, and family reunion. Ager and Strang (2008) argue that the provision of services based on social relations are key to settlement alongside the processes of integration and acculturation referred to by Berry (1992) and others. Crock et al. (2017: 2) argue that there is no single, generally accepted definition, theory, or model for refugee 'settlement' and that policy and practice across politically similar states remains diverse.

The successful settlement of refugees in Australia is an under-acknowledged narrative of social inclusion. Dominant discourses highlight trauma and the problematic victim status of refugees and contribute to a limited understanding of the diverse characteristics that make up multicultural communities. This chapter draws on Australian examples of successful settlement and highlights good practice in the context of health and social care services. It points to the foundation of collaborative interdisciplinary work and long-term commitment to inclusive practice with service user involvement. It also identifies how new approaches and innovative solutions emerge from unexpected places. This chapter will be focusing on community-based organisations (CBOs, also called nongovernment organisations, not-for-profit, or charitable organisations) that provide settlement support in Australia, but prior to that, I will briefly discuss the historical Australian immigration policy context.

Australian immigration practices: an historical overview

The British settlers declared Australia '*terra nullius*' (empty country) in 1788, despite having a diverse Indigenous population throughout the continent. The Aboriginal population was subject to genocide and dispossession of their land and traditions, and their children were removed into the 'care' of white families, Christian settlements, and other institutions. Historian scholar Klaus Neumann (2015: 4) argues that the two key themes of Australian history are Indigenous dispossession and immigration. Prior to World War Two, the majority of settlers came from Britain, with smaller groups of Irish, German, and Italian settlers who often faced hardship, hostility, and racism (Neumann 2004). Australia is one of the most ethnically diverse countries in the world (Castles and Miller 2009: 250). The most recent census in 2016 shows that nearly half (49 per cent) of Australians had either been born overseas (first-generation Australian) or one or both parents had been born overseas (second-generation Australian) (Australian Bureau of [ABS] Statistics 2017).

The British colonial administration and later the Australian federal and state governments recruited, subsidised, and encouraged immigrants from Europe. In 1901, one of the first laws passed by the new Federal Parliament was the *Immigration Restriction Act*, the so-called 'White Australia' policy. Unashamedly racist, it was designed to exclude non-Europeans with the rationale of ensuring social cohesion, cultural similarities, and political consistency. It reinforced the fears of the 'yellow peril' and the 'threat' of Asian invasion from the North. It also denied the geographical location of Australia being more Asian than European. These perceived threats are still current in contemporary political discourse (see Seccombe 2018).

After World War Two, the immigration minister, Arthur Calwell, said that there would be ten British immigrants for every 'foreigner'; however, it became clear that Australia needed additional labour. There were concerns that non-British immigration would threaten social cohesion and the dominant white colonial identity. Castles (1992) notes how in the 1950s and 1960s most migrants came from Italy, Greece, and Malta and that a two-class system of immigration developed. The first class accessed assisted passage which was available for the British (often referred to as the 'ten pound poms') and northern Europeans, who had full labour market and civil entitlements and importantly, could bring family with them. The second class of Eastern and Southern Europeans were unlikely to have assisted passage, had no right to family reunion, and were often working in low-paid and high-risk jobs. There was however, another agenda.

> There was a third, invisible class: those who were not admitted at all. The White Australia Policy kept out all non-whites and was applied so zealously that even the Asian wives of Australian soldiers who had served overseas were excluded.
>
> (Castles 1992: 551)

The postwar immigration programme emphasised the need for labour, with migrants forming the key workforce for projects to develop the infrastructure of the country. Australia has a rich literary history reflecting the struggles of the multicultural lives of these workers and their encounters with the harsh environment, the Indigenous populations, and each other. It has been suggested that the postwar time was when 'the idea of the "good" refugee was born: the one who, fleeing communist persecution, waited patiently in a camp far away to be selected as "genuine" and invited to Australia' (Moorehead 2005: 97). This theme continues today in current debates, where the authenticity of those seeking protection and asylum continues to be questioned and positioned as a risk *to* society (Masocha and Robinson 2017: 163).

In the 1970s, new measures were put in place to attract people to Australia and retain them. The Australian Labor Party's prime minister, Gough Whitlam, abolished the White Australia Policy and introduced entry criteria that did not discriminate on the basis of 'race, ethnicity, religion or national origin' (Castles 1992: 552). This was significant as history in the region was changing dramatically with the Vietnam War. In the ten years following the fall of Saigon, 95,000 displaced Vietnamese people were 'processed' to arrive in Australia, and Australia's immigration officials selected people directly from the holding camps in Malaysia, Indonesia, and China. Castles (2003) argues that it was this Indo-Chinese refugee programme that led to the demise of the White Australia policy. Moorehead (2005: 97) notes 'Australia was no longer white, but a neat and cautious system was in place'. The immigration levels fluctuated in the 1980s due to economic conditions and government policies, and there were large intakes from South East Asia, New Zealand, and Eastern Europe.

This, by no means exhaustive, summary of immigration provides a background as to what emerged in Australia in the late 1990s into the 2000s, which was an increase in policy and procedures that restricted access for those seeking protection. In effect, there were separate categories established for humanitarian arrivals and those claiming asylum outside of the systems of UNHCR. Castles and Loughna (2004: 187) describe a convergence of practice internationally in three key areas when they wrote 'Restricting access to the territory of states; discouraging asylum applications by restricting access to welfare benefits; and the replacement of permanent asylum with various forms of temporary protection'.

The HSP (introduced in October 2017) provides Specialised and Intensive Services (SIS) to support 'humanitarian entrants to build the skills and knowledge they need to become self-reliant and active members of the Australian community' (Australian Government Department of Social Services 2018). It is against this backcloth that I now go on to briefly identify some key themes in relation to social cohesion and this discourse in the context of immigration.

Social cohesion and immigration

While there is no agreed definition of social cohesion, most definitions address a sense of belonging, attachment to the group, and willingness to participate and to share outcomes. Markus and Kirpitchenko (2007) describe social cohesion at a number of levels; first it requires universal values, mutual respect, and common aspirations shared by their members. It also describes a well-functioning core group or community in which there are shared goals and responsibilities, and it finally is viewed not simply as an outcome, but a process of achieving social harmony.

Various sociological theories have developed over time to understand the processes of social integration and social cohesion, and in the context of Australian humanitarian entrants, these have moved from assimilation to integration and to multiculturalism (Spinks 2009). The Chicago School developed assimilation theory in the 1920s, and some academics argue it retains prominence today (Fozdar and Banki 2017; Modood 2007). According to this theory, a migrant went through a process of resocialisation or acculturation in order to be assimilated and effectively denounce their heritage and background. This has been widely criticised as a one-way process where the responsibility is on the migrant rather than the host society to facilitate inclusion (Modood 2007). Assimilation theory in Australia has been widely criticised in the context of the dispossession of Aboriginal land and the disregard of the human rights of Indigenous peoples (Briskman 2014; Ife 2012). Integration continues to be a problematic term and is often framed in terms of adaptation to the host country rather than understanding the complex dynamics of diversity, culture, and intersectionality (see Allweiss and Hilado 2018; Fozdar and Banki 2017).

In Australia in the 1970s, multiculturalism was embraced and supported in terms of the cultural, social, and economic rights of all members in a democratic state. Parekh (2000: 6) suggests that a multicultural society is one that responds to its cultural diversity by being welcoming and respectful and by making 'it central to its self-understanding, and respect the cultural demands of its constituent communities'. The literature on critical multiculturalism and whiteness has informed new ways of thinking about promoting inclusive practice and of framing structural disadvantage within a complex diversity discourse (Boccagni 2015; Daniel 2008; Nylund 2006). While theories and policies fluctuate according to political parties and international tensions, assimilation theory has regained popularity in dominant discourse in many countries today. It has been increasingly promoted since the 'war on terror' post-9/11 (11 September 2001 in the USA) and 7/7

(7 July 2005 in the UK) and the debates about the role of the nation-state to protect its borders and citizens. All of these measures have had a direct impact on community organisations that support refugees and they have sought to respond to these concerns in a variety of ways. Critical race theory, anti-oppressive practice, and postmodern approaches to working with diversity are current approaches to what Williams and Graham (2016) call 'embedded transformatory practice'. This positions working with diversity as the norm and not the 'other', a theme which shall be returned to in the context of the case studies in this chapter. Understanding the case studies also requires an understanding of some of the policy and practice development issues that have faced CBOs and have a direct impact on refugees seeking health and social care services.

Health and social care work and inclusive practice

Influences on the development of services

There are a number of theoretical and ideological influences on organisations, and researchers have highlighted the diverse schools of thought that have influenced refugee service provision, including mainstream healthcare approaches, multicultural mental health, sociological approaches, 'managed care', and the role of users' movements (Hilado and Lundy 2018; Neumann et al. 2014). This work has illustrated the often-conflicting policy demands on service provision to refugees and the tensions between migrant healthcare in mainstream services with that in CBOs.

Many organisations link globalism (the ideology that supports globalisation through international partnerships) with the fight for overcoming inequality and promoting human rights and have developed practices that emphasise solidarity, mutual responsibility, and social justice (Ife 2012). Historically CBOs have adopted a human rights discourse, with a focus on restorative and social justice and provide advocacy which is central to tackling inequality. Ife notes,

> The idea of human rights, by its very appeal to universally applicable ideas of the values of humanity, seems to resonate across cultures and traditions and represents an important rallying cry for those seeking to bring about a more just, peaceful and sustainable world.
>
> (Ife 2012: 9–10)

Prior to the 1980s, community organisations worked primarily with refugees as victims of state-based organised violence, most frequently political survivors of torture and dissidents from Eastern Europe, Latin America, and parts of South East Asia. In the 1980s and 1990s, the focus shifted to an emphasis on working clinically with past sufferings and trauma (Ingleby 2005: 5–6). Services were often developed in partnership with community-based organisations and sought philanthropic funds and government grants to establish programmes. For example, the London-based Medical Centre for the Care of Victims of Torture was established in 1985, and the Victorian Foundation for Survivors of Torture in Australia was established in 1987.

During the late 1990s and early 2000s, challenges from other disciplines emerged, and a reappraisal of practice based on a number of different perspectives occurred in recognition of what Watters (2001: 1713) described as 'emerging paradigms'. Central to services was the focus on social justice and human rights. *The Universal Declaration of Human Rights* (United Nations 1948), supported by the Australian government and CBOs, has promoted support for vulnerable adults and families via humanitarian programs and assistance for integration to redistribute the 'burden' from developing countries. Hatton and Maloney argue,

> Every year hundreds of thousands of people apply for political asylum, seeking sanctuary in the stable safe and secure countries of the developed world. Most of them come from poor and middle-income countries that are in the grip of civil wars or international conflicts, countries that systematically persecute minorities, or in which human rights abuses are commonplace.
>
> (Hatton and Maloney 2015: 2)

There have been ongoing debates on the use of the term trauma and post-traumatic stress disorder (PTSD) and to what extent refugees are labelled as victims or survivors, vulnerable, or resilient (Masocha and Robinson 2017). Scholars have a more developed formulation and understanding of the distinction between the pre-flight, flight, and post-arrival status of refugees (Watters 2001). There is recognition too of the increased evidence that the stressors associated with reception and resettlement are more profound than previously thought (Allweiss and Hilado 2018).

Researchers have highlighted the tension between international and national obligations to humanitarian arrivals, with the state's obligation to protect the interests of its citizens and electorate (Castles and Miller 2009). The Australian government provision of a national social welfare system is protective of scarce resources and wary of acting as a 'pull factor' in attracting refugees and asylum seekers. This has contributed to the 'othering' of refugees and asylum seekers as 'good' (deserving) or 'bad' (undeserving) in political discourse and a mechanism for pitting marginalised communities against each other (Grove and Zwi 2006; Robinson and Masocha 2016).

Finally the social model of health was another key driver in the development of health and social care services for refugees. The World Health Organization (WHO) defines health as 'a state of complete physical, mental and social well-being and not merely the absence of disease or infirmity' (WHO 1948). The *Ottawa Charter for Health Promotion* identifies five priority action areas for health promotion: build healthy public policy, create supportive environments, strengthen community action, develop personal skills, and reorient health services (WHO 1986). The social model contrasts with the medical model and argues that illness and disease are socially created by a disabling society that discriminates based on social, economic, and environmental factors. Importantly challenges and critiques emerged of dependency, personal tragedy, segregation, and stereotypes with an emphasis on empowerment, self-help, and partnership working (Marmot 2005). Advocates of the social model argue that the biomedical approach has a lack of emphasis on social inequalities and political factors. This history has played a key role and contributed to the formation of services for refugees and those affected by trauma and, in turn, settlement services.

Community development models of practice

Healthcare, social, and welfare workers work every day with refugees, those with lived experience of immigration control and separation from their home and family. Services, and the individuals who work in them, are exposed to a range of discourses that limit and define the context under which refugees arrive and obtain or are denied access to resources. As noted earlier researchers have documented how services have developed individual, community, family based and child centred approaches. Trauma informed and clinical mental health approaches have been central to the field, and many have also drawn on community development models of participation (Kenny and Connors 2017; Mitchell and Correra-Velez 2010; Westoby and Ingamells 2009).

The community development model of practice emphasises the involvement of refugee communities in the development and implementation of services. Researchers and frontline workers have advocated community development as a model to redress social exclusion of refugees experiencing war trauma (Craig and Lovel 2005; Kenny and Connors 2017). Based on collaborative work in the community involving refugees and researchers Craig and Lovel (2005) identified a framework that involved the participation of refugees in the following areas: the identification of needs, mobilization of resources, identification of intervention options, decision-making on choice of intervention, delivery of the action/ intervention, developing skills, identifying and measuring process and end-point outcomes. Drawing from this model, Mitchell and Correra-Velez (2010) document the implementation of these elements based on a project developed as an evaluation framework for services working with torture and trauma survivors in Australia. They argue that joint working is a key element of community development and professionals working with refugees and fosters empowerment 'based on the meaning and experience of the community' (Mitchell and Correra-Velez 2010: 104.). Another model advocated by Williams and Graham (2016: 14) is based on the concept of 'embedded transformatory practice' and constitutes four key domains of service provision: critical reflexive interrogation; responsiveness; rights-based advocacy; and co-production. Drawn on the principles of anti-oppressive practice, intersectionality and engagement with service users this model promotes the development of innovative and responsive services.

How refugees adjust to a new life in a new country is contingent on many different issues including the community being receptive and having access to social capital, individual personality traits, and the extent of the dislocation and trauma one has experienced (Silove 2017; Strang and Ager 2010). Research needs to be focused on assessing the benefits of current treatment options and the diverse outcomes for service users, and whether to focus on individual treatment, families, or communities or on wider systems. Allweiss and Hilado (2018) address key elements of adjustment for refugees in the context of support services that build a sense of community and overarching resilience. They emphasise housing affordability, access to a community, access to English language training or native language training, family and social support, financial and employment resources, and adequate health and mental health supports (Allweiss and Hilado 2018).

Case studies

The next part of this chapter highlights two Australian examples of transformative and inclusive practice that have specifically drawn on these models; the first works with young people from refugee backgrounds, and the second is the Victorian Refugee Health Network.

Case study one: Ucan2

Young people from refugee backgrounds experience particular stresses and challenges when they are resettling and these are often directly related to education (Correa-Velez et al. 2017). Attending school or adapting to a new environment from what was a disrupted education has a significant impact on settlement and employment. Foundation House in partnership with the Centre for Multicultural Youth (CMY) and AMES (based in Melbourne) developed a programme called Ucan2. It works in partnership with an interdisciplinary team and is delivered in various education and employment service settings.

The Ucan2 programme aims to facilitate and support the social inclusion of newly arrived young people of refugee backgrounds between the ages of 16 and 25 years. It was developed to support learning and employment pathways that connect young people of refugee backgrounds into the Australian community.

Ucan2 is underpinned by theory and evidence concerning effective ways to support recovery from trauma, integration and successful settlement. These approaches include practice based models from Foundation house and CMY (The Victorian Foundation for Survivors of Trauma 1998) and Ager and Strang's (2008) conceptual framework for understanding integration. All of these approaches draw from a human rights base, with an emphasis on social capital and trauma informed practice. Combining an integrated group work programme, work experience and mentors from major Australian employers, the programme was designed to be highly relevant for young people of refugee backgrounds, to build their social capital and to increase their access to mainstream jobs.

Evaluation findings based on surveys and interviews with young people indicate that the programme:

- Promotes English language learning;
- Supports engagement in education and employment;

- Increases the size and diversity of participants' social networks;
- Fosters wellbeing and resilience and builds confidence; and
- Builds the capacity of teachers to respond to the needs of young people of refugee backgrounds.

Over 80 per cent of those surveyed who had undertaken Ucan2 in 2016 were studying or working when contacted in 2017 and 95 per cent were actively engaged in work, study, caring responsibilities or seeking employment. Further information about the evaluation of Ucan2 can be found in Block et al. (2017).

Case study two: Victorian refugee health network

A major challenge for refugees is accessing health and social care support services. The issue of health literacy and the associated stigma in contacting services for newly arrived communities is the subject of ongoing research (Riggs et al. 2016). Linked to this is the importance of health and social care professional's knowledge of specific health issues of diverse communities. The Victorian Refugee Health Network (2018) is a case example of utilising community-based strategies to reach out to refugee communities along with service providers in health and social care. Established in June 2007, its remit is to facilitate greater coordination and collaboration amongst health and community services to provide more accessible and appropriate health services for people of refugee backgrounds. The Network aims to:

- build the capacity of the Victorian health sector to respond to health concerns experienced by people of refugee backgrounds and address health inequality through health promotion;
- support services to be more accessible to people from refugee backgrounds particularly in regional and outer metropolitan areas; and
- improve service coordination for recent arrivals and those with more complex needs.

(Victorian Refugee Health Network 2018)

In partnership with a wide range of community health, primary care and acute services, the network provides guidance, training, publications and research for those working in this area. A recent publication utilised a community development framework to consult with over 300 service users to inform best practice with refugees (Tyrrell et al. 2016). This wide-ranging consultation identified the following eight key themes:

These were: healthy eating and food security, social connectedness, opportunities for physical exercise and sport, health information and knowledge about health service systems, communication with health providers, accessibility and appropriateness of services, mental health, and income and employment.

(Tyrrell et al. 2016: 13)

This type of consultation is central to the networks philosophy of promoting good process to ensure inclusion and builds on existing policy culturally and linguistically diverse communities (see State Government of Victoria Department of Health and Human Services 2015). Further work in consultation by the network last year reviewed the organisational structure and identified a number of recommendations to improve communication in relation to local and national refugee health networks (Duell-Piening 2018). Dealing with a complex and rapidly changing sector across a number of geographical and government departments, is challenging work and requires both flexibility and clear structures for service users and providers.

Successful settlement: key elements for transformative practice

Health and social care work is a socially constructed activity and is both exposed to and shaped by the dominant discourses outlined in this chapter. Strategies that promote inclusion and minimise exclusion, and that aid successful integration are critical to a well-functioning society and are highly contested in terms of their defining features (Ager and Strang 2008). Academics have highlighted social exclusion as the result of a lack of social capital in addition to being excluded from the employment market (Taket et al. 2009). Social capital is critical for the inclusion of asylum seekers and refugees, because they are so often excluded from economic capital. The workers in these case studies demonstrate a commitment to a human rights framework, and the programmes illustrate a number of core elements that contribute to successful settlement as outlined earlier. First, they combine collaborative interdisciplinary work; that is they work across a range of sectors including health, social welfare, education, and employment services. This joint working and service user involvement drives change and facilitates co-production (Mitchell and Correra-Velez 2010; Williams and Graham 2016). They demonstrate a long-term commitment to the refugee populations they serve, and ensure that service user involvement is part of core business in the development of programmes and identification of intervention options. Third, they address racism. Tackling racism in its various forms is part of navigating the community environment when establishing programmes that promote social inclusion. Addressing discourses of risk and trauma to inform the planning and development of projects and programmes needs to take into account the tensions and contradictions that can result (Masocha and Robinson 2017). Transformative practice that addresses social justice and human rights contributes to new interpretations of cultural competence within a global context (Williams and Graham 2016).

Conclusions

This chapter illustrates some of the ways that transformative practice in refugee communities can promote long lasting and sustainable change as well as some the challenges facing the development of services in the context of a review of immigration policies. There is an important ongoing emphasis in the literature on interagency collaboration and multi-agency working in the refugee sector (UNHCR 2017). While the policy response to the needs of refugees has varied between individual treatment to community development to support newly arrived groups to address exclusion and marginalisation, the competition between services for limited funding means that joint working and partnerships are critical for future longevity.

A key element of liberal governmentality is the ability of individuals to engage in practices that challenge dominant discourses that marginalise and oppress newly arrived members of the community (Carey and Foster 2011). Activism and collaboration with refugees has been prominent in Australia and integral to the establishment of refugee organisations. Frontline workers promote opportunities for innovation in CBOs working with refugees, and engage in a range of strategies including promoting change within their organisations and the sector. Doing advocacy work with other agencies and sectors, and conducting research to document the provision of health and social care to refugees in the context of increasing immigration controls must inform the future agenda. This involves challenging the legal frameworks governing the determination of immigration status, utilising participatory methods and strategies with service users and refugee communities to reflect their needs and concerns, and working with the broader community advocating for change in attitudes and government policy. The creation of long term harmonious community relationships alongside advocacy for resources and supportive humanitarian services is critical for the development of sustainable social inclusion.

Acknowledgement

I would like to thank colleagues at Foundation House for both supporting and agreeing to the inclusion of the case studies included in this chapter.

References

Ager, A. and Strang, A. (2008) 'Understanding integration: a conceptual framework', *Journal of Refugee Studies*, 21: 166–91.

Allweiss, S. and Hilado, A. (2018) 'The context of migration. Pre-arrival, migration, and resettlement experiences', in A. Hilado and M. Lundy (eds) *Models for Practice with Immigrants and Refugees: Collaboration, Cultural Awareness, and Integrative Theory*, Thousand Oaks, CA: Sage.

Australian Bureau of Statistics [ABS] (2017) '2016 Multicultural census summary'. Available at www.abs.gov.au/ausstats/abs%40.nsf/lookup/Media%20Release3 (accessed 14 August 2018).

Australian Government (2016) 'Report to the United Nations human rights committee on the international covenant on civil and political rights'. Online. Available at http://docstore.ohchr.org/SelfServices/FilesHandler.ashx?enc=6QkG1d%2fPPRiCAqhKb7y hsoAl3%2fFsniSQx2VAmWrPA0s38oA smarter Australia: policy advice for an incoming government 2013–2016%2ba6goo6jUTK7HrJ3FD3R4XqdPcac4oLbE xZlWNPa%2bU 3q5oc32Y12yw%2boMlBa6fyhhpycej3EEb44memhTE (accessed 12 August 2018).

Australian Government Department of Social Services (2018) 'Settlement services. Humanitarian settlement factsheet February 2018'. Online. Available at www.dss.gov. au/settlement-services/programs-policy/settlement-services/humanitarian-settlement-program (accessed 15 August 2018).

Berry, J. (1992) 'Acculturation and adaptation in a new society', *International Migration*, 30(S1): 69–85.

Block, K., Young, D. and Molyneaux, R. (2017) *Ucan2: Youth Transition Support—Evaluation Report*, Melbourne: Centre for Health Equity, University of Melbourne.

Boccagni, P. (2015) '(Super)diversity and the migration-social work nexus: a new lens on the field of access and inclusion?' *Ethnic and Racial Studies*, 38: 608–20.

Briskman, L. (2014) *Social Work with Indigenous Communities: A Human Rights Approach*, 2nd edn, Annandale, NSW: The Federation Press.

Carey, M. and Foster, V. (2011) 'Introducing "deviant" social work: contextualising the limits of radical social work whilst understanding (fragmented) resistance within the social work labour process', *British Journal of Social Work*, 41: 576–93.

Castles, S. (1992) 'The Australian model of immigration and multiculturalism: is it applicable to Europe?' *International Migration Review*, 26: 549–67.

Castles, S. (2003) 'Towards a sociology of forced migration and social transformation', *Sociology*, 37: 13–34.

Castles, S. and Loughna, S. (2004) 'Globalization, migration and asylum', in V. George and R. Page (eds) *Global Social Problems and Global Social Policy*, Cambridge: Polity Press.

Castles, S. and Miller, M.J. (2009) *The Age of Migration: International Population Movements in the Modern World*, 4th edn, London: Palgrave Macmillan.

Correa-Velez, I., Gifford, S.M., McMichael, C. and Sampson, R. (2017) 'Predictors of secondary school completion among refugee youth 8 to 9 years after resettlement in Melbourne, Australia', *Journal of International Migration and Integration*, 18: 791–805.

Craig, G. and Lovel, H. (2005) 'Community development with refugees: towards a framework for action', *Community Development Journal*, 40: 131–6.

Crock, M.E., Mahony, C. and Fozdar, F. (2017) 'Introduction in a "slippery fish": the differential application of human rights obligations to the settlement of refugees', *International Journal of Migration and Border Studies*, 3: 1–4.

Daniel, C.L. (2008) 'From liberal pluralism to critical multiculturalism: the need for a paradigm shift in multicultural education for social work practice in the United States', *Journal of Progressive Human Services*, 19: 19–38.

Duell-Piening, P. (2018) 'The Victorian refugee network restructure'. Online. Available at http://refugeehealthnetwork.org.au/wp-content/uploads/Structure_2018_April_Victorian-Refugee-Health-Network.pdf (accessed 11 October 2018).

Fozdar, F. and Banki, S. (2017) 'Settling refugees in Australia: achievements and challenges', *International Journal of Migration and Border Studies*, 3: 43–66.

Grove, N.J. and Zwi, A.B. (2006) 'Our health and theirs: forced migration, othering and public health', *Social Science and Medicine*, 62: 1931–42.

Hatton, T. and Maloney, J. (2015) *Applications for Asylum in the Developing World: Modelling Asylum Claims by Origin and Destination*. Australian Government Department of Immigration and Border Protection, Research Programme Occasional Paper Series No.14. Online. Available at www.homeaffairs.gov.au/ReportsandPublications/Documents/research/hatton-applications-for-asylum.pdf (accessed 9 November 2018).

Hilado, A. and Lundy, M. (eds) (2018) *Models for Practice with Immigrants and Refugees: Collaboration, Cultural Awareness, and Integrative Theory*, Thousand Oaks, CA: Sage.

Ife, J. (2012) *Human Rights and Social Work: Towards Rights-based Practice*, Cambridge: Cambridge University Press.

Ingleby, D. (ed) (2005) *Forced Migration and Mental Health: Rethinking the Care of Refugees and Displaced Persons*, New York: Springer.

Kenny, S. and Connors, P. (2017) *Developing Communities for the Future*, 5th edn, South Melbourne: Cengage.

Markus, A. and Kirpitchenko, L. (2007) 'Conceptualising social cohesion', in J. Jupp, J. Nieuwenhuysen and E. Dawson (eds) *Social Cohesion in Australia*, Port Melbourne: Cambridge University Press.

Marmot, M. (2005) 'The social determinants of health', *The Lancet*, 365: 1099–104.

Masocha, S. and Robinson, K. (2017) 'Mental health risk, political conflict and asylum: a human rights and social justice issue', in S. Stanford, E. Sharland, N. Rovinelli Heller and J. Warner, J. (eds) *Beyond the Risk Paradigm in Mental Health Policy and Practice*, London: Palgrave Macmillan.

Mitchell, J. and Correra-Velez, I. (2010) 'Community development with survivors of trauma: an evaluation framework', *Community Development Journal*, 45: 90–110.

Modood, T. (2007) *Multiculturalism*, Cambridge: Polity Press.

Moorehead, C. (2005) *Human Cargo: A Journey Among Refugees*, London: Chatto and Windus.

Neumann, K. (2004) *Refuge Australia: Australia's Humanitarian Record*, Sydney: University of New South Wales Press Limited.

Neumann, K. (2015) *Across the Seas: Australia's Response to Refugees: A History*, Collingwood, Victoria: Black Inc.

Neumann, K., Gifford, S.M., Lems, A. and Scherr, S. (2014) 'Refugee settlement in Australia: policy, scholarship and the production of knowledge, 1952–2013', *Journal of Intercultural Studies*, 35: 1–17.

Nylund, D. (2006) 'Critical multiculturalism, whiteness and social work', *Journal of Progressive Human Services*, 17(2): 27–42.

Parekh, B. (2000) *Rethinking Multiculturalism: Cultural Diversity and Political Theory*, Basingstoke: Palgrave Macmillan.

Riggs, E., Yelland, J., Duell-Piening, P. and Brown, S.J. (2016) 'Improving health literacy in refugee populations', *Medical Journal of Australia*, 204: 9–10.

Robinson, K. and Masocha, S. (2016) 'Divergent practices in statutory and voluntary-sector settings? Social work with asylum seekers', *British Journal of Social Work*, 47: 1517–33.

Seccombe, M. (2018) 'Who is making money out of racism?' *The Saturday Paper*. Online. Available at www.thesaturdaypaper.com.au/contributor/mike-seccombe (accessed 30 August 2018).

Silove, D. (2017) 'Effective interventions and models for refugee trauma', *Refugee Transitions*, 32: 34–9.

Silove, D. and Mares, S. (2018) 'The mental health of asylum seekers in Australia and the role of psychiatrists', *BJPsych International*, 15(3): 65–8.

Spinks, H. (2009) 'Australia's settlement services for migrants and refugees', Research Paper. Parliament of Australia. Department of Parliamentary Services. Available at www.rssfeeds.aph.gov.au/binaries/library/pubs/rp/2008-09/09rp29.pdf (accessed 9 November 2018).

State Government of Victoria Department of Health and Human Services (2015) *Refugee and Asylum Seeker Health Services: Guidelines for the Community Health Program*, Melbourne: State of Victoria. Online. Available at https://www2.health.vic. gov.au/about/publications/policiesandguidelines/Refugee-and-asylum-seeker-health-services—Guidelines-for-the-community-health-program (accessed 12 October 2018).

Strang, A. and Ager, A. (2010) 'Refugee integration: emerging trends and remaining agendas', *Journal of Refugee Studies*, 23: 589–607.

Taket, A., Crisp, B.R., Nevill, A., Lamaro, G., Graham, M. and Barter-Godfrey, S. (eds) (2009) *Theorising Social Exclusion*, London: Routledge.

The Victorian Foundation for Survivors of Torture (1998) *Rebuilding Shattered Lives*. Victorian Foundation of Survivors of Torture Incl. Online. Available at https://www.foundationhouse.org.au/wp-content/uploads/2014/08/Rebuilding_Shatterd_Lives_Complete. pdf (accessed 3 March 2020).

Tyrrell, L., Duell-Piening, P., Morris, M. and Casey, S. (2016) *Talking About Health and Experiences of Using Health Services with People from Refugee Backgrounds*, Melbourne: Victorian Refugee Health Network. Online. Available at http://refugee healthnetwork.org.au/talking-about-health-and-experiences-of-using-health-services-with-people-from-refugee-backgrounds/ (accessed 12 October 2018).

UNHCR (2018a) 'Figures at a glance'. Online. Available at www.unhcr.org/en-au/figures-at-a-glance.html (accessed 12 August 2018).

UNHCR (2018b) 'Expanding partnership report 2017'. Online. Available at www.unhcr. org/en-au/publications/fundraising/5b30bbe67/unhcr-global-report-2017-expanding-partnerships.html (accessed 19 August 2018).

United Nations (1948) 'The universal declaration of human rights'. Online. Available at www.un.org/en/universal-declaration-human-rights/index.html (accessed 30 August 2018).

Victorian Refugee Health Network (2018) 'Victorian refugee health network'. Online. Available at http://refugeehealthnetwork.org.au/ (accessed 27 August 2018).

Watters, C. (2001) 'Emerging paradigms in the mental health care of refugees', *Social Science and Medicine*, 52: 1709–18.

Westoby, P. and Ingamells, A. (2009) 'A critically informed perspective of working with resettling refugee groups in Australia', *British Journal of Social Work*, 40: 1759–76.

Williams, C. and Graham, M.J. (2016) *Social Work in a Diverse Society: Transformative Practice with Black and Minority Ethnic Individuals and Communities*, Bristol: Policy Press.

World Health Organization (1948) 'Constitution of WHO principles'. Online. Available at www.who.int/about/mission/en/ (accessed 12 October 2018).

World Health Organization (1986) 'The Ottawa charter for health promotion'. Online. Available at www.who.int/healthpromotion/conferences/previous/ottawa/en/ (accessed 15 August 2018).

Part 6

Sustainable social development

17 Strengthening everyday peace formation via community development in Myanmar's Rohingya–Rakhine conflict

Vicki-Ann Ware and Anthony Ware

Introduction

To achieve sustainable outcomes, community development in deeply divided, poor societies must address the drivers of both poverty and inter-communal tension. One of the most promising recent theoretical advances examining the bridging between communities in conflict-affected situations is that of 'everyday peace', suggesting that the strengthening of everyday peace formation is crucial to both creating the space for and then maintaining community development (CD) outcomes.

This chapter examines one CD programme working in the conflict situation of Rakhine State, Myanmar, between the ethnic Rakhine Buddhists and the Rohingya Muslims. This programme operates amongst communities on the periphery of this violence, deeply impacted by conflict fears and narratives, yet remaining in their villages rather than displaced, adopting a participatory arts-based pedagogy. After outlining the context and programme, this chapter summarises the key theoretical foundations of the programme and then examines evidence that it has given rise to critical-awareness of conflict dynamics and strengthened the empowerment of local actors to advance everyday peace formation between ethnic Rakhine villages and their Rohingya neighbours in sustainable ways.

The context: conflict and poverty

Prior to the recent violence, Rakhine State, the westernmost state in Myanmar, was home to about 2 million ethnic Rakhine Buddhists, 1.3 million Rohingya Muslims, and small numbers of Burmans and other ethnic minorities (Republic of the Union of Myanmar 2015). Violence drove 720,000 Rohingya Muslims across the Bangladeshi border in 2017–18, leaving no more than 550,000 in Myanmar. The mass violence reflects very high levels of intercommunal fear and tension. Massive army operations, labelled ethnic cleansing 'with genocidal intent' by the United Nations (Human Rights Council 2018: 16), were provoked by Rohingya insurgent attacks in 2016 and 2017 and supported by ethnic Rakhine nationalist groups. However, this was not an isolated case of violence, but another episode in a long-running conflict between ethnic Rakhine Buddhists, the Rohingya, and the Burman majority (Myanmar's dominant ethnicity).

Origins of the conflict can be traced to the destruction of the old Arakan kingdom by the Burmans in 1784, the impact of colonial era (1824–1948) migration, and atrocities committed during World War II and the civil war after independence in 1948. The Rohingya, as demonstrated by recent violence, are genuinely existentially threatened. The ethnic Rakhine also hold deep existential fears that the Burmans have been attempting to destroy their culture and identity for centuries on the one hand and that they are being overrun by Muslim migration on the other. There is some truth behind the latter: while some Muslim ancestors of the Rohingya lived in Rakhine as early as the fifteenth century, the vast majority are descendants of British-sponsored colonial-era migrants. Census data shows that, as a proportion of the Northern Rakhine population, Muslims grew from 10 per cent to 38 per cent between 1826 and 1931 (Ware and Laoutides 2018). Coupled with living just across the border from one of the world's highest population densities, Bangladesh, most Rakhine feel a deep sense of existential threat from the Muslims on one side and Burmanisation on the other.

Rakhine also struggle with deep poverty for everyday survival. Recent census data paints a compelling picture of extreme poverty and underdevelopment, far worse than most of the rest of the country and almost as bad as anywhere in the world. Table 17.1 shows 2014 Census data highlighting the deep poverty in contrast with Myanmar's national averages.

The World Bank created a Wealth Ranking Index for all 330 townships in Myanmar, using the census data (World Bank 2015). Over half of Rakhine's 17 townships are amongst the 20 most impoverished in the country, and Rakhine ranked as the lowest state or region in the country. Rakhine State's low-lying coastal topography also makes it prone to extreme weather events, including frequent cyclones and floods, adding significantly to the vulnerability of the people.

Table 17.1 2014 Census data contrasting the situation of the Rakhine with all persons in Myanmar

Measure	Rakhine	All persons
	%	%
Improved drinking water	37.8	69.5
Improved sanitation	31.8	74.3
Electricity for lighting	12.8	32.4
Thatch roofing	72.5	35.1
Cook with firewood	88.9	69.2

Source: Republic of the Union of Myanmar 2015

The community development education programme

Previous research by one of us found localised, highly participatory, bottom-up approaches to community development to be an effective approach to alleviating poverty in Myanmar, even during the authoritarian military-rule period pre-2010 (Ware 2012). On this basis, in 2011 we offered the NGO *GraceWorks Myanmar* (GWM) assistance to develop the strategic design and implementation of what is now their flagship programme. The Community Development Education (CDE) programme seeks to bring empowerment and locally led change to this context of extreme poverty, political domination, and armed-plus-communal violence.

Now operating in 60 ethnic Rakhine villages in northern and central Rakhine State, the programme offers training and a limited amount of financial support to village-nominated facilitators, who lead village action. Facilitators are selected based on motivation and personal attributes rather than age, education, experience, or status, forming a diverse group. Half women and half men, they range in age from mid-20s to early-50s. Few are tertiary-trained, and many do not have secondary education. Some are already village leaders; others are not. Oral, participatory, arts-based training initially focuses on mobilising communities, asset and needs mapping, and implementing locally planned projects. Later training explores citizenship and human rights, critical analytical and creativity skills, and locally appropriate approaches to advocacy and engagement with officials. Hence, there is a focus on local agency and initiative and instituting good processes in villages.

Facilitators commit to a three-year role, with a long-term goal of building sustainability through strong, representative community committees able to facilitate ongoing, locally led development action. Work to date has focussed more directly on development than peacebuilding outcomes, with an emphasis on low-cost, largely self-funded activities that enhance long-term well-being, village life, intercommunal relations and ways to engage with authorities and official power.

We have previously analysed and documented the development aspects of this programme in depth (Ware 2013a, 2013b; Ware and Ware 2018). Three cohorts of communities have shown solid track records in achieving small-scale, self-led development outcomes, ranging from water filtration and latrines to road repairs, volunteer teachers in schools, and improved livelihoods. They are able to regularly analyse and articulate governance problems, moving from feeling dominated and powerless to starting to influence local power relations through co-option and advocacy. Increasingly, facilitators are going to local officials, to present need as an opportunity for them to be seen to help, rather than confronting them with lists of demands.

For example, in one creative demonstration of their newfound agency, in the lead-up to the 2015 elections, one village committee planned and implemented their own form of advocacy by producing a video clip on a mobile phone. They documented need and community commitment for reconstruction of a damaged local gravel road and approached the local candidate running for the military-backed party to ask for money. Not only were they successful in receiving funding before election day, but highlighting their newfound agency, they all confirmed they still chose to not vote for that candidate because of his military ties.

Yet in the context of overwhelming violence, no CD outcomes are likely to be sustained unless both poverty and conflict drivers are successfully addressed. Bouts of violence in 2012, 2016, and 2017 have unravelled decades of guarded social engagement. At the height of the violence, as frightened villagers fled state-sponsored and communal violence in nearby parts of the state, remaining communities terminated all inter-communal relations across the region. In each case, only once relative peace and order was reestablished could trust be slowly rebuilt and relationships slowly, very cautiously resumed. After multiple rounds of violence, the extreme narratives about 'the other' have played deeply on fears and created deep obstacles to any sense of social cohesion or inclusion.

Commencing from late 2015, the programme has sought to subtly introduce elements to combat conflict-fuelled narratives and strengthen peace formation, using an arts-based pedagogy. The average education level in Rakhine is only Grade 4 (Republic of the Union of Myanmar 2015). In such low-literacy settings, we have found songs, stories, and poems aided retention and transmission of concepts and supported the uptake of skills in villages. But since 2016, arts have also been incorporated to provide safe, nonthreatening spaces to engage in discussion of sensitive issues. Arts-based activities have good potential to extend critical awareness-raising to understanding of conflict dynamics and explore the agency of individuals and communities in either perpetuating conflict or developing peace at local levels. At the time of writing, a three-year action research project has just been concluded, into the efficacy of arts-based CDE facilitator pedagogy in supporting everyday peace formation. Data on the arts-based pedagogy is being reported in detail elsewhere (Ware et al. under review). This chapter demonstrates strengthened everyday peace formation between ethnic Rakhine villages and their Rohingya neighbours by the development of intracommunal conflict resolution skills, helping imagine alternative futures, and building empathy toward 'the Other', resulting in increased intercommunal engagement.

Key concepts underpinning CDE's CD and peacebuilding components

Before more detailed examination of the case study, this section briefly reviews the key theoretical concepts underpinning the CDE approach to both CD and peacebuilding, explaining how they contribute to sustainably enhancing social inclusion. In particular, this section provides an overview of asset-based community development, the notion of 'everyday peace', and the potential of arts-based pedagogy in attitudinal and behavioural change to sustain development and social inclusion.

Asset-based CD and conscientisation

We designed GWM's CDE programme in 2010–11, primarily around the concepts of Asset-Based Community Development (ABCD) and *conscientisation*. ABCD starts with the premise that recognition of personal and local assets, resources, and strengths is more likely to inspire empowered action than a focus on problems, needs, and deficits. The tangible and social assets communities already possess thus become the basis for self-managing development, relying upon community leadership, social networks, and advocacy to bring about substantial change (Kretzmann and McKnight 1993; Mathie and Cunningham 2003). ABCD requires two dimensions of work with a community, one to create and seize contextual opportunities for locally led sustainable development and the other being to help them leverage outside assistance or claim their rights and entitlements as state and global citizens. In practice, this replaces professional, external development workers with the training of local individuals to facilitate participatory community processes and whole-community or representative decision-making and empowerment of community members to participate actively.

Freire's (1972) concept of *conscientisation* seeks to facilitate people to become aware in social groups of their subjugated economic or sociopolitical position, its causes, and the means available to take action against oppressive and dehumanising elements of that reality. According to Freire, economic and/or sociopolitical oppression has a dehumanising effect, which 'submerges' people until they internalise power inequalities and surrender autonomous thought and agency, becoming the objects of other's will rather than being self-determining subjects.

The solution Freire proposes is for oppressed groups to rediscover their agency through critical reflection, in so doing regaining a sense of their own humanity and agency to act upon their world. Critical-awareness raising or conscientisation is a process of facilitated self-discovery, helping people reject the internalised and dehumanising self-image imposed upon them and begin to generate personal responsibility and agency for their own condition. To Freire, this process of becoming aware of one's own oppressed condition cannot be done for others by outsiders; rather it must be won through personal struggle. However, Freire argues that neither can it be done alone; it can only occur through group dialogical encounters with others, usually requiring skilled facilitation.

Hence, CDE is designed around the principle of empowering marginalised, powerless, and poor people to overcome submergence by developing individual and communal agency and with a focus on the resources and positive attributes already existing as the basis for locally led action. Evidence from our previous research points to the greater sustainability of outcomes from such an approach (Ware 2013a, 2013b; Ware and Ware 2018). This requires helping people achieve new awareness of their circumstances, imagine their world differently, and become more empowered to take action to change their circumstances. The programme therefore does not prescribe local projects, nor bring in external experts to impart 'advanced' knowledge unless requested. Rather it trains community members to be able to facilitate community processes, to discover their own situation, context, realities, resources, and plans for change.

'Everyday peace'

The 'everyday' has been a staple in social theory for years, drawn from the ideas of philosophers and scholars, including Lefebvre, De Certeau, Foucault, Bourdieu, and even Adam Smith, Durkheim, Marx, and Engels. MacGinty (2014) proposed the concept of 'everyday peace' from this, by which he refers to the means by which individuals and groups navigate everyday life in deeply divided societies in ways that seek to avoid and minimise conflict or awkward situations, at both inter- and intra-group levels. It is thus an analytical concept based on observation of post-conflict contexts.

Based on the literature and his own field research, MacGinty has identified and elaborated five types of local action emerging post-conflict, contributing to the nonviolent reengagement of 'everyday peace', namely avoidance, ambiguity, ritualised politeness, telling, and blame deferring. At the most minimalist end of the spectrum, everyday peace may be simply eking out safe space where a façade of normality prevails, despite the conflict. At this level, it could be seen as the first and last peace: the first peace in that it can be the first inter-group contact made after violence and the last peace in the sense of being the last remaining social capital before total rupture. Noting 'everyday peace' involves considerable innovation, creativity, and improvisation, he argues it displays considerable agency in the face of overwhelming power and thus constitutes a form of resistance involving sociality, solidarity, and reciprocity. MacGinty thus conceives of 'everyday peace' as something which ruptures totalising ideas of conflict and division and thus holds potential to contribute to peace formation through the pooling of micro-solidarities. MacGinty thus argues 'everyday peace' as an important component to sustain peace initiatives and advocates for 'enhanced . . . everyday diplomacy' to complement formal approaches.

'Everyday peace' is not, however, something ever deliberately operationalised prior to this programme. Building on ABCD and *conscientisation*, since late 2015, the CDE programme has sought to introduce elements into trainings to combat conflict narratives and strengthen bottom-up peacebuilding agency. Increasingly, workshops have drawn on MacGinty's ideas in efforts to strengthen everyday peace formation.

Arts-based pedagogy

CDE facilitator training has utilised arts-based activities since its inception to allow functionally semi-literate facilitators to capture key lessons in memorable format and to celebrate progress along the way. Arts-based processes have been foundational to incorporating peacebuilding into facilitator training because arts provide safer spaces for being confronted and exploring alternative points of view.

Particularly during intractable conflicts (protracted conflict with no solution or end in sight), creativity and critical thinking are actively stifled by dominant voices, and identities become narrowed and rigid (Bar-Tal 2013). Progress toward peace formation is not possible until people can 'unfreeze' these rigid thought-patterns, consider other perspectives, and reimagine alternative futures (Cummings et al. 2016). The arts are ideal for this, providing an important, less-threatening mechanism for confrontation and change (Burnes and Cook 2013; Ware et al. under review).

By nature, the arts are symbolic and rely upon metaphor to portray complex ideas. They are widely used to shock and confront, to allow participants to distance themselves while considering sensitive or painful issues, and to express thoughts and feelings difficult to articulate verbally (Schirch 2005). They also allow multiple interpretations of an issue to exist side by side, supporting people's ability to deal with ambiguity. Arts activities can thus provide safe, nonthreatening liminal spaces, outside everyday life, which are crucial for the challenging work of exploring issues from multiple angles, healing trauma, recognising one's own role in perpetuating conflict, and imagining new ways of thinking to support peace (Hanley 2013; Hunter 2008; Shank and Schirch 2008; Schapiro 2009). The arts can create an intermediary, or liminal, space between what was and what could be.

Arts-based activities are also ideal because they facilitate broader participation, due to low skill levels required for entry to activities. They do not presume the literacy that undergirds most other approaches to peacebuilding, and the pleasurable nature of activities sustains deep engagement with subject matter (Bergh 2010). They are ideal for communities with limited literacy and potentially promote wider uptake of new ideas by allowing greater numbers of people to participate in formulating new, peace-oriented thinking and action. Bergh (2010), however, found that one-off arts-based interventions are unlikely to produce genuine change. Hence, CDE adopts a three-year process with multiple workshops to address issues in prolonged fashion for sustained change.

Case study: strengthening everyday peace formation

Central to efforts at strengthening everyday peace formation is a need to counter narrow, exclusionary conflict narratives, views of identity and 'the Other', and the lack of empathy they engender. This section offers several snapshots highlighting how we have attempted to address these and facilitate critical awareness-raising around local conflict dynamics, building participants' capacity to respond differently and contribute toward everyday peace formation. It provides narrative accounts of some of the series of workshops we have run over the past three years, presenting empirical data (translated) collected during this action research project, to highlight ways in which activities supported the development of new attitudes and reported behaviours.

Process and evidence

The first workshop, in early 2016, started with an introduction to songwriting, poetry, and storytelling and a discussion of how these might be used as learning spaces in training and in the villages. Commencing this engagement, most facilitators clearly displayed narrow, highly prejudiced views. Early songs and poems clearly focussed solely on the need for peace and development so the ethnic Rakhine could prosper and that Rakhine State belonged to the ethnic Rakhine. Occasionally throughout the three years, sentiment has been expressed that they wished the Muslims would just 'go away', clearly reflecting powerful macro-conflict narratives. Until the final year, they universally denied that they contributed to the conflict in any manner, blaming the Muslims, government, or international community for causing and perpetuating conflict. An evolution of views is clearly apparent, however, for most facilitators, as documented later.

We followed the initial workshop with an emphasis on human rights and advocacy, and human rights has become the foundation for talking about the conflict. Training commenced by reading the entire United Nations (1948) *Universal Declaration of Human Rights* as a group and discussing its implications for themselves and their Muslim neighbours. This was followed by practical training on using rights as a basis for advocating to authorities, to seek much-needed development support. In June 2017, we began to explore identities, seeking to combat the narrow discourses created by intractable conflict—i.e. 'I am Rakhine, I am Buddhist, I am good. You are Muslim, you don't belong, you are dangerous'. Through a series of activities, we began to explore the multifaceted nature of each facilitator's identity and the ways in which these different facets could become the entry point to a large number of different social groupings.

Songs written in this workshop about identity conveyed messages such as:

> We are different colours, but we're the same. Our gods are different, but we're all human beings.

Feedback at the end of the workshop included comments such as:

> We are different, but also the same. If we have peace, we can work together.

> Now I realise I have many different identities and things in common with other people around the world:

> Perspectives—look at our own and try to look from other's perspectives.

> I came to realise peace and development need to go hand in hand.

Stories written toward the end of this identities workshop showed how they were beginning to look beyond narrowly defined conflict narratives of identity and see the need for cooperation with the 'Other':

> Once there was a village, where villagers followed several different religions, and they were aggressive towards each other. At the eastern end of the village there is a deep hole. One day when the children were playing, a Muslim boy fell into the hole and died. Because it was a Muslim boy, the Christians and Buddhists said 'Oh well, let the Muslim boy die'. Then later Christian and Buddhist boys fell down the hole and died. So even though the religious leaders were fighting against each other, the villagers realised they were the ones losing their children. So they came and worked together to build a fence around the hole, to protect all of their children.

Distinctions remained sharp, however, with only partial acceptance and continued expressions implying blame, such as 'The Muslims can stay here, but only if they abide by our laws and customs'.

Feedback during the following workshop suggested they had reflected further on the identities workshop and begun to further change their own attitudes and behaviour as facilitators in their villages.

> My professional work is as a village medic. I need to show the people how I have compassion for others, and other people show the respect to me. Personally speaking, I was very selfish. But after joining this training, I realised I have different identities. I need to be humble and I need to be pleasant for others as well.

The outbreak of significant violence in August 2017, with the displacement of hundreds of thousands from townships adjacent to the areas we work, set back the process significantly. While none of our facilitators was directly affected by violence, many were in the path of Rakhine refugees fleeing south, and some villages hosted numbers of displaced for short periods, placing additional strain on already limited resources and exposing them to extreme narratives of grief and violence from just one side.

The December 2017 workshop therefore became a space for expressing that pain, fear, humiliation, and stress. Some extreme emotions were expressed, but facilitators also requested training in conflict resolution, expressing a desire to learn how trust could be rebuilt after such violence. This became an opportunity to explore the idea that there is good and bad in every person, even their enemies, underscoring their agency at local levels in a live conflict setting. If we had a perspective we hoped to convey, it was that regardless of what was happening around them, they maintained the ability to choose how to respond and that their 'enemy' is still human and needs to be perceived as such.

One poem written at this workshop illustrates their response to these ideas:

The Good and the Bad

> We can't differentiate if a person is good or bad
> by looking at their physical appearance.
> If you think a good person is human,
> Then understand that a bad person is also still human.
> Only if we interact and get to know them,
> we will know what they are thinking and planning
> Then we can decide if they are a good person or a bad person

They also began to talk about the need for compassion, tolerance, and forgiveness, as illustrated by this comment on a story shared in the workshop.

> I was impressed by the Little Frog, she forgave those who hurt her. Even though we are still in a conflict, we can love [our enemies].

By June 2018, we ran a two-day workshop for selected facilitators and community leaders, introducing the concept of everyday peace and discussing how they might be able to facilitate everyday peace formation in their local regions. We followed this by two more days of arts-based activities focusing on practical conflict resolution skills, while an October 2018 workshop re-examined the question of how seeing other people as human beings affects the way we treat them. Participant feedback shows how they were beginning to regulate their responses to the violence around them, to begin building greater social cohesion within villages as well as beginning to promote nondiscrimination and even cooperation with Muslim communities around them:

> Everybody has problems. So when being a mediator, I noticed that it's also very important to be aware of what kind of words and tone I use when I am dealing with these people. The way I do this can create the problem or can solve it.
>
> (June 2018)

A poem written in the June 2018 workshop illustrates how they processed and synthesised ideas about delaying anger and responding quietly and taking charge of their own responses to conflict.

Poem: Fire of Anger

Fiery anger can't be calmed
Greed can't be killed
Love fading
No more truth . . . Fiery anger.
Put love first
Have gratitude
Put away anger
Keep on walking with truth
The angry fire be calmed

The final 2018 workshop culminated in a large group discussion about the Rakhine-Rohingya conflict. While several vocal group members persisted in talking about the Rohingya in derogatory terms and many raised persistent concerns about Muslims coming into their villages and stealing from them (a common stereotype), approximately two thirds of the facilitators actively discussed proposals to work on everyday peace formation and voiced active support for building greater harmony with their Muslim neighbours. Some began to accept responsibility for their role in conflict and talk about what they needed to do to smooth things over with other people in order to build peace and cohesion, as illustrated by these song lyrics.

> What should I do—I've thought about it
> I can't struggle out of this darkness

Please help me my dearest friends
I think about it and I'm scared . . .

It's easy . . . They said that it's easy
Just admit your fault
Apologise and solve the problem
It will be alright . . .
Please forgive—I'm sorry . . .

I'm sorry if I did something wrong . . .
We are neighbours
I really want to talk and chat just like before
Please don't act frostily to me
I apologise for my fault
I'm sorry . . . I apologise and wish you would give me another chance to be with you like before

However, applying theory in practice is not easy. One focus group participant in June 2018 noted quite candidly that

> We learn about different identities, and we practise trying to build reconcili-
> ation between two groups, particularly Rakhine and Muslims. We learn this
> theoretically, but it's hard to implement.
>
> (June 2018)

Impacts in villages

Despite these difficulties, in June and October 2018, we began to collect detailed data from facilitators who had begun to actively promote social cohesion and inclusion in their own Rohingya–Rakhine village contexts. Many related stories of already having begun to approach Rohingya neighbours and begin rebuilding relationships as well as promoting their human rights and peacebuilding to their own communities.

There are numerous villages in central and northern Rakhine State in which Rohingya and Rakhine communities reside side by side in almost mixed villages. One of these, in Minbya township, central Rakhine State, even has a single village name, with the Rohingya and Rakhine only separated by 20 feet or so, living on either side of a small creek. The proximity only heightened fears during the height of the conflict. Indeed, tensions were so great when the intercommunal violence first erupted back in 2012 that despite the proximity, the two communities cut off all relations for two years. Rakhine refused to go into the Rohingya village, and the Rohingya did not go into the Rakhine village. Trade and other connec-tion between the two were minimal. So while there was a slow re-engagement by about 2014, the eruption of violence again in August 2017 shattered relations once again.

Yet even in such a fragile context, as early as March 2018, while refugees were still fleeing to Bangladesh, and based in large part on the CDE workshops and his new critical awareness of conflict dynamics, the CDE facilitator initiated community meetings to discuss how to rebuild trust. It was a courageous move, but he reports it led to a rapid resumption of business, even social relationships, during the course of 2018. Now, Rohingya and Rakhine are doing business together, hiring one another to work in the fields, working alongside one another in road construction, and so on. The women have set up a market at the bridge between villages to buy fish, fruit, and vegetables from one another. It was initially agreed that villagers should meet one another only at this bridge between the villages to make arrangements, hire, or trade, but by late 2018, Rohingya and Rakhine were drinking together in teashops and socialising there as much as making business arrangements. The most serious issues faced have been a few accusations of theft, but they have been investigated and resolved without serious quarrel between community members and certainly no violence all year. Village leaders are now expressing a desire to put all animosities aside and return to 'peaceful and harmonious' relations. These are small steps, but signs of real progress.

A similar mixed village in Kyauktaw Township, central Rakhine State, half Rohingya and half Rakhine, has reopened their small bazaar between the villages. Even as violence and chaos reigned in northern Rakhine, just 20 miles from them, late last year, the facilitator helped initiate discussions, and the two communities reconnected and cautiously resumed trade. Villagers now come from neighbouring Rakhine and Rohingya villages to do business daily. The Rakhine, being Buddhist, rely on the Muslims to butcher their meat, for example, but even the women come out to buy and sell from one another. The bazaar is bringing Rohingya and Rakhine into contact, facilitating conversations. Suspicion and hesitation remain, but village leaders now see the macro-violence issues as related to national-level dynamics that have little to do with their local relationships.

The situation in northern Rakhine State, where violence was experienced firsthand, remains tenser. Buddhist and Rohingya villagers from Maungdaw and Buthidaung districts, who witnessed neighbouring villages being burned in August 2017 and contemplated fleeing their homes, remain cautious, yet are reestablishing links. As the violence raged, Buddhist and Muslim leaders in one part of Buthidaung encouraged the Rohingya to stay, resulting in about a third of the local Rohingya population remaining. Informants from three local villages, on different sides of Buthidaung town, all concur that Rohingya, Rakhine, and other local minorities such as the Daignet, regularly visit one another's villages for trade and labour hire. They usually travel in groups rather than alone, and the women do not go after dark, but Rohingya, Rakhine, and other minority women all do go to one another's villages to buy and sell regularly. Trade, civility, and a semblance of suspicious normality are returning. Yet highlighting the high level of caution that remains when around members of the other community they do not personally know, one Buddhist villager described going into the main township at Maungdaw for trade recently and feeling threatened by some of the Rohingya traders who seemed to act aggressively toward them as a group. The re-emergence of interaction comes with a lack of ease and some deep suspicions, but it is re-emerging.

Back in central Rakhine state though, in Minbya township some 50 miles from where the violence occurred in 2017, perhaps the most remarkable incident occurred in yet another mixed Rakhine-Rohingya community. As the August 2017 violence raged, a group of 43 ethnic Rakhine displaced by the violence arrived in the village. The CDE facilitator, an ethnic Rakhine leader, was away in Yangon at the time, so on being notified, he phoned his good friend to seek help—a local Rohingya religious leader. The Rohingya community immediately provided about USD 120 worth of food to help these internally displaced people (equivalent to three to four months' wages for one labourer). Relations are such between the communities in this village by the end of 2018, Rohingya and Rakhine community members regularly eat and drink together, and the women from both communities come out and trade even late into the evening, hours after dark. In this community, they not only trade and work together, but Rakhine even lend money to Rohingya community members and vice versa, as need arises. The Rakhine village leaders have openly spoken to the local Rohingya, saying they should stay together in this land, that there is no need for them to leave, and urging good relationships since they have lived like brothers for a very long time. The Rakhine village leaders have also conducted village meetings urging their own ethnic community members not to discriminate against the Rohingya in any way. They are now discussing ways of embarking on livelihood and education projects together, in cooperation.

These may not be the majority of cases in Rakhine, but neither are they are rare occurrences. On the surface, given the scale of conflict, not much has changed. Some 1.1 million Rohingya Muslim refugees still shelter in Bangladesh after what the UN has labelled ethnic cleansing, and narrow conflict narratives continue to dominate social media and the public discourse. Deep fears continue to permeate both communities, and animosities run deep. There is no magic bullet. There are copious examples of poor relations, extreme fear, and even hatred of the Other, and there have been calls by some Rohingya nationalist groups to isolate the remaining Rohingya from trade and services, to drive them all out of the country by means of total social exclusion. Yet local peace is returning to some villages, and some local attitudes are changing. Some of this appears linked to the CDE programme's attempts to strengthen everyday peace formation through workshops attempting to facilitate critical awareness about conflict dynamics, by doing things like exploring the nature of human rights, re-examining identities, building empathy, and re-imagining alternative futures.

How sustainable are these changes? It is hard to say. Yet they are grounded in sustained engagement with communities through a community development approach, which is built on empowerment. The earlier evidence suggests the changes are grounded in attitudinal shifts and new understandings rather than conformity to the expectations of the external organisation. It would appear that the arts-based pedagogy has led to the 'unfreezing' (aka Lewin's model) of conflict attitudes for many participants and allowed them to critically explore new ideas and modes of operating than to 'refreeze' new behaviours and attitudes. In other words, progress in everyday peace formation appears to be sustainable based on personal attitudinal change and new critical awareness of social and conflict dynamics.

References

Bar-Tal, D. (2013) *Intractable Conflicts: Socio-psychological Foundations and Dynamics*, Cambridge: Cambridge University Press.

Bergh, A. (2010) 'I'd like to teach the world to sing: music and conflict transformation', unpublished PhD Thesis, University of Exeter.

Burnes, B. and Cooke, B. (2013) 'Kurt Lewin's field theory: a review and re-evaluation', *International Journal of Management Reviews*, 15: 408–25.

Cummings, S., Bridgman, T. and Brown, K.G. (2016) 'Unfreezing change as three steps: rethinking Kurt Lewin's legacy for change management', *Human Relations*, 69: 33–60.

Freire, P. (1972) *Pedagogy of the Oppressed*, Harmondsworth: Penguin.

Hanley, M.S. (2013) 'Introduction: culturally relevant arts education for social justice', in M.S. Hanley, G.W. Noblit, G.L. Sheppard and T. Barone (eds) *Culturally Relevant Arts Education for Social Justice*, New York: Routledge.

Human Rights Council (2018) *Report of the Independent International Fact-Finding Mission on Myanmar, A/HRC/39/64*. Online. Available at www.ohchr.org/Documents/HRBodies/HRCouncil/FFM-Myanmar/A_HRC_39_64.pdf (accessed 26 February 2019).

Hunter, M.A. (2008) 'Cultivating the art of safe space', *Research in Drama Education*, 13: 5–21.

Kretzmann, J. and McKnight, J.P. (1993) *Building Communities from the Inside Out*, Chicago: ACTA Publications.

MacGinty, R. (2014) 'Everyday peace: bottom-up and local agency in conflict-affected societies', *Security Dialogue*, 45: 548–64.

Mathie, A. and Cunningham, G. (2003) 'From clients to citizens: asset-based community development as a strategy for community-driven development', *Development in Practice*, 13: 474–86.

Republic of the Union of Myanmar (2015) *The 2014 Myanmar Population and Housing Census, Rakhine State Report, Census Report Volume 3—K*, Naypyitaw: Department of Population, Ministry of Immigration and Population, Republic of the Union of Myanmar.

Schapiro, S.A. (2009. 'A crucible for transformation: the alchemy of student-centered education for adults at midlife', in B. Fisher-Yoshida, K.G. Geller and S.A. Schapiro (eds) *Innovations in Transformative Learning: Space, Culture, and the Arts*, New York: Peter Lang.

Schirch, L. (2005) *Ritual and Symbol in Peacebuilding*, Boulder: Kumarian Press.

Shank, M. and Schirch, L. (2008) 'Strategic arts-based peacebuilding', *Peace and Change*, 33: 217–42.

United Nations (1948) 'Universal declaration of human rights'. Online. Available at www.refworld.org/docid/3ae6b3712c.html (accessed 4 November 2019).

Ware, A. (2012) *Context-Sensitive Development: How International NGOs Operate in Myanmar*, Sterling, VA: Kumarian Press.

Ware, A. (2013a) 'An assessment of empowerment through highly participatory asset-based community development in Myanmar', *Development Bulletin*, 75: 110–14.

Ware, A. (2013b) 'Asset-based community development in Myanmar: theory, fit and practice', in L. Brennan, L. Parker, T.A. Watne, J. Fien, D.T. Hue and M.A. Doan (eds) *Growing Sustainable Communities: A Development Guide for Southeast Asia*, Prahran, Victoria: Tilde University Press.

Ware, V.A. and Laoutides, C. (2018) *Myanmar's 'Rohingya' Conflict*, London: Hurst.

Ware, V.A., Lauterjung-Kelly, J. and McSolvin, S. (under review) 'Arts as learning space in conflict transformation: the contribution of the arts-based workshop to attitudinal and behaviour change'.

Ware, V.A. and Ware, V.A. (2018) 'Critical consciousness-raising amongst poor Rakhine villages in rural Myanmar', in N. Yu (ed) *Consciousness-Raising: Critical Pedagogy and Practice for Social Change*, London: Routledge.

World Bank (2015) *Data Wealth Ranking World Bank*, Yangon: MIMU Myanmar Information Management Unit. Online. Available at www.themimu.info/search/node/World%20 Bank%20Wealth%20Ranking (accessed 26 February 2019).

18 Sustaining inclusion through work

Livelihoods experience of rural Indonesian villagers with disability

Ekawati Liu, Yuhda Wahyu Pradana, Irfan Kortschak, Hezti Insriani and Erin Wilson

Introduction

Despite the prolonged rainy season, the skies on this particular Saturday were clear. The research team gathered in the yard of what is said to be the oldest primary school in the village of Sidorejo, a 50-minute drive to the south of Yogyakarta. The research team had arrived in a jovial mood, but this turned to a sense of chaos when they saw that the classrooms for the focus group discussion were filled with rows of desks and benches with extra desks and benches stacked to the ceiling against the wall. This layout was completely unsuitable for the planned activity. Candy wrappers, scrap paper, bottle caps, broken pencils, straws, and a torn plastic fan from yesterday's school sessions littered the floor. The team hurriedly rearranged the seating to create the necessary space, swept the floor clean, and checked the width of the doors to ensure that everyone would be able to enter. There was no point talking about ideas like 'universal access' if people in wheelchairs couldn't even get in the door. Before the research team members could catch their breath, two female participants with disabilities arrived early with baskets of rempeyek (peanut and anchovies crackers). 'Can we sell these here?' they asked opportunistically. On pieces of scrap paper, they wrote 'AYO BELI! ["Come and buy!"] Rp 3000'. Filled with hope, they left their baskets of wares on the already crowded registration desk. Within half an hour, the laughter and voices of participants with a diverse range of disabilities from six villages filled the main hall. Some of them had been dropped off; others were accompanied by family members. Some came with other participants who used modified three-wheeled motorbikes. Some came with their children. Some walked. They had come to discuss issues related to economic and social inclusion for people with disabilities, a subject dear to their hearts. Amongst other burning issues, they were there to address these questions: How can we make ends meet? How can we cope with precarity and insecure livelihood conditions? How does our disability, gender, and age influence livelihoods access, choice, and expansion? In what ways does our participation or nonparticipation in formal or informal economic activities shape our social roles and degree of acceptance in community?

This chapter describes a research project conducted in rural Indonesia that used collaborative and multi-methods participatory approaches to explore and address issues related to the livelihoods of people with disabilities. While this chapter aims to highlight the value and process of collaborative and participatory inquiry to understanding the livelihoods experiences and situations of villagers with disability, it also aims to provide insights into how the participation or nonparticipation of people with disabilities in formal or informal economic activities shape their social role and their degree of acceptance in the community. Our findings remind us that social and economic inclusion are interdependent phenomena and a sustainable development approach must recognise and build on this complex relationship.

The economic exclusion of people with disabilities

Facilitating the equal social inclusion of people with disabilities is an explicit goal of the *Convention on the Rights of Persons with Disabilities* (United Nations 2006). This *Convention* reaffirms the right of people with disabilities to economic participation, particularly the right to work or to otherwise generate a livelihood on 'an equal basis to others' (Article 27). Despite this intention, the worldwide unemployment rate for people with disabilities in developing countries remains a significant issue, with unemployment levels as high as 80 per cent for some groups (United Nations 2007; World Health Organization and World Bank 2011). In addition, the experiences of people with disability in the areas of livelihoods and economic participation in developing countries have received only relatively recent and ad hoc inclusion in policy design and intervention strategies (Lepper 2007). Past and current approaches to economic development and the inclusion of people with disabilities still focus narrowly on people with disabilities' participation in the labour market; access to decent work; and formal employment (Hanass-Hancock and Mitra 2016; Lepper 2007). In particular, they tend to overlook crucial challenges related to the realities that people face in the area of livelihoods in the Global South, most particularly in rural areas (Grech and Soldatic 2016).

The concept of livelihoods is a complex one and beyond the scope of this chapter. An enormous body of work on livelihoods (mostly focusing on Sub-Saharan Africa and South Asia) utilises a broad understanding of livelihoods, as exemplified by the definition proposed by Chambers and Conway.

> A livelihood comprises the capabilities, assets (stores, resources, claims and access) and activities required for a means of living: a livelihood is sustainable which can cope with and recover from stress and shocks, maintain or enhance its capabilities and assets, and provide sustainable livelihood opportunities for the next generation; and which contributes net benefits to other livelihoods at the local and global levels and in the short and long term.
>
> (Chambers and Conway 1992: 7–8)

For the purpose of this chapter, the concept of *livelihoods* is focused on *work or labour performed either at home or in the community to provide either goods or services to others and to meet the needs of the individual and his or her family.* When focusing on issues related to livelihoods in rural areas in the Global South, there is often a dangerous and misguided assumption that people in these areas rely solely on strategies involving the use of land and other natural resources for their livelihoods. This assumption fails to recognise the importance of non-agricultural and non-resource-based activities in these areas, thus leading to failed interventions. Bebbington (1999) proposes a broader conceptual framework that recognises the importance of these activities. Basing his argument on studies on access to resources, he states that people's livelihoods shift from a dependence on natural resources to 'livelihoods based on a range of assets, income sources, product and labor markets' (Bebbington 1999: 2023). Thus, he argues, there is a need for an expanded conceptual framework that recognises five different types of capital assets as being significant to the livelihood experiences of people in rural areas, these being *produced, human, natural, social*, and *cultural* capital. Such an understanding begins to foreshadow the interconnection between social and economic development.

Similarly, an exploration of the meaning of 'work' also recognises the relationship between work, culture, and social identity. The concept of work is a highly fluid one, as suggested by the prominent economic anthropologist, Karl Polanyi (1944, 1977), who argued that work and labour can be considered as activities embedded in community and culture, often based on exchange and reciprocity. This conception of work has broad implications for how work and type of work affects cultural and community status. The relationship between work (either paid or unpaid) and social identity has been highlighted by sociologists and academic scholars since the 1950s, with a number of recent studies on precarious work and unemployment demonstrating the subliminal dimension of work, which recognises that work provides a space to make individual lives meaningful and dignified (Kwon and Lane 2016), as judged both by the individual and the broader community. This set of understandings suggests that the manner in which people with disabilities are perceived and the degree to which they are accepted in the broader community is significantly affected by their access to and the nature of their work or livelihoods.

Although it has been claimed that livelihoods and enterprise activities are effective strategies to address the social exclusion, as well as poverty, of people with disabilities in developing countries, the evidence for this conclusion remains weak. This is largely because researchers have not specifically sought to address the particular needs of people with disabilities, particularly those in rural areas (Grech 2016; Hanass-Hancock and Mitra 2016). Gustafson and Brunger (2014: 999) argue that this omission is partly due to a dominant paradigm that regards people with disability as 'abnormal, deficient, deviant, and in need of fixing or treatment and paternalistic protection'. This paradigm perpetuates an approach that strongly emphasises initiatives to *rehabilitate* people with disability rather than programs that allow them to meet their own needs on a sustainable basis by ensuring their access to economic and livelihoods opportunities that meet their specific needs and that are suited to their individual circumstances.

In recognition of the relationship between social and economic inclusion, increasing the degree of participation of people with disabilities in development programs that focus on improving livelihoods and economic development could facilitate both a reduction in poverty as well as a transformation in public opinion regarding people with disabilities who are often perceived as being a burden on society (Colbran 2010). Economic development programs, including disability-specific and non-disability-specific initiatives (such as general poverty reduction and social protection programs), should therefore include measures not only to provide some measure of financial support to people with disability, but also to increase inclusion and promote the economic, social, and political participation of those with disabilities (Department for International Development [DFID] 2018). However, further evidence is needed to ensure that these ideas inform the development and implementation of poverty reduction and/or inclusion practice. The study discussed later specifically explores the inter-relationship between social and economic inclusion through a focus on the livelihood experiences of rural Indonesians with a disability.

The Indonesian context: the emerging power of the village for the economic inclusion of marginalised groups

In recent decades, Indonesia has implemented a massive decentralisation initiative that has devolved power from the central level of government to local levels, often involving extremely high levels of community participation. At the same time, the paradigm for international development has also evolved, with increased demand for cross-cutting approaches, particularly with the active involvement of civil society organisations and people with disability in informing and driving poverty reduction and inclusion efforts. Examples of this new paradigm can be found in *Transforming our World: the 2030 Agenda for Sustainable Development* (United Nations 2015) and the *2018 Disability Global Summit* (UK Government 2018). The manner in which Indonesian poverty reduction initiatives have been conceptualised, designed, and implemented provides an excellent example of the confluence of these agendas.

Since 1997, Indonesia has implemented an extensive rural poverty reduction effort through a community-driven development programme, particularly through an umbrella programme known as *Programme Nasional Pemberdayaan Masyarakat* (PNPM). The programme is implemented by providing block grants to communities to enable them to determine their own priorities and plans. To develop these priorities and plans, communities are provided with technical assistance by village facilitators, who guide and train the communities to develop basic skills in participatory planning, community self-management, capacity building, and oversight. With small initial pilot studies commencing less than two decades ago, the community-driven approach has now been formally adopted as

Indonesia's principal national strategy for poverty reduction. In 2011, this programme was refined and enhanced to focus more specifically on marginalised groups. In recognition of the low level of participation of marginalised groups in village meetings and decision-making process, the Indonesian government launched a large-scale pilot to support civil society organisations (including disability-specific organisations) involved in poverty reduction, social justice, and inclusion on the basis that these organisations had the specific skills and capacities to reach marginalised segments of communities.

Building on the recognised success of this programme, the Indonesian government sought to incorporate the programme's principles and practices more broadly into governance systems across the country. In January 2014, Indonesia's Parliament enacted the *Village Law*, which was intended to provide villages with an unprecedented high level of autonomy and authority. This *Village Law* is expected to significantly impact the lives of marginalised groups, including persons with disabilities, because it provides villages with a far greater degree of autonomy to determine their governance structures, development priorities, and natural resources management, among other issues, at the local level (Antlöv et al. 2016). According to this law, up to 10 per cent of the national budget is allocated for disbursement to village-level institutions, with the use of these funds to be determined through a highly participatory process. Although this will result in a significant increase to the value of funds available to villages, mechanisms to involve marginalised groups in villages (including people with disability) in governance planning and decision-making processes are still nascent.

Following the enactment of the *Village Law*, SIGAB (a local organisation advocating for the rights of people with disability based in the district of Sleman) convened a three-day community meeting with representatives from a coalition of grassroots disability organisations, neighbouring villagers, and community leaders. The meeting resulted in a high level of public and political support for the implementation of the Inclusive Village Model (*Rintisan Desa Inklusi*, usually referred to as RINDI). Following a mapping of the conditions of people with disability and related service gaps at subsequent village-level consultations, RINDI was launched in June 2015 in eight villages. The Inclusive Village initiative envisions the creation of a range of village models, each with accessible and inclusive services and resources that are available for everyone ('universal access'). It is intended that these models should be easily replicated so they can be adopted by other villages. The strategies adopted involved cultural approaches, increased access to communication facilities and other resources (including livelihoods and savings and loan programs), and measures to establish networks between people with disabilities and other marginalised groups.

Given the lack of evidence about relevant and sustainable economic development initiatives for people with disability in the Global South and in this Indonesian initiative in particular, a research project was established to explore the experiences of rural villagers with disability in six villages participating in the Inclusive Village initiative. The project and its results are described as follows.

Exploring the voices and livelihood choices of villagers with disability in Indonesia

To better understand the lived experiences of people with disability and to achieve better informed policy development and interventions, scholars involved in disability studies have advocated a critical (Rioux and Bach 1994; Grech 2016), participatory (Gustafson and Brunger 2014; Oden et al. 2010; Vaughan et al. 2015), and interdisciplinary (Fisher et al. 2016) approach to research. They have also emphasised that both the process and product of research need to be of practical utility for the participants (Shore 2007). This emerging trend also aligns with a broader conceptual framework proposed by Scoones (2009, 2015) and Bebbington (1999) for approaches to livelihoods and poverty. Recent discussions in the field of critical disability emphasise the need for holistic and nuanced disability-oriented livelihoods frameworks to assess the livelihoods situation of people with disability in the Global South and for an interdisciplinary and participatory approach to deepen the research base. Hanass-Hancock and Mitra (2016) point out that excessive emphasis in the area of disability studies on isolated components (e.g. malnutrition, inaccessible working conditions, barriers to financial capital, income, health, and education) are associated with the failure of livelihoods interventions and insufficient evidence on the effectiveness of livelihoods programs of Community-Based Rehabilitation (CBR).

This context shaped the design of this research project which emphasised an exploration of the lived reality of villagers with disability regarding their livelihoods choices within the Inclusive Village initiative, with the findings informing strategies for sustainable economic and social inclusion. The research process and the outcomes of this process are intended to improve the general level of understanding of the nature of people with disability's economic participation and the interactions between disability, gender, age, and social capital in determining their social and economic inclusion or exclusion.

Research was conducted in the period from November 2017 to May 2018 in six villages in Kulon Progo district, these being Bumirejo, Gulurejo, Ngentakrejo, Wahyuharjo, Jatirejo, and Sidorejo, and in two villages in Sleman district, these being Sendangadi and Sendangtirto. All eight villages had been involved in the Inclusive Village Initiative (RINDI) since 2015. The research project was conducted in collaboration with SIGAB, with funding provided through the Asia Foundation's Peduli Programme and a research scholarship from the Australian Department of Foreign Affairs and Trade.

Stages of collaborative research

The disability rights movement has embraced a paradigm that proposes the full participation of people with disability in all aspects of community life, but most particularly in the conceptualisation, formulation, and implementation of disability policy, practice, and research ('Nothing about Us, Without Us'). The involvement of people with disability in research underpins emancipatory and participatory methodologies as well as intersecting with a disability rights framework, where participatory research can be understood as both a practical and political tool. A key goal is to create space for people with disability to facilitate transformative changes, both at the personal and community level. In addition, given that a central critique of the decentralised model in Indonesia was the lack of participation of people with disability in the deliberative space (for example, in village governance and decision-making regarding decentralised funds), a participatory approach in this project also aimed to explore and potentially model increased deliberative roles for people with disability.

The design and approach of collaborative and participatory livelihoods research described in this chapter was also shaped by intersectional thinking that sees disability as a complex phenomenon involving widely varying personal experiences and responses. Each person deals with disability differently: the unique experiences and perspectives of each person with disability is strongly influenced by factors such as age, gender, belief, geography, and socioeconomic backgrounds.

With the adoption of a participatory approach, this study involved 13 Indonesian researchers from a diverse range of backgrounds and abilities. In addition, villagers with disability were invited to participate in village-level discussion groups and individual interviews and also in creating public theatre performances. The research was conducted in stages, with the processes and findings from each stage informing the subsequent design and approaches of the next stage, as described later.

Stage one

SIGAB facilitated the recruitment process for researchers in mid-October 2017, resulting in the recruitment of a team of 13 Indonesian researchers with diverse backgrounds and abilities. The gender and disability to non-disability composition of the team mirrored the reality in the field, with five females and eight males, and five researchers with disability and eight without disability. The principal researcher from Deakin University and the research supervisors from SIGAB conducted briefings and research capacity training for a week prior to the data collection process. The training aimed to equip the researchers with interviewing skills and knowledge regarding disability, including the etiquette for dealing with people with disability and research ethics. Throughout this training process, all members worked on building rapport and developing relationships between the team through ongoing discussions and debates on real-life disability issues. They were also given the opportunity to apply the knowledge and skills they had learned related to the livelihoods situations of marginalised groups through engaging in mock focus group discussions and role-plays. These hands-on activities were also part of a participatory strategy to ensure that all members of the team remained actively engaged in the learning process. Time was allocated for the team to practice interviewing and probing skills using research instruments with SIGAB staff members and visitors. All members provided input on the types of data to be collected and revised the interview instruments prior to the data collection process. Due to the widely varying backgrounds and abilities of the researchers, novice researchers were paired with experienced researchers in the field to create opportunities for a transfer of skills and knowledge between researchers; to facilitate improved communication; and to maintain a positive work ethic.

Data was collected through in-depth interviews with 157 people with disability, with the subjects aged from 20 to 65-plus (116 adults in Kulon Progo and 41 adults in Sleman). In addition, three focus group sessions were held in each district, with the groups consisting of women with disability, men with disability, and a deaf-only group.

To facilitate communication between two deaf researchers, deaf respondents in the villages, and those without proficiency in sign, local sign language interpreters were deployed, and real-time captioning was used. For respondents identified as having intellectual disability (with cognitive limitations and/or communication difficulties), the team utilised a paired interviewing strategy, in which individual respondents were interviewed together with someone they interacted and communicated with on a daily basis.

Stage two

The team analysed the collected data using a participatory data analysis approach. The team members had widely varying levels of educational attainment, some with high school diplomas, most with undergraduate degrees, and three with masters-level qualifications. Thus, to ensure the effective participation of all members of the team, the team's learning approach for processes related to data analysis was experiential and conversational to support team members to reflect on findings. Over nearly two months, all interview and focus group transcripts were coded, with an intensive process of discussion to identify themes before formally conducting the concept mapping process of overall findings.

During this data analysis stage, the research team and SIGAB also coordinated with local theatre activists to design training modules to facilitate People's Theatre workshops for 12 interested research participants. Preliminary findings generated from the collaborative data analysis process served to provide material for discussion to be included in the People's Theatre workshop sessions. This approach allowed research participants to verify and revise the findings. At the workshop, they learned a range of different communication techniques, including through body movement, facial expressions, and voice. They also developed the confidence and courage to perform in front of an audience, with these performances including the highly personal sharing of their stories, thoughts, and memories related to making a living, being rejected, and/or accepted by others and their hopes for themselves and society more generally. With support from the facilitators, the performers created plays and dialogues.

Those involved in the project did not anticipate the level of support and interest expressed by the general public, particularly in the People's Theatre performances. A large number of audience members became actively involved in discussions on alternative outcomes to scenarios performed. These discussions were held immediately after the plays were performed, providing feedback and input directly to the performers.

Stage three

The process of writing and disseminating the report involved half of the research team, as half had no interest or ability in these processes. The remaining six-member team collectively wrote the research report, developed an accompanying infographic, and assisted the local community visual ethnography team, Ethnoreflika, on the video-related documentation of the People's Theatre workshop and play sessions. Three team members joined the Ethnoreflika team and returned to research sites to document the daily lives and economic activities of villagers to produce a documentary film, which was not part of the research project, rather part of research dissemination. SIGAB also conducted workshops with officers from local government agencies to discuss research findings and to incorporate their proposed solutions and feedback in a final report to the funding agency.

Findings and discussion

The study found that seven in every ten participants in rural areas and five in ten in peri-urban areas engaged in informal work activities. Almost half of them engaged in more than one livelihood activity to meet daily needs or income needs. The majority of villagers with disability engaged in livelihoods diversification and participated in the informal economy as tofu factory workers, goat or chicken farmers, mechanics, garbage collectors, home-based food business owners, broom makers, masseuses, shopkeepers, tailors, restaurant clerks, batik makers, carpenters, toy sellers, and *angkringan* (a popular light-bite hawker).

Financial inclusion and financial literacy as crucial steps to social (and economic) inclusion

In the absence of access to the labour market and limited employment opportunities, loans can be considered as a key enabling factor for people with disability to become self-employed or to promote their inclusion in the labour market. Loans in this context refer to financial services that include the formal provision of money or capital to people with low earnings/limited assets or informal self-organised credit/saving within a group or community. Participants in focus group discussions obtained money from either formal institutions or informal networks. They did not experience significant barriers in accessing loans and used certificates of land and/or vehicle ownership as collateral. Although the role of social networks and trust with regard to sponsorship and lending behaviours was left largely unexplored during focus group discussions, we noted that those lacking the minimum to meet asset requirements for loans but who had viable livelihoods were able to obtain loans through informal channels (such as by joining group rotating savings and credit in their villages, attending yasinan[1], and borrowing from family/relatives/friends and village heads) and Islamic microfinance. Under the sponsorship of family members, some research participants who had no and/ or low assets were able to access formal loans. Those who had performed well with their efforts tended to have their loans increased by formal institutions in subsequent years. Interestingly, our findings relating to the usage of loans are consistent with the literature (e.g. Banerjee et al. 2015), where access to credit is beneficial and has a positive effect on measures of well-being, investment, and daily needs. The participants used the loans to improve their housing conditions, such as installing electricity or adding a roof on the house, purchase a motorbike to work or deliver their products, pay for their child's school uniform and fees, for general consumption (food purchases), and community giving. While this is a positive finding evidencing people with disability's access to formal credit, it also highlights the importance of social capital in the provision of informal finance, identifying a significant barrier to finance for those without adequate or relevant social networks.

Three reasons were given by those who did not use financial services. The first was fear of inability to repay the loans. Such fear is warranted as villagers reported hearing stories of other people unable to pay back loans in their villages due to not having regular income. As a result, some participants hesitated to take out loans or seek information pertaining to flexible repayment arrangements from loan and saving institutions. Second, borrowing money with interest is considered to be *riba*, a violation of the Islamic code of conduct. Third, participants did not see the need for business loans due to reliance on informal social safety nets or support from parents or relatives to meet their basic needs, cope with household hardship, obtain occasional one-off job offers or purchase orders, or obtain chickens and goats.

It is worth noting that the majority of informants with disability displayed a low level of financial knowledge and understanding. Many did not keep records on their household budget and income. More than half of the respondents we interviewed allowed non-disabled family members to hold the saving accounts and make financial decisions on their behalf. Such limited understanding of finances or lack of financial skills had considerable impact on utilisation of financial services as well as independence/self-sufficiency.

Microfinance generally has proven successful both throughout Indonesia and elsewhere. It has the potential to support assets building, ease financial burdens of households with disability, cushion individuals with disability and their families from economic shocks, and improve children's well-being and health outcomes (DeLoach and Lamanna 2011; Posso and Athukorala 2018). However, the majority of microfinance programs have limited or no outreach to people with disability. While several online lending platforms (people to people or group to people) exist in Indonesia, the low literacy and technology usage among those in rural or peri-urban areas, including people with disability, means that such platforms automatically and inadvertently exclude these groups. Our research strongly suggests that there is a niche opportunity for a microfinance programme focused on people with disability, particularly if offered in tandem with small business training. The establishment of a microfinance programme structured to adapt to the unique circumstances of people with disability would open up opportunities for both lenders and borrowers. There would be, perhaps, space to invest in people with disability beginning a new business, through this initiative and, contingent on success, bridging opportunities to transition into standard existing microfinance programs, increasing the inclusion of people with disability in the mainstream economy.

Economic roles and labour of women with disability are largely unacknowledged

Various factors influenced the participation of women with disability in livelihoods and economic activities. From women-only focus group discussions, we learned women who worked prior to becoming disabled choose not to work after they became disabled. These women felt that their disability affects their mobility and capacity to work. They also dealt with disability-related health issues (i.e. they were easily tired or frequently sick). Interestingly, gender roles were also a factor in women ceasing income-generating activities, as some reported giving up their role as the primary breadwinner in order to care for a sick child or parent.

When women with disability were asked for their reasons for engaging in employment or economic activities, some cited working as their obligation to the family. 'As long as I'm able to work, I will work' is the attitude adopted by those who wished to remain productive and avoid unemployment. Some mentioned they enjoyed working, feeling useful, and not burdening others. Those not participating in employment or income-generating activities tended to do unpaid work around the house, like parenting, caretaking of sick family members, housekeeping, and cooking for other family members. In addition to (physical) disability, their lack of skills, and start-up capital, as well as a mismatch between their skills and work opportunities, were reasons why they stayed home. In some instances, previous failure to maintain livelihoods resulted in less motivation to try again, also affecting the participation of women with disability in economic activities.

Within international development and the recent *Millennium* and *Sustainable Development Goals* debates, gender has been considered as an essential component in a broader poverty reduction agenda (Chen et al. 2004; Molyneux 2002); however, the economic roles and labour of women with disability remain neglected and not well understood. Our research identifies the need for future research to explore how women with disability can expand their economic participation and work choices to improve life quality. Such research needs to encompass what specific challenges they face and strategies utilised to manage competing demands of work, family, and personal illness (stemming from disability).

Social capital and disability inclusion: 'I work to earn money. When I have money, I can give to the community and be accepted'

One unexpected finding from the research process related to the importance of establishing networks and social capital through giving to the community. During the focus group discussions, a large number of participants agreed that donating food, money, labour, and time was vital to facilitate their inclusion in the community. 'Even if I didn't have enough to eat or any money to give, I would borrow money to donate my fair share', stated one informant. Others added that one of the reasons they worked was to be able to donate and thus to ensure this acceptance within the community. For example:

> I work hard so I can donate my fair share. I worry that if I didn't donate and I got sick, no one would help me. Thus, whenever members of the community solicit donations for wedding, medical treatment, or community events in this village, I donate my fair share. It doesn't matter if I don't have enough to feed myself. I'd borrow money to make sure that I could make a contribution to neighbor and community.
>
> (Person with disability who works as garbage collector)

Participants of both genders expressed these sentiments. They saw working as a means not only to meet their needs, but to establish their value to the community and to benefit from a sense of belonging. This finding carries important theoretical and practical implications regarding disability inclusion and merits further exploration.

Reflections and conclusions

As discussed previously, work is a complex phenomenon with more than financial gain at stake. This research identifies that most rural villagers with disability are engaged in informal work, with many piecing together a series of economic activities into a livelihood. A focus on formal work and participation in the labour market, a cornerstone of much economic development policy, would appear to have little relevance in this context. By contrast, a focus on building the skills and knowledge of rural villagers with disability around small business management, markets, business setup and incorporation, business technology, and establishing networks would provide a relevant response to encourage livelihood development as well as support its longevity.

Kwon and Lane (2016: 7) suggest that 'work produces value—material, moral, symbolic, and social—and constitutes ways of life and forms of individual and collective identity as well as exclusion'. Consistent with this, the experience of research participants identifies an iterative relationship between economic participation and social inclusion: the ability to economically contribute to community activities (through donations) builds social capital, whilst social capital is necessary to support livelihood development via loans and other forms of support. This points to a key element of successful and sustainable social development—that social and economic inclusion cannot be treated separately but need to be attended to as two parts of a whole.

Economic and social inclusion for rural Indonesian villagers with disability are dependent on participation in key deliberative mechanisms of the village and of wider social and economic programs (such as *Village Law*). This participation is fundamentally linked to attitudes toward people with disability and constructions of disability. The process of participating in research, and in particular the public theatre performance was a mechanism to change the way disability is viewed, challenge exclusive social relations, and open up opportunities for discussion of economic participation for people with disability. In this context, villagers with disability came to be seen as valued community members with the desire and potential for equal roles in economic participation as well as village decision-making about this.

Overall this research highlights the complex nature of economic and social inclusion, even within an explicitly inclusive and deliberative structural change programme in Indonesia, that of *Village Law* and the Inclusive Village Model (*Rintisan Desa Inklusi*, RINDI). The findings from rural Indonesia demonstrate that no single circumstance produces economic inclusion: it is based on social networks, access to finance, religious, and social supports, economic opportunities and capabilities, social roles and gender, and attitudes to disability, all occurring within a social policy setting that offers opportunity to shape funding support to meet local needs. In this context, sustainable social development for people with disability requires a set of structural, social, cultural, and economic conditions that are responsive to the complexity and diversity of the lives of people with disability.

Note

1 Yasinan derived its name from Yasin, one chapter in the Qur'an. It is one of traditional religious practices common in rural areas and mostly done once a week on Thursday night. It is sort of community gathering with religious purposes where the Yasin chapter is read out loud together.

References

Antlöv, H., Wetterberg, A. and Dharmawan, L. (2016) 'Village governance, community life, and the 2014 village law in Indonesia', *Bulletin of Indonesian Economic Studies*, 52: 161–83.

Banerjee, A., Karlan, D. and Zinman, J. (2015) 'Six randomized evaluations of micro-credit: introduction and further steps', *American Economic Journal: Applied Economics*, 7: 1–21.

Bebbington, A. (1999) 'Capitals and capabilities: a framework for analyzing peasant viability, rural livelihoods and poverty', *World Development*, 27: 2021–44.

Chambers, R. and Conway, G. (1992) *IDS Discussion Paper 296. Sustainable Rural Livelihoods: Practical Concepts for the 21st Century*, Brighton: Institute of Development Studies. Online. Available at www.ids.ac.uk/publications/sustainable-rural-livelihoods-practical-concepts-for-the-21st-century/ (accessed 14 March 2019).

Chen, M.A., Vanek, J. and Carr, M. (2004) *Mainstreaming Informal Employment and Gender in Poverty Reduction: A Handbook for Policy-makers and Other Stakeholders*, London: Commonwealth Secretariat. Online. Available at www.wiego.org/sites/default/files/publications/files/Chen-Mainstreaming-Informal-Employment-and-Gender.pdf (accessed 13 March 2019).

Colbran, N. (2010) *Access to Justice Persons with Disabilities Indonesia: Background Assessment Report*. Report submitted to AUSAID. Online. Available at www.ilo.org/wcmsp5/groups/public/@asia/@ro-bangkok/@ilo-jakarta/documents/publication/wcms_160337.pdf (accessed 14 March 2019).

DeLoach, S.B. and Lamanna, E. (2011) 'Measuring the impact of microfinance on child health outcomes in Indonesia', *World Development*, 39: 1808–19.

Department for International Development [DFID] (2018) *DFID's Strategy for Disability Inclusive Development 2018–23*, London: DFID. Online. Available at https://assets.publishing.service.gov.uk/government/uploads/system/uploads/attachment_data/file/760997/Disability-Inclusion-Strategy.pdf (accessed 27 February 2019).

Fisher, K.R., Shang, X. and Xie, J. (2016) 'Global south—north partnerships: intercultural methodologies in disability research', in S. Grech and K. Soldatic (eds) *Disability in the Global South*, Cham: Springer.

Grech, S. (2016) 'Disability and development: critical connections, gaps and contradictions', in S. Grech and K. Soldatic (eds) *Disability in the Global South*, Cham: Springer.

Grech, S and Soldatic, K. (eds) (2016) *Disability in the Global South*, Cham: Springer.

Gustafson, D.L. and Brunger, F. (2014) 'Ethics, "vulnerability," and feminist participatory action research with a disability community', *Qualitative Health Research*, 24: 997–1005.

Hanass-Hancock, J. and Mitra, S. (2016) 'Livelihoods and disability: the complexities of work in the global south', in S. Grech and K. Soldatic (eds) *Disability in the Global South*, Cham: Springer.

Kwon, J.B. and Lane, C.M. (eds) (2016) *Anthropologies of Unemployment: New Perspectives on Work and Its Absence*, Ithaca: Cornell University Press.

Lepper, F. (2007) *The Employment Situation of People with Disabilities: Towards Improved Statistical Information*, Geneva: International Labour Office. Online. Available at www.ilo.org/wcmsp5/groups/public/—ed_emp/—ifp_skills/documents/publication/wcms_173498.pdf (accessed 27 February 2019).

Molyneux, M. (2002) 'Gender and the silences of social capital: lessons from Latin America', *Development and Change*, 33: 167–88.

Oden, K., Hernandez, B. and Hidalgo, M. (2010) 'Payoffs of participatory action research: racial and ethnic minorities with disabilities reflect on their research experiences', *Community Development*, 41: 21–31.

Polanyi, K. (1944) *The Great Transformation*, New York: Farrar and Rinehart.

Polanyi, K. (1977) *Livelihoods of Man: Studies in Social Discontinuity*, New York: Academic Press.

Posso, A. and Athukorala, P.C. (2018) 'Microfinance and child mortality', *Applied Economics*, 50: 2313–24.

Rioux, M.H. and Bach, M. (1994) *Disability Is Not Measles: New Research Paradigms in Disability*, Canada: L'Institut Roeher.

Scoones, I. (2009) 'Livelihoods perspectives and rural development', *The Journal of Peasant Studies*, 36: 171–96.

Scoones, I. (2015) *Sustainable Livelihoods and Rural Development*, Rugby: Practical Action Publishing.

Shore, N. (2007) 'Community-based participatory research and the ethics review process', *Journal of Empirical Research on Human Research Ethics*, 2: 31–41.

UK Government (2018) 'Global disability summit 2018'. Online. Available at www.gov.uk/government/topical-events/global-disability-summit-2018 (accessed 24 November 2019).

United Nations (2006) 'Convention on the rights of persons with disabilities'. Online. Available at www.un.org/development/desa/disabilities/convention-on-the-rights-of-persons-with-disabilities/convention-on-the-rights-of-persons-with-disabilities-2.html (accessed 4 November 2019).

United Nations (2007) *Fact Sheet: Employment of Persons with Disabilities*, Geneva: United Nations Department of Public Information. Online. Available at www.un.org/disabilities/documents/toolaction/employmentfs.pdf (accessed 12 March 2019).

United Nations (2015) 'Transforming our world: the 2030 agenda for sustainable development'. Online. Available at https://sustainabledevelopment.un.org/post2015/transformingourworld/publication (accessed 4 November 2019).

Vaughan, C., Zayas, J., Devine, A., Gill-Atkinson, L., Marella, M., Garcia, J., Bisda, K., Salgado, J., Sobritchea, C., Edmonds, T. and Baker, S. (2015) 'W-DARE: a three-year program of participatory action research to improve the sexual and reproductive health of women with disabilities in the Philippines', *BMC Public Health*, 15: 984.

World Health Organization and World Bank (2011) *World Report on Disability*, Washington: World Health Organization. Online. Available at www.who.int/disabilities/world_report/2011/report.pdf?ua=1 (accessed 14 March 2019).

19 The potential of Information and Communication Technology (ICT) to create sustainable caring communities

Zsolt Bugarszki

Caring communities in a network society

Traditionally, a community is considered as a small or large social unit, whose members know each other, share common values or interests and a sense of place, and which is situated in a given geographical area where they do things together (Bell and Newby 1972). Another important element of communities is described in the classic work of Ferdinand Tönnies (2012) *Gemeinschaft und Gesellschaft*. Tönnies describes Gemeinshaft (in English: community) as something characterised by a natural will. Community relations are governed by natural ties and friendship, neighbourhood, and old habits. Informal bounds are more important in communities than institutionalised or protocolised formal relations.

The fostering element of communities became more relevant in the work of American scientist Robert Putnam, who emphasised the idea of social capital in his book *Bowling Alone: The Collapse and Revival of American Community*.

> Whereas physical capital refers to physical objects and human capital refers to the properties of individuals, social capital refers to connections among individuals—social networks and the norms of reciprocity and trustworthiness that arise from them.
>
> (Putnam 2000: 19)

Putnam concluded that traditional communities that are characterised by strong social bonds and are connected to specific geographical locations that are disappearing. He empirically demonstrates a drop in social capital in the contemporary United States, pointing out that, while in 1975 the average American entertained friends at home 15 times per year, the equivalent figure in 1998 was barely half that. Family dinners dropped by 43 per cent and attending club meetings by 58 per cent (Putnam 2000).

Parallel to the decline of traditional communities, the 'network society' as described by urban sociologist and social movement researcher Manuel Castells (2009) has become more important. Castells investigated the connection between technology, economy and society and how these were reflected in urban structure.

He defines 'network' explicitly as a set of interconnected nodes, emphasising that networks do not have one centre but are characterised by decentralised structures and decision-making patterns. The existence of networks is determined by the utility of the nodes of the network.

Castells further highlights that technological development is the most important precondition for the resurge of networks. The emergence of networks as an efficient form of social organisation is the result of three features that have proved their usefulness in the emerging techno-economic environment (Anttiroiko 2015):

1   Flexibility: they can reconfigure, keeping their goals while changing their components. They go around blocking points of communication channels to find new connections.
2   Scalability: they can expand or shrink in size with little disruption.
3   Survivability: because they have no centre and can operate in a wide range of configurations, they can resist attacks to their nodes and codes because the codes of the network are contained in multiple nodes that can reproduce the instructions and find new ways to perform (Castells et al. 2004).

While Putnam (2000) warned us that our traditional, local communities are vanishing and called for a renewed civic engineering, Castells emphasised the raise of the network society where technological development has an important role in creating new types of communities which replace or complement the functions of traditional ones. The main question is whether those communities emerging in the network society are also able to develop the caring, containing character of traditional communities. When Putnam discussed social capital, he referred not purely to the connections between individuals but how these connections develop the atmosphere of reciprocity and trustworthiness.

The principle of reciprocity was described by Karl Polányi as one of the distribution schemes in the economy with a very strong social element through a claimed mutual dependency. He defined reciprocity as the mutual exchange of goods or services as part of long-term relationships (Servet 2007). In this long-term relationship, economic activities are embedded and enmeshed in social relations instead of relying on formal institutions. In this way, economic actors are not atomised and utilitarian individuals, but are in fact positioned within specific historical contexts in various social networks (Ghezzi and Mingione 2007).

Drawing on Castells' concept of network society, we were particularly interested in communities emerging from networks created by modern information and communication technology tools. Our pilot project aimed to explore if these new types of communities are able to develop a caring element that makes them able to contain and hold vulnerable people, contributing to their independent life in the community. We assumed that if these elements can appear in modern networks, then the new form of communities generated within a network society might have a chance to be sustainable as they meet their members' needs and are able to reproduce themselves.

The importance of community connections in disability and mental health care

Contemporary social and health care services in the fields of disability and mental health care are typically community-based, emphasising the participation of these people in community activities as a fundamental human right. Article 19 of the United Nations (2006) *Convention on the Rights of Persons with Disabilities* sets out the right of all disabled people to 'live in the community, with choices equal to others', requiring participating states to enable disabled people to be fully included and participate in society. The European Coalition for Community Living (ECCL) has interpreted this to mean:

> Community living refers to people with disabilities being able to live in their local communities as equal citizens, with the support that they need to participate in every-day life. This includes living in their own homes or with their families, going to work, going to school and taking part in community activities. To ensure that disabled people have the same choice, control and freedom as any other citizen, any practical assistance provided to them should be based on their own choices and aspirations.
>
> (ECCL 2009)

People with a disability often have difficulties engaging in the wider community. They face fewer opportunities than other citizens due to stigma, discrimination, and poverty (World Health Organization 2011). In a European research project about participation in the community of persons with psychosocial disabilities, we discovered that there are many different obstacles to participation (Wilken et al. 2014). The research project explored how, in Estonia, Hungary, and the Netherlands, the community participation of people with disabilities is perceived. The current reality of social and mental health care services is that the main focus is on individuals and categorical groups. For many people using these services, professionals and peers form their 'community'. From our research, we concluded that the bonds with the neighbourhood where people live vary considerably. The difficulty is that community in this sense is interpreted and valued in very different ways (Wilken et al. 2018).

In Estonia and Hungary, community as a social entity disappeared during the communist era. We conclude that in post-communist countries, the 'community' is not considered a manifestation of social capital and that therefore social cohesion in society as a whole has a poor quality. This is a big obstacle for people with disabilities since it hinders the possibilities for community participation and integration (Wilken et al. 2018).

By way of contrast, in the Netherlands, the notion of community has eroded over the years due to increasing mobility and individualisation. People do not connect anymore to the neighbourhood; therefore they often remain strangers. Another obstacle for community connections is, paradoxically, the well-established welfare state of the Netherlands. In the welfare state that developed following World War Two, the state took care of the needs of its citizens. The quality of services was generally very high, but a disadvantage of this system was that vulnerable people became invisible to society. They had their own 'community', a separated area containing housing, food, work, and leisure facilities, all within the framework of the formal care system (Wilken et al. 2018).

The state provided all kinds of services for people who needed social care, with the result that formal care became strongly separated from informal communities (Pfau-Effinger 2005). Now there is a tendency to repair the connection between the two, emphasising and valuing all kinds of informal care. At the same time, the traditional Dutch welfare state schemes had become unsustainable and out-dated. King Willem-Alexander's Speech from the Throne on 17 September 2013, signalled the formal political aim to transform the Dutch welfare state into a par-ticipation society.

> It is an undeniable reality that in today's network and information society people are both more assertive and more independent than in the past. This combined with the need to reduce the budget deficit, means that the classical welfare state is slowly but surely evolving into a participation society. Eve-ryone who is able will be asked to take responsibility for their own lives and immediate surroundings.
>
> (in Delsen 2016: 11)

It is important to emphasise that the participation society is not the same as the abolition of the welfare state, but stands for a different distribution of collective and individual responsibilities (Delsen 2016). The Dutch welfare system reform provided inspiration to our ICT-based pilot as it suggested that emerging Eastern European countries should explore new approaches instead of replicating the tra-ditional solutions of well-established welfare states.

The notion of a digital society

E-Governance in Estonia

Estonia, with a population of 1.3 million, is a Baltic country in Northeast Europe that gained political and economic independence from the Soviet Union in 1991. The first Estonian government after independence wanted to build a modern nation. This moment provided a great opportunity to integrate services across governmental departments and to invest in common technological infrastruc-tures. Estonia has had remarkable success in promoting a technology-based infor-mation society and especially with establishing the principles of e-government (Kalvet 2007).

E-government is defined as the use of information and communication tech-nologies in public administration, combined with organisational change and new skills, to improve public services and democratic processes and to strengthen support for public policies (European Commission 2003). E-governance has been a strategic choice for Estonia to improve the competitiveness of the state and increase the well-being of its people. Ninety-nine per cent of public services are now available to citizens as e-services. The public sector plays an active role in the uptake of innovative solutions and investments in new technologies. In principle, the internet is accessible nearly everywhere in Estonia; the fixed broadband coverage was 98 per cent in 2018. In 2017, the internet was used by 88 per cent of individuals aged 16 to 74 years. This means that the majority of Estonians are motivated to use the internet and have the necessary skills to do so (Ministry of Economic Affairs and Communications n.d.).

The United Nations' *Transforming our World: the 2030 Agenda for Sustainable Development* underlines the strategic benefits offered by the technology revolution.

> The spread of information and communications technology and global interconnectedness have great potential to accelerate human progress to bridge the digital divide and to develop knowledge societies, as does scientific and technological innovation across areas as diverse as medicine and energy.
>
> (United Nations 2015)

The 2018 United Nations E-Government Survey provided a new analysis to further utilise the potential of e-government to support the 2030 Agenda. The Survey examined how governments can use e-government and information technologies to build sustainable and resilient societies. The Survey highlighted, with many examples, how ICTs overall can enable personalised medicine and education, support vulnerable populations, predict and manage shocks and disasters, promote social and political inclusion, improve sanitation, provide identity for unregistered persons, and reduce environmental toxicity through better monitoring (United Nations 2018).

Estonia considers itself as one of the first digital societies that tends to solve its economic and societal issues by integrating information and communication technologies at all levels. Another important phenomenon of Estonian society today is the emphasis on entrepreneurship and especially on the technology driven start-up scene in their development policies. In this context, entrepreneurship is a societal phenomenon as it has become a fundamental tool to overcome the learned dependence of its citizens in a totalitarian regime, encouraging entrepreneurship as a precondition of (economically, legally, and politically) independent citizenship.

Start-ups and other entrepreneurship development programmes took an important role in the new developments in moving toward an innovative knowledge-based society (Ministry of Economic Affairs and Communications 2011). Several entrepreneurial start-up programmes were launched by the government and by large universities (Mets 2017).

The Helpific pilot project

The Estonian Ministry of Social Affairs (hereafter 'The Ministry') has initiated a new form of service development which combines the solutions of the vibrant start-up scene, the innovative nature of information and communication technologies, and the strong value proposition of the welfare sector. In cooperation with the creative hubs of Tallinn, the Ministry organised special hackathon events dedicated to societal issues.

A hackathon is typically an event in which computer programmers and other professionals such as graphic designers, project managers, and business developers are involved in intensive collaboration to develop software or hardware projects. In Estonia, hackathon events are connected not only to traditional IT topics, but they are organised around relevant economic or social issues. In Autumn 2014, an 'Enable Hackathon' was organised in Tallinn with the support of the Ministry, with the aim of developing creative ICT-based projects to increase the quality of life of disabled people in the country (Alapoikela and Bugarszki 2016).

The Helpific platform was developed by a multidisciplinary group of professionals with the involvement of people with disabilities and became one of the pioneer initiatives in the country to extend the achievements of a digital society to the welfare system. The platform connects people with disabilities with fellow citizens in order to create informal support networks around vulnerable people in local neighbourhoods.

Tallinn University has participated in this development process from the very beginning, contributing to the development work using the Learning by Developing (LBD) action model and monitoring the pilot period between June 2015 and March 2018. The LBD action model focuses on the development process. In that model, students not only absorb knowledge intellectually but learn primarily from the process of creative development itself. Individual learning is combined with creative, multidisciplinary teamwork, where the knowledge and experience of social and health professionals are combined with business development and IT skills (Raij 2014).

The prototype of the platform was created in November 2014, and after many adjustments and preparation work, it began operations in June 2015 under the domain www.helpific.com. The first version of the platform was created in Estonian and English. The Hungarian and Ukrainian version started to work in 2016, while the Croatian version of the website went live in 2017.

The Helpific platform offered a peer-to-peer solution where people with disabilities or mental health problems can post a help request related to their everyday life, and fellow citizens in their neighbourhood can respond to these requests. It was also possible to post help offers that people in need can respond to. There was no restriction that only qualified professionals could register to the platform; we encouraged people to have encounters involving help in very basic, everyday situations. We predefined six categories, but we did not restrict the actual content of the help requests:

* Transportation—giving a ride to someone or carrying items to somewhere;
* Personal assistance—physical help and personal help;

- Household tasks—cleaning, shopping, gardening, and a little help around the household;
- Accompanying—going out with someone, being a gym buddy, participating in leisure or cultural events, and accompanying them to offices;
- Tuition, education—teaching computer skills, language, helping with school tasks, and preparing for exams; and
- Other.

The primary aim of the platform was to provide relevant support for vulnerable people to help them maintain their independent life in the community. During the pilot period, we wanted to explore the following questions:

1 Is an ICT-based platform a relevant tool for vulnerable people? Do they have access to internet, and can they use the required devices?
2 How can people build trust in an online platform to create encounters that possibly lead to developing small networks?
3 Are these connections increasing the social capital of vulnerable people?

Methodology

In Estonia, Ukraine, and Hungary, partner universities had an opportunity to participate in different stages of the development process, and a special research team was established that analysed the pilot's results based on Helpific's server data and by conducting interviews with relevant stakeholders. In Croatia, a local social service provider contributed to the operation of the Helpific platform, and their customer relation team provided information to our research team for our analysis (Bugarszki et al. 2018).

For the pilot period, each partner organisation set up a team that followed and analysed each encounter, conducting interviews and focus group conversations with the active members and different stakeholders around the platform. In Estonia, this was Tallinn University's School of Governance, Law and Society; in Ukraine, Kiev State University's Faculty of Psychology; in Hungary, ELTE University, Faculty of Social Sciences and the Faculty of Special Education; while in Croatia, Susret Association, a local service provider in the mental health field, participated in the pilot project.

More than 4,000 messages exchanged by registered members were analysed. Helpific server's data also provided us with the opportunity to analyse the strength of connections between the registered members.

Pilot results

Altogether, 5,925 people have registered on the Helpific platform during the pilot period. In each country, most members were from the capital city. The platform performed mainly in large urban environments. Due to the longer period of operation and to the better resources, the Estonian version of the platform had the most registered members (4,585 people), followed by Ukraine (598 people), Hungary (474 people), and Croatia (268 people).

Due to data protection requirements and in order to increase the safety and security of the platform, only registered members were able to see the posted help requests and help offers. In order to avoid people using the platform as traditional social media (browsing among users and chatting with them), personal profiles were not displayed on the website. People only saw (after registration) incoming help requests or help offers and the profiles connected to them, while the only action they could do was to answer a request/offer or to post their own one.

This simplified operation decreased the quality of user experience but helped us considerably in measuring the core activity (creating connections with vulnerable people in the neighbourhood) without being misled by not-relevant activities (i.e. members chatting with each other as they do on a general messenger). Our aim was not to have a rapid growth to reach tens of thousands of people; we preferred to follow the activity of our active users manually, getting relevant information about their experience with an online tool targeting a very specific, vulnerable group of citizens.

Between 2015 June and 2018 March, we identified 447 help requests and help offers that were relevant for our analysis. Three hundred and eighteen of them were posted in Estonia, 31 in Hungary, 23 in Croatia, and 13 in Ukraine.

We identified 597 people who became active users of the platform. People connected each other by using the platform. In its internal message system, more than 4,000 messages were exchanged during the pilot period, but not this was the only method of communication. Sixty per cent of the active users managed to meet after two to five messages being exchanged online.

If we examine the proportion of different type of help requests and help offers, we find that each of the offered categories were relevant to both help seekers and helpers. Providing help in everyday activities became a good occasion for new encounters, while these activities were in line with the personal needs of help seekers, contributing to their independent life in the community.

In the case of personal assistance, we found the largest difference between the requests and offers. Providing personal assistance to someone requires a sense of intimacy which might be out of the comfort zone of many helpers, whereas helping around the household, giving a ride, or explaining a school task are more natural activities familiar to fellow citizens without any specific professional background:

> Indrek (A 30 year old man with physical disability) needed personal assistance in the mornings before he left for work. He lived independently in a

Table 19.1 Percentage of requests and offers for help on the Helpific platform

	Transportation	Personal assistance	Accompanying	Household task	Tuition/ Education	Other	Total
Request	14	28	17	16	7	18	100
Offer	19	13	16	21	13	18	100

rented property, 300 kms away from his parents and other family members. He managed to get a job and was able to use public transportation, but as he was not able to use his hands at all, every morning and evening he needed personal assistance for dressing, help with personal hygiene, and for small tasks like closing the door of his apartment. The local municipality provided him with a small personal budget that he could use to hire a personal assistant, and his flatmate also helped him. However, it became clear to him that the social benefit he received from the local government covered only about 60 per cent of his needs and his flatmate was not always around to help. He decided to use the Helpific platform to request help for specific mornings. People living in his area started to respond his request and he managed to build a network of 5–6 people in his neighbourhood who were capable of helping him occasionally.

Both help seekers and helpers were looking for opportunities to participate in community events, cultural, sport, or social activities. In general, we can state that those activities were the most effective method to create new encounters, as none of the partners had to do make much extra effort out of their comfort zone, and this was beneficial for both of them.

Eszter (a 22 year old lady using a wheelchair) posted a help request on the Helpific platform explaining that she wanted to go to a rock concert in Kaposvár, Hungary. She needed a person to accompany her, helping in an area where she was not familiar with the environment and accessibility. A young lady, interested in the same concert, responded to her request, offering her company during the concert.

A crucial question was the way in which way people build trust in an online environment and what strategies they use to build a personal relationship. Surprisingly, we did not encounter major issues around registration or access to the internet and to the required devices. The platform has been developed so that it works well on all types of devices, including PCs, laptops, tablets, and smartphones. Registration was very simple via existing social media profiles or via email. The system did not require a sophisticated registration process but transferred personal profile data from social media (Facebook or Google profiles). This helped many people with physical disabilities to enter the system easily while the link to existing social media profiles increased reliability. One of the most frequent strategies to check new encounters was to search for social media profiles or have an introductory phone call/video call via Skype or mobile phone. People also paid attention to organizing first meetings at public places. In some countries, we managed to involve friendly cafés run by NGOs as social enterprises, that served as 'safe places' for a first personal meeting. In most of the cases, users preferred to check the identity and reliability of their responders by themselves, but in case of uncertainty, different community members could be involved. Helpific team members responsible for customer relations contacted local service providers (social workers or other helping professionals), community leaders, pastors or church members, and also existing helpers, personal assistants, or family members could be present to ensure safety and security for a first meeting.

> Tanya (a thirty-nine-year-old lady from Kiev, Ukraine) posted a cheerful help offer that she was ready to meet persons who needed accompanying in leisure time, going out at times, having a cup of coffee and a nice conversation. Igor, a young gentleman with severe physical disabilities, answered her offer and the first meeting occurred with the help of volunteering social work students from Kiev State University.

Frequently after the first personal meeting, people continued their communication on multiple channels, adding each other as 'friends' on Facebook or other social media sites, exchanging phone numbers or meeting in person on a regular basis. Encounters were rather individual. In the middle of a network was the help seeker, and the platform helped them to build up a personal support network around themselves, with five to six or even more potential contacts that they could mobilise in case of need or, as in any other natural relations, keep in touch as new friends or neighbours. For this, reciprocity between network members was very important.

> Aul (a 42 year old visually impaired woman from Tallinn, Estonia) needed help in her household and kept in touch with eight different people on the Helpific platform who occasionally went over to her place to fix things or help with packing and cleaning. However, the relationship between them was not restricted to this help only. Aul has good computer skills and she started to help her new 'friends' by installing software on their laptops, solving technical problems or teaching them new skills.

The original intention was to create an opportunity to receive help on a voluntary basis, but very early it became clear that many participants prefer to involve monetary compensation. During our focus group conversations with target group members, we found that in the long term they prefer to pay for help. Being continuously dependent on someone and repeatedly asking for favours is rather humiliating and does not help to develop relationships on an equal level. Paying a fee, even if it is under the market rate, created a completely new situation where help seekers became customers. Forty-one per cent of the regular users were offering or requesting monetary compensation, and the average offered amount was €8 for a one-time help (ranging between €3 and €40). Those who wanted regular help (mostly personal assistance) offered an average amount of €185 per month. Involving monetary compensation helped not only to balance the relationship between helpers and help seekers but also contributed to the sustainability of the platform and created a way to turn platform users into micro-entrepreneurs.

> Marko (a 35 year old man from Keila, Estonia) started to offer web design and computer related services for a reasonable price. Marko suffers from

mental health problems; his health condition and social phobia are obstacles to him taking a regular job, but as a web designer, working from his home office helped him to establish a revenue stream. In his case, Helpific became a potential market place where he could find new customers for himself.

In the pilot period, the Helpific platform did not charge people with commission or other fees, but for the future operation, the appearance of monetary compensation in the system gave the opportunity to take the initiative to set up a business plan, making the platform sustainable as a social enterprise that connects people for voluntary help completely free of charge, but generates income from transactions where monetary compensation is involved.

Conclusion

The platform's aim was to create new encounters in urban neighbourhoods where traditional, natural communities do not exist anymore or are very weak in order to support vulnerable people. Our target group were people with disabilities and mental health problems who had additional challenges due to their isolation. In the involved countries (Estonia, Ukraine, Hungary, and Croatia), this target group were usually institutionalised in large care homes or lived almost completely isolated with their family members, far away from general communities. The process of deinstitutionalisation was begun a couple of years ago in these countries, when people started to move (back) to local communities without any ties and connections to their neighbourhoods, with a very low level of social capital.

The platform's function was to create initial encounters with fellow (non-professional) citizens, and we wanted to explore if an ICT tool were able to create these encounters, leading to new social bonds and the creation of support networks and caring communities around vulnerable people. We were concerned as to whether our target group would have access to the internet and to the required devices for ICT-based communication and if they have the relevant skills to use them. We found that for our target group members, digital solutions and modern technology represent a potential breakthrough from their isolation, and they used ICT tools with more confidence than the many helping professionals around them. For many people with disabilities or mental health problems, their online presence is the main connection to the outside world, and using e-services or e-government solutions gives them an opportunity to participate in activities that were not previously accessible. ICT tools have become relatively cheaper over the last few years, especially in countries where access to the internet is subsidised (in Estonia, access to the internet is a constitutional right); a presence in the digital life is now an available option even for low-income households.

On the other hand, we had difficulties in motivating and mobilising people living in 24-hour support housing facilities or institutions. This group of people are still surrounded by caregivers and other helping professionals, covering almost all of their needs, and the platform was not appealing for them. We also experienced how professionals working in these facilities were suspicious toward the online platform, protecting their users from potentially dangerous encounters with the outside world. Obviously we also could not reach those people who had no resources or skills to get access to technology or refused to use them.

People started to use the Helpific platform when they were already on their personal journey to build their own life in the community. Usually they were at a certain stage of their recovery process, or they had already reached a certain level of independent life. These people lived on their own or with their family members or friends or else were using small, integrated housing services whereby they needed to face challenges on a daily basis and were eager to find solutions to their problems. Access to technology and the motivation to find solutions to everyday challenges opened the way to successful network building on the Helpific platform. Fellow citizens (helpers) also emphasised the easy access and rapid solutions. The Helpific platform created an opportunity to help someone in a simpler way than any traditional form of voluntary activity. Receiving a peer-to-peer notification to the smartphone about a help request in the neighbourhood created the opportunity for instant action instead of a long, formal process of joining a voluntary organisation.

The platform turned out to be a useful tool for creating first encounters, but the ICT tool itself is only an entry point for building a network. The development to become a network and the process of building a sense of community have been embedded into a diverse structure combining different methods of communications. We found that successful help seekers created a support network around themselves, keeping touch with a small group of people (the range was between 4 and 15 people) where individual group members could be replaced but the network itself remained functional over a long time by running new campaigns on the platform if additional members were needed. Reciprocity, the atmosphere of mutual help and the potential involvement of monetary compensation, helped to balance the relationship. Many help-seekers found it very important that they also wanted to help or be useful, which contributed to a more integrated role in the community beyond their disability status or any other vulnerable position.

This potential we find to be the most important feature of the Helpific platform. The ICT tool and the use of modern technology helped to create encounters between people who would hardly meet otherwise, while the occasion of (little) help served as a perfect entry point for a subsequently more complex network, where the roles and relations became more than one-dimensional. Helpific platform is not a tool that replaces the functions of professional help (social work, psychotherapy, physiotherapy, vocational rehabilitation, etc.) but seems to be a sustainable way to create new relations in an urban environment where traditional communities are vanishing, but technology-driven networks offer new potential to revitalise missing connections.

References

Alapoikela, M. and Bugarszki, Z. (2016) 'Teaching e-service competence with the learning by developing (LBD) action model in Finland and Estonia', in T-A. Aholaakko,

K. Komulainen, A. Majakulma and S. Niinistö-Sivuranta (eds) *Crossing Borders and Creating Future Competences*, Helsinki: Laurea University of Applied Sciences, Laurea Publications.

Anttiroiko, A. (2015) *Networks in Manuel Castells' Theory of the Network Society*, Munich Personal RePEc Archive. Online. Available at https://mpra.ub.uni-muenchen.de/65617/ (accessed 18 October 2018).

Bell, C. and Newby, H. (1972) *Community Studies: An Introduction to the Sociology of the Local Community*, New York: Preager.

Bugarszki, Z., Barna, I., Diez, P.A., Lombo, C.F., Veloy, N.M. and Iglesias, S.H. (2018) *Analysis of the Results of a Sharing Economy Based ICT Tool Supporting Vulnerable People in Eastern-European Urban Environments*, Tallinn: Tallinn University.

Castells, M. (2009) *The Rise of the Network Society*, 2nd edn, Oxford: Wiley-Blackwell.

Castells, M. Fernández-Ardévol, M., Linchuan Qiu, J. and Sey, A. (2004) *The Mobile Communication Society: A Cross-cultural Analysis of Available Evidence on the Social Uses of Wireless Communication Technology*, Los Angeles: University of Southern California, Annenberg School for Communication. Online. Available at http://citeseerx.ist.psu.edu/viewdoc/download?doi=10.1.1.109.3872&rep=rep1&type=pdf (accessed 18 October 2018).

Delsen, L. (2016) *The Realisation of the Participation Society: Welfare State Reform in the Netherlands: 2010–2015*, Nijmegen: Radboud University, Institute for Management Research. Working paper. Available at www.ru.nl/publish/pages/516298/nice_16-02.pdf (accessed 18 October 2018).

European Coalition for Community Living (ECCL) (2009) 'The right to live in the community: ECCL briefing on Article 19 of the UN convention on the rights of persons with disabilities', in *Focus on Article 19 of the UN Convention on the Rights of Persons*. Online. Available at http://community-living.info/wp-content/uploads/2014/02/ECCL-Focus-Report-2009-final-WEB.pdf (accessed 18 October 2018).

European Commission (2003) *The Role of eGovernment for Europe's Future: COM (2003)567*, Brussels: European Commission. Online. Available at http://ec.europa.eu/transparency/regdoc/rep/2/2003/EN/2-2003-1038-EN-1-1.PDF (accessed 18 October 2018).

Ghezzi, S. and Mingione, E. (2007) 'Embeddedness, path dependency and social institutions: an economic sociology approach', *Current Sociology*, 55: 11–23.

Kalvet, T. (2007) 'The Estonian information society developments since the 1990s', Working Paper No. 29, Tallinn: Praxis Centre for Policy Studies and Tallinn University of Technology. Online. Available at http://praxis.ee/wp-content/uploads/2014/03/2007-Estonian-information-society-developments.pdf (accessed 18 October 2018).

Mets, T. (2017) 'Entrepreneurship in Estonia: combination of Political and entrepreneurial agenda', in A. Sauka and A. Chepurenko (eds) *Entrepreneurship in Transition Economies: Diversity, Trends and Perspectives*, Berlin: Springer.

Ministry of Economic Affairs and Communications (2011) 'Start-up Eesti 2011–2013: Tegevuskava innovaatiliste start-up ettevo˜tete arendamiseks (Action plan for development of innovative startups)'. Online. Available at www.riigikantselei.ee/valitsus/valitsus/et/ . . . ja. . . /Start-up.doc (accessed 18 October 2018).

Ministry of Economic Affairs and Communications (n.d.) *Digital Agenda 2020 for Estonia*. Online. Available at www.mkm.ee/sites/default/files/digital_agenda_2020_estonia_engf.pdf. (accessed 13 August 2018).

Pfau-Effinger, B. (2005) 'Welfare state policies and the development of care arrangements', *European Societies*, 7: 321–47.

Putnam, R.D. (2000) *Bowling Alone: The Collapse and Revival of American Community*, New York: Simon and Schuster.

Raij, K. (ed) (2014) *Learning by Developing Action Model*, Vantaa, Finland: Laurea University of Applied Sciences.

Servet, J-M. (2007) 'The principle of reciprocity by Karl Polanyi: contributions to a definition of solidarity-based economy', *Revue Tiers Monde* (2): 255–73.

Tönnies, F. (2012) 'Community and society', in J. Lin and C. Mele (eds) *The Urban Sociology Reader*, 2nd edn, London: Routledge.

United Nations (2006) 'Convention on the rights of persons with disabilities'. Online. Available at www.un.org/development/desa/disabilities/convention-on-the-rights-of-persons-with-disabilities/convention-on-the-rights-of-persons-with-disabilities-2.html (accessed 4 November 2019).

United Nations (2015) 'Transforming our world: the 2030 agenda for sustainable development'. Online. Available at https://sustainabledevelopment.un.org/post2015/transformingourworld/publication (accessed 4 November 2019).

United Nations (2018) 'United Nations e-Government survey 2018: gearing e-Government to support transformation towards sustainable and resilient societies'. Online. Available at www.unescap.org/resources/e-government-survey-2018-gearing-e-government-support-transformation-towards-sustainable (accessed 31 October 2018).

Wilken, J.P., Bugarszki, Z., Hanga, K., Narusson, D., Saia, K. and Medar, M. (2018) 'Community orientation of services for persons with a psychiatric disability: comparison between Estonia, Hungary and the Netherlands', *European Journal of Social Work*, 21: 509–20.

Wilken, J.P., Medar, M., Bugarszki, Z. and Leenders, F. (2014) 'Community support and participation among persons with disabilities: a study in three European countries', *Journal of Social Intervention: Theory and Practice*, 23: 44–59.

World Health Organization (2011) 'World report on disability'. Online. Available at www.who.int/disabilities/world_report/2011/en/ (accessed 31 October 2018).

20 Building an accessible and inclusive city

Richard Tucker, Patsie Frawley, David Kelly,
Louise Johnson, Fiona Andrews and
Kevin Murfitt

Introduction

This chapter describes an approach to investigating what is required to establish and sustain a provincial city in Victoria, Australia, as a leading accessible and inclusive city created by the authors who are members of Deakin University's HOME Research Hub. This is a transdisciplinary research group which collaborates with a range of stakeholders, including disability advocates, to deliver well-designed, sustainable, and connected communities for all. We define an accessible and inclusive city as one that can be accessed, understood, and used to the greatest extent possible by all people. The strategies described were intended to form a collective impact approach based on the premise that for sustainable change to large-scale social inclusion problems (Burchardt et al. 2002), the drawing together of key stakeholders to work together toward a common goal is more powerful than individual organisations working toward similar goals in isolation (Kania and Kramer 2011).

Our vision of an accessible and inclusive city is one that is designed to provide equitable opportunities for connectivity (spatial and digital), economic participation, employment, education, housing, and community and social infrastructure that meet the needs and aspirations of all. However, addressing inclusive city-design holistically is difficult when there is such complexity, diversity, and individuality of citizens' needs. This requires a methodological approach that accounts for the needs of community members by working in partnership with them in order to support and sustain the planning, design, and decision-making processes.

Accessible and inclusive cities

Accessibility is a 'broad and flexible concept that can be defined as the ability to approach something by someone' (La Rosa et al. 2018). In practical terms, accessibility can be perceived from a variety of perspectives, including economic, physical, information, and communication to health and community services. Concerning people with disability, accessibility reflects the ability to access and use a particular environment, product, service, or information (Burchardt et al.

2002). It represents a strong tool for empowering citizens with disability to live an everyday life like any other citizen. Accessibility is thus a precondition for inclusive cities and societies. In the project described here, the terms 'accessibility' and 'inclusion' primarily, but not exclusively, refer to: 1) *accessibility* of public spaces, community services, and infrastructure and economic participation; and 2) *inclusive* urban planning, design governance, and employment practices.

Becoming an accessible and inclusive city requires lasting structural and attitudinal change. Global case studies and benchmarks for what constitutes an accessible and inclusive city broadly conceive it as a place that proactively fosters equitable access to and participation in the social life of the city for all. Based on a cross-section of a wide range of peer-reviewed and grey literature, we suggest five (composite) domains to which an accessible and inclusive city would attend:

1   connectivity (spatial and digital);
2   economic participation, employment, and education;
3   housing;
4   community and social infrastructure; and
5   processes of engagement and inclusion.

Improving inclusivity and accessibility across these five domains requires, we argue, commitment and intervention across eight overlapping spheres: 1) technology, 2) policy processes, 3) rating systems, 4) the built environment, 5) employment programs, 6) grant programs, 7) community awareness, 8) and legislation and policy.

While globally, as in Australia, legislation, policy, and the underlying mechanisms that drive contemporary city forms across all five domains commonly aspire to principles of access and inclusion, rarely in practice do outcomes live up to these aspirations. Prioritising accessibility and inclusivity at a city scale necessitate a solid understanding of existing conditions and the key structural, social, economic, and political processes that drive change. Our project aimed, therefore, to influence policy from the ground up: initiated through multi-entity, multisector engagement with influential stakeholders. It was intended that such an approach would provide more complete and mutual understanding of current obstacles and thus clear a pathway for longer-lasting structural and attitudinal changes for sustaining social inclusion through these changes and the processes used for identifying and implementing them.

Extending and delivering social inclusion in cities to people with disabilities

Documenting the processes by which the disadvantaged are segregated in the cities of the United States, theorists such as Peter Marcuse (Iveson 2011), Don Mitchell (2003), and David Harvey (2008) not only detail the structural and institutional means by which these patterns occur but also demanded change—a 'right to the city' for those excluded from its most desirable neighbourhoods, best services, political institutions, and public spaces (Mitchell 2003). Pragmatic responses to exclusion in cities have moved beyond their sociostructural foundations to invoke ethics and broader principles of inclusion at the same time as concern for the socially marginal has been extended to those with disabilities.

This work has focused on the definition of disability and the political economy of exclusion (for example, Butler and Bowlby 1997; Butler and Parr 1999; Dyck 1995). Robert Imrie (1996) has detailed the processes by which the urban environment erects barriers to marginalise and impoverish people with disabilities. Imrie joins others—such as Reg Golledge (1991), Brendan Gleeson (1997, 2001, 2002), and Jos Boys (2017)—to unpack the links between disability and the built environment. Here the social-cultural and political processes are highlighted that underpin the social construction and reproduction of disability as a state of marginalisation and oppression in the city (Imrie 1996, 2001). Such an approach directs attention to how the built environment is riddled with barriers that create a geography of disability as the city expresses assumptions about the able bodies within it (Hall 2005, 2010; Imrie 2001). Furthermore, Milner and Mirfin-Veitch (2016: 87) have noted that attempts to 'fit people with disabilities', and in particular people with intellectual disabilities, 'into the mainstream' have 'left untroubled the socio-economic and social ordering of spaces' that have always and more subtly excluded people with intellectual disabilities. The city therefore has spaces and process of exclusion that create powerlessness (Imrie 1996).

Imrie (1996) also invokes the notion of embodiment and how the 'disabled' body is variously demonised, medicalised, and not planned for or accommodated in the city (see also Butler and Bowlby 1997; Butler and Parr 1999; Teather 2005). Cameron Duff (2017) introduces the notion of 'affect' to studies of homelessness, which can also be added as a key dimension in the experiences of those with disability as they attempt to negotiate spaces and places built for the able-bodied.

A focus of research addressing social exclusion has been on widening participation in the decision-making processes that determine the built form of the city, including housing, public spaces, and mobility. Other areas of inclusivity research have concentrated on employment and economic participation, especially the marginalisation and economic vulnerability of those with a disability. Although Hall (2010: 51) cautioned that 'diagnosis of the marginalised social position of people with intellectual disabilities as "social exclusion" has generated a very limited and even damaging discourse and set of policy responses' that are underpinned by an 'economic and moral expectation' to work and to participate in 'normal activities' and contribute to society, he argues that at least equally there needs to be a consideration of the relational context of inclusion, which he poses as being best articulated through the idea of 'belonging'. He suggests that understanding 'belonging' is at the heart of understanding 'inclusion' and this is best understood when we look at the 'self-authored' spaces, places and experiences where people with disabilities feel and perhaps 'know' they belong.

This attitude to inclusion underpins the approaches adopted in the project described in this chapter, which, furthermore, acknowledge the importance of a political voice, pride, and representation of those often left out and who feel 'unwelcome' within places, spaces, and activities to have a voice in developing what access and inclusion looks and feels like (Aitken et al. 2019; Bigby 2008; Fudge Schormans et al. 2019; Harrison 2004; Tually et al. 2011).

Disability researcher Paul Milner and his colleagues, in their work in New Zealand spanning two decades, have developed a theoretical framework for understanding social inclusion informed by the lived experiences of people with disabilities. In this work, people with disabilities have 'told' the researchers (indicating the privileging of the voices of people with disabilities in the research) that it was not 'so much *where* they were that mattered it was *how* they were in place that counted toward whether or not they felt a sense of belonging' (Milner and Mirfin-Veitch 2016: 76). Furthermore, it is not the spatial indicators of inclusion that are set out in policy that are the best markers of inclusion, but relational markers that more closely align with their experiences of inclusion and belonging. From this research, they have developed five qualitative attributes of social inclusion. These attributes, which are summarised later and reorientated to our interest about 'the accessible and inclusive city', provide a theoretical and pragmatic way of thinking about social inclusion that can be used to shape the way we think about sustainable social inclusion in the spaces and places of a city. We include them here because they are formed from the perspective of those who are most at risk of exclusion or having their inclusion signposted and determined by others' perspectives. These qualitative markers of social inclusion can be summarised as:

1   Autobiographic—people can participate [in the city] in ways that best tell who they are allow them to communicate their sense of self [not a predetermined sense e.g. worker or independent traveller];

2   Social identity—people find themselves represented in the social history of a place as a member and contribute to the way a community [city] sees itself;

3   Reciprocity—people are aware of and strengthen relationships [with others in the city] that humanise relationships—through acts of kindness and consideration as social exchange;

4   Insider—when 'in place' people experience an insider's sense of psychological safety—sharing spaces, places, and experiences with others they trust; and

5   Expectation—people are met by expectations that they contribute to the wellbeing of other members of the community (see Milner and Mirfin-Veitch 2016).

Systems thinking for collective social impact

The short project lead-time required an inclusive research approach able to concentrate the collection of a broad range of opinions, viewpoints, and ideas. Broad-level nonintrusive consultations with community stakeholders were developed in the form of group systems-thinking workshops designed with representatives from two consultative stakeholder groups: a project steering committee and a project task force. The steering committee, which consisted of representatives of the research funding body, research project leaders, local government planning department civic servants, disability representative organisations, and elected members of a project task force who had lived experience of disability, had a formal guidance role that included approval of staged deliverables. The task force, which provided more informal feedback at regular intervals, was championed and assembled by a state member of parliament and consisted of representatives from disability stakeholder groups, many of whom had personal lived experience of disability.

Workshop participants

People who identify as having a disability were specifically included because 'access and inclusion' is central to the lived experience of disability. Here the diversity of ability and disability must be noted: many people who identify as having a disability do not have reduced capacity to consent but rather experience disability due to issues related to physical or sensory impairment, age, or environmental/social barriers. Additionally it was also recognised that some participants who are stakeholders in their professional capacity, such as architects, educators, policy and project workers, or advocates, may at the same time identify themselves as having a disability.

In contrast to many research projects in which people with disabilities are considered as 'vulnerable', in this project they were considered as active and informed participants in civic decision-making processes. This stance follows Article 12 of the *Convention on the Rights of Persons with Disabilities* (United Nations 2006) in upholding the rights of persons with disability, recognising 'that persons with disability enjoy legal capacity on an equal basis with others in all aspects of life'. Similarly, local Indigenous community groups provided input. In actively recruiting persons and representative bodies with lived professional and personal knowledge on issues of accessibility and inclusion, an incidental level of participation of non-targeted groups was assumed.

Systems thinking in community knowledge exchange

The *Systems Thinking in Community Knowledge Exchange* (STICKE) tool (Deakin University 2019) was used in workshops to allow diverse stakeholders to express a broad range of views. STICKE is based on the Group Model Building (GMB) methodology (Peck 1998), which guides participants through a series of tasks (guided activities), facilitated by a small team of trained researchers, to examine their mental models (cognitive representations of interdependent causes and effects) of a given situation or problem. During the guided activities, participants are introduced to the nature and scope of the problem being investigated, worked to identify the various factors contributing to the problem over time, and finally identified the interconnections between those factors. Throughout the discussions, researchers make notes of the general discussion and points raised by participants.

Crucial to the tool's success is the mix of participants, which should ensure representation of diversity of experience and expertise across the system network under consideration. Recognising the complexity of accessibility and inclusivity issues, three workshops were held that each concentrated on a separate 'sub-system' were held. These subsystems reflected the separate foci identified by the funders and the five domains of accessibility identified at the project outset, but in a collapsed form:

1   Building, planning, and building regulations to make this a world-class accessible and inclusive city within the next five years;
2   Community infrastructure to make this a world-class accessible and inclusive city within the next five years; and
3   Employment and economic participation to make this a world-class accessible and inclusive city within the next ten years.

Participant numbers ranged between eleven and twenty-five. Each workshop lasted one day during which participants engaged in the four sequential steps of the STICKE process: 1) Group model building, 2) Model review and development, 3) Confirm systems map and generate action ideas, and 4) dissemination. The day was structured in two halves with a break between sessions.

Step 1: Group Model Building

A GMB session was conducted for three hours with key stakeholders to produce an initial causal loop diagram of the accessibility and inclusivity of a city system. Here, participants developed a setting-specific system map of what would make a world-class accessible city. The group identified six key areas that gave rise to obstacles to accessibility and inclusion: 1) lack of affordable and appropriate *housing*, 2) poor access to *buildings, facilities, and public spaces*, 3) systemwide negative and misinformed *attitudes towards access and inclusion*, 4) inadequate *transportation* infrastructure, 5) lack of high-quality policy interventions from *government*, and (6) poor access to *services*. Table 20.1 provides further detail as to the issues identified in each area.

A system is a representation of the sources of influence over a particular problem and the individual relationships between these components. During this initial session, participants' input was used to develop a visual representation of the various sources of influence over the problem under investigation and the many relationships between those influences, known as a 'causal loop diagram' (Tip 2011). The causal loop diagram aids in the visualising of how different variables in a system are interrelated. The diagram consists of a set of nodes and edges: nodes represent the variables, and edges are the links that represent a connection or a relation between the two variables. Participants' ideas were used here in real time, via input into graphic software, to visually represent the various sources of influence over the problem under investigation and the many relationships between those influences. At the conclusion of this step, participants were invited back for the second session to further refine the map.

Table 20.1 Obstacles to accessibility and inclusion in the built environment identified by participants in the STICKE workshop

Area	Contributing factors
Attitudes about access and inclusion	Attitude toward inclusion/access; Attitudes toward progressive development; Education about access/inclusivity; Engagement for people who don't have a voice; Timely communication avenues to report access issues
Buildings, facilities, and public spaces	Access to buildings, facilities, public spaces, tourism, and major events (parks, public amenities, and others); Accessible bathrooms; Accessibility of buildings, facilities, public spaces, tourism, major events, and wayfinding (parks, public amenities, and others); Updating entrances of existing buildings
Governance	Accessibility requirements for all housing; Accessibility requirements for new housing; Coordinated planning for accessibility; Desire for profit; Inclusionary rezoning; Integration of inclusivity into planning; Meeting minimum standards rather than championing; Modernisation of regulation standards; Quality of policy interventions; Understanding of existing accessibility infrastructure
Housing	Affordable and appropriate housing; Costs of housing; Demand for housing; Efficiency of housing; Living with people you are compatible with; Rent cost; Suitable housing for all
Services	Access to information; Access to services; Aged services; Disability services; Support from the National Disability Insurance Scheme (NDIS)
Transport	Accessible charge points and interactive technology; Accessible parking; Accessible taxi network; Accessible transport by buses/public transport; Accessible transport premises/infrastructure; Clear wayfinding; Coverage of public transport; Quality of signage

Step 2: Model review and development

The diagram created during Step 1 was further developed and refined by the participants, supported by the workshop organisers, first visually clarifying the initial model and then reviewing the content based on the written workshop notes to ensure that the content of the model accurately reflects participants' discussion. This process ensures that any discussion points that are not captured during the initial in-workshop modelling (from Step 1) can be retrospectively added into the model.

Step 3: Confirm systems map and generate action ideas

At the beginning of the second session, participants were led through an abbreviated version of the Step 1 process to validate and finalise the revised map from Step

2 and also to identify any gaps that remained. After participants were next given ideas on how to identify potential points for intervention within causal loop diagrams, they then generated and prioritised actions that might be taken to improve the accessibility and inclusivity of their city. The actions were prioritised via the consensus of the participants according to their perceived impact and feasibility.

At the culmination of the workshops, teams of stakeholders are formed that might work together to implement the identified actions. Participants are informed that they can sign up to be members of working groups that have emerged. This is not a binding agreement, but an indication that participants are interested in the ideas and would like to be involved in discussing how they can move forward with support from a local backbone group. Finally the facilitator explained the next steps, including who the local backbone group is, the support-on offer to the working groups going forward, and plans to support the working groups in establishing a first meeting.

Step 4: Dissemination

An interim report was then created in consultation with the participating stakeholder groups that summarised the STICKE workshop process and presented the finalised model of each workshop, along with prioritised actions for making a world-class accessible and inclusive city within five years. The interim report (unpublished) formed the basis for discussions with stakeholder groups, including focus group people with disability who are members of these groups.

Analysis: prioritising the actions

During Step 3 of the STICKE workshops, participants generated 109 actions that could be taken to improve the accessibility and inclusivity of their city. Of these, 37 were identified as priority actions and were ranked by participants according to their perceived impact and feasibility. These priority actions were then taken by the research team and further analysed according to systems-thinking principles.

Meadows' (1999) framework of 'leverage points' in systems analysis was used to evaluate the 37 priority actions. Here, 12 leverage points denote places within a complex system where interventions can be staged. Meadows (1999: 1) terms these 'points of power'. Each priority action was presented to the research team during an analysis workshop and allocated a value between 12 and 1, from tinkering to paradigm shifting. Importantly, no hierarchy or continuum is indicated by the leverage-point allocated, for the actions can be, and often are, interdependent. After all actions were allocated a value, they were further synthesised into themes that can be narrated and disseminated back to the stakeholders and research participants. Malhi et al.'s (2009) 'intervention level framework' was used to perform this synthesis, in which the 12 leverage points used in the initial analysis were collapsed into five corresponding intervention levels. These five intervention levels—paradigm, goals, systems structure, feedback and delays, and structural elements—were used to categorise all priority actions. At the time of writing, further work with stakeholders and participants was occurring to refine and translate these priorities into a policy agenda.

Validating the priorities: focus groups with people with disabilities

The eight researchers that acted as facilitators in the STICKE workshops noted that low representation in the workshops of people with lived experience of disability— around 20 per cent—had impacted the process and results and, moreover, meant the approach fell short of inclusive and participatory research principles. The low numbers were largely because attending all-day workshops for people with disabilities was challenging, especially for those who relied on paid support to attend, including people with complex needs or with intellectual impairment and/or mental health issues; as was reaching and recruiting such participants. To redress this lack of representation, three two-hour focus groups were added to the research programme to evaluate the key priority actions developed in the STICKE workshops. Each focus group was made up of members of the local community and consisted almost exclusively of people with lived experience of disability. These groups included: a service user reference group for a disability support provider (12 participants); local members of a support group for survivors of stroke and acquired brain injuries (six participants); and seven representatives from the project task force.

Each focus group included five themes of discussion, based on the five intervention levels in systems analysis offered by Malhi et al. (2009). These themes were reconstituted to form five focussed narratives that incorporated the 37 priority actions produced in the STICKE workshops. The narratives took the form of vocally delivered descriptions that allowed the participants who were unable to attend the STICKE workshops, and thus who had not experienced the group development of the actions, to easily comprehend the evolution and intent of the actions. Thus, through these vocally delivered descriptions and facilitation from the project team, participants were made aware of how the actions linked to obstacles identified in the STICKE workshops. The narratives had to both reflect and simplify the complexity of the system context that informed the actions. Each of the five narrative themes corresponded to the effectiveness of intervention in the given system. Nine priority actions were used as examples, chosen because they were identified in the STICKE workshops as key actions and were seen by the research team as representative of each intervention level. The narratives constructed included:

1 Paradigm level which targets deeply held beliefs: Change the entire system all at once, involves completely altering how things are done and how disability is imagined. In changing these structural elements, we need to fundamentally change how we think and how we act.
2 Goals and targets of a system: There are issues around access and inclusion that, if addressed, can rethink our current aims and way of doing things. These actions don't necessarily have to shift attitudes. If we set new aims, goals, and targets here, we can eventually shift how the whole system works.

3   Structure across the system: Change the relationship between many small things. If we act at this level, we can change the entire system, but we have to change how the small everyday things relate to each other.
4   Feedback and delays, loop dynamics: Create new or reshape old ways that relationships between people and organisations work. The types of actions that the community recommended here will not bring about massive changes to the overall system but will change how information is transferred between things. What we are trying to do here is break the cycle between problems by changing how they speak to each other.
5   System elements that are subsystem-specific: The most complex way of making change is to change many small factors over time. If we think of the physical things in our daily lives, such as catching a bus or using the restroom, changing how these things work will be an example of one small change in a larger system. These changes will change small aspects of our lives, so it will take many actions at this level to create wider change.

After presentation of each of the narratives participants were asked three questions: 1) what is missing here in the narrative; 2) what would you like to add to the narrative to include your own lived experience; and 3) what do you think about the validity, feasibility, and potential impacts of the actions suggested? The aim in these questions was to enable participants to compare their own lived experiences to the solutions envisaged by the wider community. The discussions around these affirmed the importance of the prioritised actions and proved to be a key step in the data collection phase of the project, ensuring the actions recommended were refined to be participant-driven.

Each group of actions were evaluated during the session using a variation of a semantic differential scale (ranging from most effective in bringing about systemic change, to least effective). The evaluation was arrived at by the all participants in the focus group via consensus. Here each action was represented in the form of a graphic pictogram illustrating the action, with the pictogram physically placed on a scale on a pin-board by the researcher as directed by the group of participants. Each action evaluated closely resembled the distribution of impact scores during the STICKE workshop phase and analysis phase where levels of intervention were used to construct the vocally delivered descriptions. Actions conformed across three phases of data collection and evaluation—STICKE workshop, level of intervention analysis, and focus group evaluation—therefore confirming the perceived level of impact that these priority actions might have of bringing about meaningful and sustainable change in access and inclusion.

Conclusion

This chapter described a feasibility study that investigated what is required to establish and sustain a provincial city in Victoria, Australia, as a leading accessible and inclusive city. The study has informed a collective plan of action supported by a wide range of community stakeholders. Systems-thinking is presented as an approach successfully used in the study that allowed for a wide range of stakeholders to identify actions to address the causes of obstacles to accessibility and social inclusion in their city.

A theoretical framework on inclusion informed this approach that 1) builds on social model ideas about addressing disability barriers; 2) extends beyond spatial and place-based conceptions of inclusion to add a relational context; and 3) positions collective impact approaches for the continued research, implementation, and evaluation of the actions identified by the project to overcome barriers to accessibility and inclusion.

While the systems-thinking workshops informed strong pathways to actions to address accessibility and social inclusion obstacles and were almost universally positively viewed by participants and researchers alike, the approach had shortcomings. A primary issue was the relatively low representation of people with lived experience of disability due to the difficulties of taking part in an all-day workshop. In other words, the complexity of approach resulted in a methodology that, counter to the fundamental aim of the research, was inaccessible and exclusionary for many people with disability. Moreover, it was found that the lower the proportion of people with lived experience of disability in the workshops, the less user-centred were the actions identified. The tone thereby shifted from user empowerment to support, and the actions identified seemed less able to inform attitudinal shift—a key aim identified across stakeholders as necessary for sustaining change toward greater social inclusion.

To redress the systems-thinking shortcomings, short-duration focus groups were added to the project that were more accessible to people with lived experience of disability. The focus groups evaluated the outputs from the systems-thinking workshops via the translation of these findings into narratives that allowed participants to overlay their own lived experiences on to the solutions envisaged by the wider community. The focus groups proved the key step for ensuring actions were more user-centred, user-created, and user-managed, thus increasing the visibility and engagement of people with disability and, in doing so, informing change able to catalyse community-wide attitudinal shift. However, if the process were to be undertaken again, the workshop may need to be adapted to consider the needs of participants with a disability.

It is concluded that multimethod inclusive consultative approaches with systems-thinking as its centre can provide a conceptual, ethical, and methodological starting point for the identification of the accessibility and inclusivity issues that face cities. However, while systems-thinking methods might inform pivotal solutions that have stakeholder-wide consensus, these solutions can lack the recognition of lived experience of social exclusion. Furthermore, as a result of such an ongoing foundation and co-development of systematic solutions with those in government and service providers, these changes will be more sustainable. In sum, to sustain such change, people with disabilities must be at the centre of co-developing, co-evaluating, co-researching actions for change that, as a consequence, are founded on a context of inclusion that is relational.

References

Aitken, Z., Baker, E., Badland, H., Mason, K., Bentley, R., Beer, A. and Kavanagh, A.M. (2019) 'Precariously placed: housing affordability, quality and satisfaction of Australians with disabilities', *Disability and Society*, 34: 121–42.

Bigby, C. (2008) 'Beset by obstacles: a review of Australian policy development to support aging in place for people with intellectual disability', *Journal of International Development and Disability*, 33: 76–84.

Boys, J. (ed) (2017) *Disability, Space, Architecture: A Reader*, London and New York: Routledge.

Burchardt, T., Le Grand, J. and Piachaud, D. (2002) 'Degrees of exclusion: developing a dynamic, multidimensional measure', in J. Hills, J. Le Grand and D. Piachaud (eds) *Understanding Social Exclusion*, Oxford: Oxford University Press.

Butler, R.E. and Bowlby, S. (1997) 'Bodies and spaces: an exploration of disabled people's experiences of public spaces', *Environment and Planning D*, 15: 411–33.

Butler, R.E. and Parr, H. (1999) (eds) *Mind and Body Spaces: Geographies of Impairment, Illness and Disability*, London: Routledge.

Deakin University (2019) 'STICKE: systems thinking in community knowledge exchange'. Online. Available at https://sticke2.deakin.edu.au/ (accessed 14 August 2019).

Duff, C. (2017) 'The affective right to the city', *Transactions of the Institute of British Geographers*, 42: 516–29.

Dyck, I. (1995) 'Hidden geographies: the changing lifeworlds of women with multiple sclerosis', *Social Science and Medicine*, 40: 307–20.

Fudge Schormans, A., Wilton, R. and Marquis, N. (2019) 'Building collaboration in the co-production of knowledge with people with intellectual disabilities about their everyday use of city space', *Area*, 51: 415–22.

Gleeson, B. (1997) 'The regulation of environmental accessibility in New Zealand', *International Planning Studies*, 2: 367–90.

Gleeson, B. (2001) 'Disability and the open city', *Urban Studies*, 38: 251–65.

Gleeson, B. (2002) *Geographies of Disability*, London and New York: Routledge.

Golledge, R.G. (1991) 'Cognition of physical and built environments', in T. Gärling and, G.W. Evans (Eds) *Environment, Cognition, and Action: An Integrated Approach*, New York: Oxford University Press.

Hall, E. (2005) 'The entangled geographies of social exclusion/ inclusion for people with learning disabilities', *Health and Place*, 11: 107–15.

Hall, E. (2010) 'Spaces of social inclusion and belonging for people with intellectual disabilities', *Journal of Intellectual Disability Research*, 54(S1): 48–57.

Harrison, M. (2004) 'Defining housing quality and environment: disability, standards and social factors', *Housing Studies*, 19: 691–708.

Harvey, D. (2008) 'The right to the city', *New Left Review*, 53: 23–40.

Imrie, R.F. (1996) *Disability and the City: International Perspectives*, London: Paul Chapman Publishing.

Imrie, R.F. (2001) 'Barriered and bounded places and the spatialities of disability', *Urban Studies*, 38: 231–7.

Iveson, K. (2011) 'Social or spatial justice? Marcuse and Soja on the right to the city', *City*, 15: 250–9.

Kania, J. and Kramer, M. (2011) 'Collective impact', *Stanford Social Innovation Review*, 9(1): 36–41.

La Rosa, D., Takatori, C., Shimizu, H. and Privitera, R. (2018) 'A planning framework to evaluate demands and preferences by different social groups for accessibility to urban greenspaces', *Sustainable Cities and Society*, 36: 346–62.

Malhi, L., Karanfil, Ö., Merth, T., Acheson, M., Palmer, A. and Finegood, D.T. (2009) 'Places to intervene to make complex food systems more healthy, green, fair, and affordable', *Journal of Hunger and Environmental Nutrition*, 4: 466–76.

Meadows, D.H. (1999) *Leverage Points: Places to Intervene in a System*, Hartland, VT: Sustainability Institute.

Milner, P. and Mirfin-Veitch, B. (2016) 'Making a space for the lost histories of inclusion', in R. Jackson (ed) *Community Care and Inclusion for People with an Intellectual Disability*, Edinburgh: Floris Books.

Mitchell, D. (2003) *The Right to the City: Social Justice and the Fight for Public Space*, New York: Guilford Press.

Peck, S. (1998) 'Group model building: facilitating team learning using system dynamics', *Journal of the Operational Research Society*, 49: 766–7.

Teather, E.K. (2005) *Embodied Geographies: Spaces, Bodies and Rites of Passage*, London: Routledge.

Tip, T. (2011) 'Guidelines for drawing causal loop diagrams', *Systems Thinker*, 22(1): 5–7.

Tually, S., Beer, A. and McLoughlin, P. (2011) *Housing Assistance, Social Inclusion and People Living with Disability*, AHURI Final Report No.178, Melbourne: Australian Housing and Urban Research Institute. Online. Available at www.ahuri.edu.au/publica tions/download/ahuri_40585_fr (accessed 15 August 2019).

United Nations (2006) 'Convention on the rights of persons with disabilities'. Online. Available at www.un.org/development/desa/disabilities/convention-on-the-rights-of-persons-with-disabilities/convention-on-the-rights-of-persons-with-disabilities-2.html (accessed 4 November 2019).

21 Theatre-based programmes

Promoting empathy and engagement

Ann Taket

Introduction

The creation and maintenance of social inclusion in different spheres of life requires recognising and respecting diversity, along with appropriate prosocial bystander action to interrupt discriminatory or demeaning speech and behaviour directed at particular individuals or groups based on some sociodemographic characteristic, plus action to create supportive and inclusive institutions and structures within society. One key factor supporting the creation of prosocial bystander or wider social action is empathic understanding across diversity. Alongside this, understanding of helpful and unhelpful ways of providing support and countering discrimination is also important. Theatre is an important medium for promoting both empathy and understanding and is becoming more widely used in health promotion and for stimulating positive social change. This chapter first introduces some of the literature on theatre, empathy, and social change before presenting two case studies. The first of these, *That Uppity Theatre*, overviews a 30-year body of work and looks briefly at two particular projects: the *DisAbility* project and *Dance the Vote*. The second case study, of the theatre-based education programme *Being Frank*, explores the participatory process by which such programmes can be developed and presents some of the feedback from participants. The chapter concludes with a short section highlighting some key points.

Theatre, empathy, and social change

> Narrative theater asks us to stand inside, to identify with the characters at the heart of the story, to see those characters in ourselves and ourselves in them. . . . When we empathize, the wall between self and other, between us and them, begins to disintegrate. We can no longer view the other as an abstraction or an object—we have to experience the other as human; as human as ourselves.
>
> (Blank and Jensen 2005: 19)

The quote succinctly captures the reasoning behind the role of empathy in bringing about the social change necessary for sustained social inclusion. Blank and Jensen (2005) describe the process of creation of their play *The Exonerated*, which focuses on the experience of wrongfully convicted death row inmates in the United States. In 2002, they were contacted by the Center on Wrongful Convictions at Northwestern University, an organisation they had worked with in researching their play. The Center asked for the play to be performed in Chicago for the then-governor as part of his decision-making process about proposed legislative reform. Proposals being considered included commuting death sentences to life in prison to remove the possibility of the wrongfully convicted being executed. The Chicago audience included the governor, members of the legislature, and about 50 exonerated death row inmates and was followed with intense discussion. A month later the governor announced his decision to commute all death row sentences before leaving office. Reports made to Bank and Jensen credit the play with making a real difference in this context, and attorney Larry Marshall from the Centre on Wrongful Convictions said he would 'never again doubt the power of art to effect social change' (quoted in Blank and Jensen 2005: 21).

Not all the research, however, finds a straightforward link between empathy and prosocial inclusive behaviour (Eisenberg and Strayer 1987). As Cummings' (2016) brief review notes, many factors intervene, and empathic skills may find an exploitive use in a con man or sadist. Cummings point to the importance of what she calls dialogic empathy, that is, empathy that recognises difference:

> not as making the other worthy of concern because she is like me, or even developing feelings of kindness or warmth toward another, but of critically expanding our understanding of how others experience the world so that we might work collaboratively toward solutions that benefit more people in a more democratic way.
>
> (Cummings 2016: 33)

Empathy is generally divided into two major types, independent of one another, affective and cognitive empathy (Jolliffe and Farrington 2006), where affective empathy is the capacity to experience the emotions of another, while cognitive empathy is the capacity to understand another's emotions. There has been a large amount of research on the links between empathy and prosocial action (Eisenberg and Strayer 1987) showing positive relationships between the two, but not always in an entirely straightforward fashion. So for example, a recent review of 40 studies of empathy and involvement in bullying in children and adolescents (van Noorden et al. 2014) found that defending (taking prosocial action) was positively associated with both types of empathy; however, being a nonactive bystander showed less consistent relationships with both cognitive and affective empathy. Turning to more recent single studies, António et al. (2017) showed that, for heterosexual adolescents, having friends who have gay friends and greater affective empathy (but not cognitive empathy), improved prosocial action intentions (i.e. intentions of helping victims of homophobic bullying). This is consistent with earlier findings that greater intergroup contact is associated with greater prosocial action (Abbott and Cameron 2014; Poteat and Vecho 2016). In contrast, for cyberbullying, Barlińska et al. (2018) found that cognitive empathy, but not affective empathy, is significant in promoting prosocial action, while Machackova and Pfetsch (2016) found affective empathy predicted support in cyberbullying while both types of empathy were important in offline bullying. Van der Ploeg et al. (2017) found affective empathy predictive of intervention in bullying, but not cognitive empathy.

Theatre-based approaches are one way of overcoming problems of low engagement, involving the ability of art to move people emotionally, and develop an empathic understanding of the challenges faced by those who experience social exclusion, as well as directly promoting inclusion of those facing various disadvantages. As Singhal et al. (2004) describe, there has been extensive work in 'education entertainment' involving drama of various types for different health promotion and social change purposes. They demonstrate that suitably constructed drama can foster engagement of the participants/audience in the subject matter to positive effect. Much of this work has taken place in low-income countries in the context of international community development (Sloman 2011). One recent example is that of work using theatre and dance for maternal health promotion in rural Zambia (Massar et al. 2018). Ayreek et al. (2018) discuss *Hamdeli* (Empathy), a pilot for a larger programme to be implemented by Afghanistan's National Programme for Culture and Creative Economy. The programme is intended to facilitate the social integration, social cohesion, and peaceful coexistence of Internally Displaced Persons (IDPs) between returnees and host communities in two major provinces of Afghanistan that are experiencing a high influx of displaced populations. In the pilot, male children and adolescents in two IDP settlements in the city of Herat were involved in participatory theatre over a period of seven months and worked with artists from the host community. The group was split by age, and the older group worked with a short half-hour play based on their own experiences (*Hamdeli*), while the younger group performed a play based on the novel *The Little Prince* (de Saint-Exupéry 1945) rewritten to reflect their experiences. Performances took place in a variety of schools and venues across the city. Ayreek et al. (2018) describe the process followed in detail and document the outcomes from the pilot based on a series of interviews and testimonials from both actor and audiences. Audiences showed high levels of appreciation and enthusiasm for the performances, with several noting that this was the first time they had interacted with IDPs. Healthy communication between IDPs and host communities was fostered by helping the IDPs and youths to find their voice and by using culture to approach host communities. The young people who participated gained in self-confidence and became ready to question tradition, for example, defying the orders they were given by children of the heads of tribes who wanted them to withdraw their participation. They also challenged some clerics who argued that theatre is an act of infidels. Initial resistance from the conservative leadership of the two IDP settlements changed into strong support through the consultations over the course of the programme's design and management. A short video was produced to document the pilot (https://youtu.be/fcOmd8dFtP4). The scale-up of the programme is underway at time of writing.

Jensen and Bonde's (2018) review of participatory arts activities and clinical arts interventions as a tool for improving mental health well-being concludes that these can be used as interventions to promote public health and well-being. Taket and Plourde (2018) explore this in relation to gender equity and gender-based violence, one source and manifestation of social exclusion. The two case studies presented later illustrate further diversity in the issues addressed and speak further to the ability of theatre to build empathy and social engagement for the purposes of social change.

That Uppity Theatre—theatre for social change

Participatory theatre is exemplified by a lot of the work of *That Uppity Theatre*, based in St Louis, Missouri, and founded in 1989 with nearly 30 years of activism to date: 'Our name reflects who we are: bold, brave, willing to step outside the status quo in order to instigate social change, promote civic dialogue and produce transformative theatrical art of the highest quality for people of all ages' (That Uppity Theatre Company n.d.). Their early years are described by founder Joan Lipkin in an interview (Lipkin 1993), and currently they focus on commissioned work about social issues as well as pairing amateur actors and seasoned professionals to create work about the lives of underrepresented populations (people with disabilities, gay, lesbian, bisexual, and transgendered adults and youth, people with Alzheimer's and early onset dementia, women with cancer, survivors of suicide, supporters of reproductive choice, at-risk youth, and university students). This particularly interesting case study demonstrates the possibilities of achieving a varied and creative programme of work supporting social inclusion that has been sustained over decades. Below just two examples of their work are presented; the first, *The DisAbility Project*, is an example of a longstanding programme of work first initiated in the late 1990s and still running today, and the second *Dance the Vote*, created more recently, encourages people to register to vote and commit to vote in American elections.

The DisAbility Project

One of *That Uppity Theatre*'s most longstanding piece of work is the *DisAbility Project* (DisAbility Project n.d.). Comprised of people with and without disabilities to model inclusion, the project creates and tours original material about the culture of disability. The group involved is diverse in age, race, ethnicity, class, occupation, education, religion, sexual orientation, physical ability, and performance experience. Weekly workshops/rehearsals, most open to the public, allow ensemble members to work up specific pieces that are presented at educational institutions, conferences, special events, festivals, religious and civic groups, and corporations.

Lipkin and Fox (2001) described the participatory process used in detail. The project seeks to construct theatre pieces that extend how theatre, dis/ability and community have been defined, making the stage 'an avenue of empowerment for the disabled community, rather than one more sideshow' (Lipkin and Fox 2001: 121). As Patty Clay, one of the original participants explained,

> It has meant so much to listen to others' stories and feel free to tell my own. . . . Sometimes it means tears, when things are tough. Then comes an inspiration for a haiku, or someone else's story, or a fun theatre exercise. As serious as the situations and histories are with our disabilities, we are able to find humor, and to "humanize" disability to the point that others without disabilities can relate their own experiences and their parallels.
>
> (quoted in Lipkin and Fox 2001: 127–8)

Dance the vote

The second example was work created specifically to encourage people to register to vote in the American elections and to encourage them to commit to vote on Election Day (Lipkin 2016; Vennhaus 2018). The project was initiated by theatre artist and social activist Joan Lipkin, artistic director of That Uppity Theatre Company, and Ashley Tate, artistic director of Ashleyliane Dance Company. The choreography is based on various themes of the voting experience, including the experience of African Americans, women, Latinx, and people with disabilities around voting, voting rights, voter suppression, and voting in other countries, among other themes. Lipkin (2016) explained that the motivation behind the creation of *Dance the Vote* lay in the low participation of eligible citizens in the 2012 presidential election and the 2016 primaries and caucuses. She worked to create an intergenerational group of four women, millennial to baby boomer, two white women and two women of colour. She describes how the project was created and successfully used to create community through making work about voting and the act of voting itself. Their initial ideas included performing pieces outside in free public spaces to reach diverse audiences and bypass traditional limited ticketing procedures and using dance and the spoken word to give focus to performing bodies and single voices and avoid the need for complicated sound systems. Each performance included a number of short pieces, alternating dance and the spoken word, giving a diversity of voices and work. As the project developed, artists came forward asking to participate, including seasoned professionals, college professors, and community teaching artists. Performers were rotated through different settings to share opportunities and work with people's other commitments. At each event, voter registration was provided in partnership with St. Louis Voter Registration Group. Nonpartisan voter registration opportunities were available on location to interested voters.

For the 2018 midterm elections, the group again formed, this time with a much longer lead time, securing a wider range of venues to deliver the work (Vennhaus 2018). *Dance the Vote* events were also held in other cities like Chicago, Boise, Idaho, as well as a wider range of places in Missouri, and other similar projects took place elsewhere in the United States (Antone 2018). Emily Underwood, director of community programmes for the Missouri Historical Society, which hosted one of the events in October 2018, explained,

> The history of our region and country is made up of choices that were made at the polls, as well as the struggle to be included in those choices. . . . Regardless of which candidates you support, voting is an important way to play a part in the continuing story of our community.
>
> (quoted in Staff 2018)

With reference to the 2018 work, Lipkin explains,

> As this is arguably one of the most important elections of our lifetime, we have to come together as artists to offer our talents, vision, and passion to actively participate in promoting voting and voter registration. The range of participating artists reflects much of the diversity in the St Louis community and offers creative and exciting perspectives on why voting is crucial and a precious right.
>
> (Joan Lipkin quoted in Vennhaus 2018)

A case study of co-creation: *Being Frank*

Being Frank is the third in a series of theatre-based programmes produced by Deakin University. What these programmes have in common is addressing the question of promoting empathy and understanding around particular issues, increasing the willingness of the audience to engage in prosocial action to interrupt discriminatory, abusive, or demeaning speech or behaviour. Programmes are delivered into different settings—schools, universities, sports clubs, workplaces, and communities. The programmes follow a common format, consisting of a 30- to 35-minute theatre piece delivered by a single actor, plus a small set of props, playing multiple roles, followed by a moderated panel discussion. The theatre piece is designed carefully to deliver accurate information and authentically depict different perspectives on the issues involving realistic story arcs. In panel discussion, issues raised are explored in further detail and questions answered, consolidating knowledge and understanding and further exploring what constitutes prosocial action. Panel members include those with responsibility for the issue in the setting concerned, so the discussion also services to strengthen positive supportive networks and capacities in the community concerned. A resource pack is provided to help guide local organisers through the process of planning and preparing for local delivery of the programme, and backup telephone and email support is available from the producer.

The first two programmes we adapted for use originated in the United States, where they have been in use since the early 2000s, *The Thin Line* which deals with eating disorders, and *You the Man*, which deals with dating violence and sexual assault. Both of these were written, directed, and produced in the United

States by Cathy Plourde and are documented elsewhere (Plourde 2017, 2018). The process by which *You the Man* was originally developed and the cultural translation to produce the Australian version are described in Plourde et al. (2014). A three-year longitudinal study of the impact of *You the Man* in schools has been carried out in the United States (Plourde et al. 2016); this demonstrated positive impacts on students' social norms, attitudes, and perceptions concerning dating violence and their intentions and behaviour when concerns of dating violence are noted.

The sections that follow, describing the development process for *Being Frank*, give a brief overview of the theatre piece and major discussion points, followed by an overview of the feedback obtained from the previews and first season. The final section then offers a summary of the main concluding points.

The development process

Being Frank was developed and is provided through a partnership between Deakin University and Transgender Victoria. The production team, producer Ann Taket, director Suzanne Chaundy, and writer Chris Summers facilitated a process of co-creation together with an advisory group. The stages in development of *Being Frank* are shown in Figure 21.1. The advisory group contained a diversity of members drawn from the trans communities as well as those with expertise in education, theatre, and health promotion. Organisations represented included Transgender Victoria (voluntary organisation promoting social justice, equity, and health for transgender people, their partners, families, and friends), Y Gender (peer-led social support and advocacy group for trans/gender diverse young people), and Minus 18 (youth-driven network for LGBTIQ youth). The advisory group was a diverse group in terms of age, ethnicity, religion, and gender identity, and all were paid for their input into the work.

The key principles on which the development of the programme were based were those used by Plourde in the development of the American programmes, namely to work to ensure that the programme serves survivors/victims; strengthens community capacity; provides good information without replicating oppression; transcends stereotypes; and validates honesty, urgency, and agency.

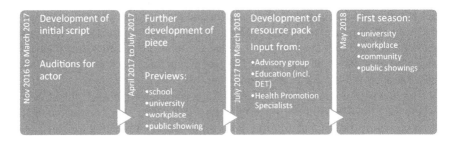

Figure 21.1 Stages in development of *Being Frank*

Intensive discussions at the first advisory group workshop provided a number of key messages for our writer as well as a wealth of detailed suggestions and points. Key messages from the advisory group were 'don't be gloomy', 'present positives as well as challenges', 'use humour', and 'convey the diversity of the community'. Once an initial script was produced and an actor/dramaturg cast, we took the work back to our advisory group at different points to further its development until we were ready to try it out in a limited number of previews, deliberately chosen to include the range of settings in which we wanted to deliver the programme. Unlike the *You the Man* and *The Thin Line*, we decided it was important to ensure that the panel includes at least one member with lived experience of trans or gender-diverse issues. This is necessary both for safety and to provide an optimal educational experience for the audience. As part of our partnership with Transgender Victoria, a suitable panel member is provided as part of the programme package. This is because we think it is important that local trans and gender-diverse people should not have to feel any pressure to sit on the panel; they should have the choice of contributing in whatever way they feel comfortable.

Following the previews, we used the feedback and other sources to compile a resource pack to support local organisers in setting up and running the programme. This resource pack went through successive drafts following feedback from our advisory group and a range of educationalists, health promotion specialists, and people involved in the previews. The first season then took place in May 2018.

Being frank: synopsis and discussion points

Being Frank is a 30- to 35-minute one-actor play. It features five main characters: Frank (Frankie/Francesca); Marco—Frank's best friend; Gita—Frank's mum; Hutch—Frank's dad; and Noor (Jenny Der), a young transwoman. Great care has been taken with the script to give accurate information in a way that does not judge but instead illustrates the emotional issues experienced by a young person coming out as transgender as well as by their family and friends. This programme promotes empathy, acceptance, and understanding for all involved.

What follows is a description of the story and action in *Being Frank*. The actor switches simply and quickly from one character to the next, assisted by minimal props.

Frank is a vlogger and invites us to be part of his very personal experience of coming out as a transgender young person. He does this via his regular Facebook videos, preferring this method to informing his parents and friends personally. Throughout the play, we follow Frank through the school year and learn a bit about the challenges and difficulties he faces, and we see Frank evolve and discover that being 'trans' is more complex and dynamic than he originally thought.

Marco is so enthusiastic and determined to be the perfect best friend and support person for Frank, but in his efforts to feel included, he tends to be overbearing and loses sight of the emotional pain and turmoil Frank is experiencing, causing Frank to pull away. He convenes the LGBTIQ Allies group at school and is dismayed to find that not all people are supportive and his well-meaning efforts to draw attention to issues and encourage dialogue may also have the effect of unearthing intolerance and discrimination.

Noor is a young transwomen who knows Frank through his Facebook video and invites him to be involved in the local trans community. She is making a documentary on being transgender and shows a romantic interest in Frank.

Gita, Frank's mother, loves her child and offers unconditional support. She is the one who takes Frank to medical appointments to facilitate hormone treatment, even though she is scared of what they may do to him. She is also privately mourning the loss of her daughter.

Hutch actually has no speaking part throughout the play, but we come to know him through Frank's and Gita's eyes and their interactions. Hutch loved and supported his daughter, Francesca, and wants to show the same to his son, Frank. But he's struggling with his own confusion, his grief over the loss of a daughter, and how to best express his feelings for Frank.

Corresponding to the different parts in the piece are multiple discussion points that can be drawn out in the panel discussion. (A discussion guide is also provided as part of the resource pack.) The path to discovering your own personal truth may be fraught with unexpected roadblocks and speed bumps, but the support of friends and family smooths the journey. Also unexpected and practical issues like uniforms and infrastructure concerns such as gender-based bathrooms emerge. Empathy, understanding, and appreciation are needed when supporting a trans or gender-diverse person. Support may not always look how we imagine, and friends need support too. Gender diversity or questioning does not stop you being a normal teenager who can be 'into' or romantically attracted to another teenager. Family members and friends need to acknowledge they may need support too. There are cultural contradictions between masculinity and fatherhood. We hear about Hutch discovering ways of supporting his child that are outside the traditional male role.

What did participants think?

During both the previews and first season, we took a variety of measures to gather feedback from audience and panel members about the programme, using a short anonymous online survey distributed at least one week after the event. The timing of one week after was deliberately chosen to give people a chance to have reflected on the programme. The survey was anonymous to prevent people feeling inhibited about offering feedback, particularly negative. It is worth noting, however, that none of the feedback was negative or hostile. We also received unsolicited feedback throughout. Table 21.1 summarises the sources of feedback and survey response rates for the previews and first season.

A number of important areas were emphasised. First of all, audience members reported that the programme helped them identify what they could do to support transgender people in their setting. For example, a student teacher responded, 'It made me think about toilets, uniforms, relationships with others, their name,

Table 21.1 Sources of feedback from previews and first season

Setting	Number attending	Survey responses	Response rate	Additional feedback
	N	N	%	
School	60	41	68	Yes—Post-it notes
University	86	23	27	Yes—email and verbal
Workplace	32	10	31	Yes—email
Community	85	30	35	Yes—email and verbal
Total	263	104	40	

providing support and how I would support transgender students in my classroom'. Secondly, the programme presented information in an accessible and relatable format. Three quotes illustrate this, the first from a health professional who said,

> the "play" tended to steer clear of jargon and instead focused on the emotional impact of discovery (for Frank) but also some of the experiences of those people around him, which I feel is really important. I feel like this is such an innovative and provocative way to provide education to kids and adults, that isn't "dumbed" down.

The second quote, from a year nine student, typical of many responses, summarised what they had learnt.

> Transgender people may label themselves as female or male or they may feel neither label fits them and it is important to respect their change and transitioning stage. In order for them to express themselves, no matter what, everyone should respect on another and not be treated any different.

Thirdly a school nurse reported, 'The acting was great and brought across the angst of the mum and friend, and of the person undergoing the experience'. Participants also appreciated the presence of someone with trans lived experience on the panel. One school student expressed it this way, 'I also would like to send a thanks for the guest that came in and shared his trans-journey with us. He was very patient, open minded and honest with us and we really appreciated that.'

Also important was feedback from trans participants that they found the programme useful and positive. One university audience member said, 'I love this performance, and as a young trans person, I feel that it has the potential to really connect with youth and change attitudes within schools and other areas!' Another commented, 'As a young trans person myself, I found some of the mother's comments quite emotionally challenging, however I think this was necessary and important.' Participants also reported that they thought the programme created a safe space for discussion.

What did participants report they learnt?

Analysing responses to the questions on what people learnt from the programme revealed a number of important areas where they had increased their knowledge. They talked about the importance of inclusivity for everyone and the diversity of journeys and destinations that are included in the spectrum of human possibilities. The reported that they had learnt about multiple perspectives of the trans person themselves but also friends and family members. Support was another area where participants talked about what they had learnt, the importance of offering support, but thinking carefully about how to offer support and about asking people what they would like. They also talked about the importance of practical things— toilets, uniforms, pronouns, etc.—and stressed that schools, workplaces, and other settings and venues need to be made welcoming to and inclusive of all.

Our main conclusions were that the feedback indicated that participants found the programme interesting and engaging. It was successful in increasing people's knowledge, empathy, and understanding. Participants expressed their willingness to offer support, and no evidence of hostility was found. The programme created safe space for discussion. The participative process of programme development, co-creation, allowed the emergence of a programme that provided participants with knowledge about trans and gender-diverse issues, introducing a range of different perspectives: that of the young trans person themselves, their parents, friends, and peers. The feedback from *Being Frank* participants demonstrated the programme's success in developing cognitive empathy in the sense described earlier and in highlighting helpful ways of providing support as well as what is unhelpful.

In conclusion

None of the previously mentioned should be taken to imply that the use of theatre is unproblematic and straightforward and necessarily serves the cause of prosocial action. Funders can alter and amend the agendas served, as critiques by Scharinger (2013) of work in Timor-Leste and Mundrawala (2007) of work in Pakistan have demonstrated. The discussion, however, does serve to illustrate what is possible.

The case studies demonstrate a number of issues. The first is the sheer variety of groups that can be engaged through the medium of theatre. The case studies are both from high-income countries, but it is important to recognise that this choice is one of convenience to the author, knowing of the work of the first case study and being involved herself in the second. As the first section of the chapter discussed, there is a long history of the use of theatre for positive social change in low- and middle-income countries and the Global South.

What the case studies demonstrate is that as well as engaging, theatre also leads to real changes in communities, as when formerly disenfranchised people vote (*Dance the Vote*) and when inclusion becomes a way of life (*The DisAbility Project*). Projects explore not only what is different but that those who are excluded have much in common with their non-excluded peers (e.g. Frank is a vlogger, as are many teenagers). Whereas sympathy is often short term and situational, empathy is potentially long term and about engaging with the essence of being human and seeing that as more important than the differences which divide.

Acknowledgements

The development and delivery of *Being Frank* would not have been possible without the partnership between the production team at Deakin University (Director: Suzanne Chaundy; Writer: Chris Summers; Dramaturg: Genevieve Giuffre; Videographer: Pier Carthew; and Producer: Ann Taket) and at Transgender Victoria (Andrew Eklund and Michelle McNamara). We also gratefully acknowledge input from a large number of other people who worked with our team at various points:

- The members of Advisory Group, drawn from the trans and gender-diverse community, as well as friends and family of trans people who provided very important guidance on the content of the play and its performance in the first stage of the project;
- The people who hosted the programme in the 2017 preview season, which enabled us to deliver the play in a variety of settings—school, tertiary education, and workplace—and to fine-tune its delivery;
- The people from different sectors, including education, health, and welfare services and the arts who have contributed by commenting on drafts of the resource pack and providing helpful suggestions for its further development; and
- Chris Varney-Clark, who undertook the production of the first drafts of the resource pack for delivery in schools as her final year project in the Masters of Public Health over 2017–2018.

References

Abbott, N. and Cameron, L. (2014) 'What makes a young assertive bystander? The effect of intergroup contact, empathy, cultural openness, and in-group bias on assertive bystander intervention intentions', *Journal of Social Issues*, 70(1): 167–82.

Antone, T. (2018) 'Getting Out the Vote: Theatres and Civic Responsibility', Howlaround Theatre Commons. Online. Available at https://howlround.com/getting-out-vote (accessed 15 November 2018).

António, R., Guerra, R. and Moleiro, C. (2017) 'Having friends with gay friends, the role of extended contact, empathy and threat on assertive bystanders behavioral intentions', *Psicologia*, 31(2): 15–24.

Ayreek, K., Noshadi, S. and Guggenheim, S. (2018) 'Hamdeli: theater, culture, and displacement in Afghanistan', unpublished report.

Barlińska, J., Szuster, A. and Winiewski, M. (2018) 'Cyberbullying among adolescent bystanders: role of affective versus cognitive empathy in increasing prosocial cyberbystander behavior', *Frontiers in Psychology*, 9: 799, DOI: 10.3389/fpsyg.2018.00799.

Blank, J. and Jensen, E. (2005) 'The uses of empathy: theatre and the real world', *Theatre History Studies*, 25: 15–22.

Cummings, L.B. (2016) *Empathy as Dialogue in Theatre and Performance*, Basingstoke: Palgrave Macmillan.

de Saint-Exupéry, A. (1945) *The Little Prince*, tr. K. Woods, London: W. Heinemann.

DisAbility Project (n.d.) 'The disability project'. Online. Available at www.uppityco.com/about-1/ (accessed 14 November 2018).

Eisenberg, N. and Strayer, J. (eds) (1987) *Empathy and Its Development*, Cambridge and New York: Cambridge University Press.

Jensen, A. and Bonde, L.O. (2018) 'The use of arts interventions for mental health and wellbeing in health settings', *Perspectives in Public Health*, 138: 208–14.

Jolliffe, D. and Farrington, D.P. (2006) 'Development and validation of the basic empathy scale', *Journal of Adolescence*, 29: 589–611.

Lipkin, J. (1993) 'Rabble-rousing in St Louis with *that uppity theatre*', *New Theatre Quarterly*, 9: 367–78.

Lipkin, J. (2016) '*Dance the Vote: on rapid response, performance, the election, and civic engagement*', Howlaround Theatre Commons. Online. Available at https://howlround.com/dance-vote (accessed 14 November 2018).

Lipkin, J. and Fox, A. (2001) 'The *DisAbility project*: toward an aesthetic of access', *Contemporary Theatre Review*, 11: 119–36.

Machackova, H. and Pfetsch, J. (2016) 'Bystanders' responses to offline bullying and cyberbullying: the role of empathy and normative beliefs about aggression', *Scandinavian Journal of Psychology*, 57: 169–76.

Massar, K., Sialubanje, C., Maltagliati, I. and Ruiter, R.A.C. (2018) 'Exploring the perceived effectiveness of applied theater as a maternal health promotion tool in rural Zambia', *Qualitative Health Research*, 28: 1933–43.

Mundrawala, A. (2007) 'Fitting the bill: commissioned theatre projects on human rights in Pakistan: the work of Karachi-based theatre group *Tehrik e Niswan*', *Research in Drama Education*, 12: 149–61.

Plourde, C. (2017) *The Thin Line: A Play on Coping with Eating Disorders*, Pawtucket, RI: Addverb Productions.

Plourde, C. (2018) *You the Man: A One-man Performance Addressing Bystanders*, Pawtucket, RI: Addverb Productions.

Plourde, C., Shore, N., Herrick, P., Morrill, A., Cattabriga, G., Bottino, L., Orme, E. and Stromgren, C. (2016) 'You the man: theater as bystander education in dating violence', *Arts and Health*, 8: 229–47.

Plourde, C., Taket, A., Murray, V. and van der Werf, P. (2014) 'The development and cultural translation of a brief theatre-based program for the promotion of bystander engagement and violence prevention', *Journal of Applied Arts and Health*, 5: 377–92.

Poteat, V.P. and Vecho, O. (2016) 'Who intervenes against homophobic behavior? Attributes that distinguish active bystanders', *Journal of School Psychology*, 54: 17–28.

Scharinger, J. (2013) 'Participatory theater, is it really? A critical examination of practices in Timor-Leste', *ASEAS Österreichische Zeitschrift für Südostasienwissenschaften*, 6(1): 102–19. Online. Available at https://doi.org/10.4232/10.ASEAS-6.1-6 (accessed 15 November 2018).

Singhal, A., Cody, M.J., Rogers, E. and Sabido, M. (eds) (2004) *Entertainment Education and Social Change: History, Research and Practice*, Mahwah, NJ: Lawrence Erlbaum Associates.

Sloman, A. (2011) 'Using participatory theatre in international community development', *Community Development Journal*, 47: 42–57.

Staff (2018) 'Poll dancing: unique partnership uses choreography as campaign for voting, civic engagement', *The St Louis American*. Online. Available at www.stlamerican.com/entertainment/living_it/poll-dancing-unique-partnership-uses-choreography-as-campaign-for-voting/article_fe53b534-c78f-11e8-9f23-97857d3f81d7.html (accessed 15 November 2018).

Taket, A. and Plourde, C. (2018) 'Engaging bystanders in violence prevention', in A. Taket and B.R. Crisp (eds) *Eliminating Gender-Based Violence*, London: Routledge.

That Uppity Theatre Company (n.d.) 'Welcome to That Uppity Theatre'. Online. Available at www.uppityco.com/#current-section (accessed 14 November 2018).

van der Ploeg, R., Kretschmer, T., Salmivalli, C. and Veenstra, R. (2017) 'Defending victims: what does it take to intervene in bullying and how is it rewarded by peers?' *Journal of School Psychology*, 65: 1–10.

van Noorden, T.H.J., Haselager, G.J.T., Cillessen, A.H.N. and Bukowski, W.M. (2014) 'Empathy and involvement in bullying in children and adolescents: a systematic review', *Journal of Youth and Adolescence*, 44: 637–57.

Vennhaus, L. (2018) '*Dance the Vote! Arts community to promote registration, awareness,*' St Louis Limelight. Online. Available at https://stllimelight.com/2018/09/19/dance-the-vote-arts-community-to-promote-registration-awareness/ (accessed 14 November 2018).

Part 7

Conclusions

22 Strategies for sustaining social inclusion

Beth R. Crisp and Ann Taket

Introduction

As many of the chapters in this volume attest, sustaining social inclusion includes rejection of pain and suffering as having to be experienced by individuals as a privatised matter. Rather,

> The message of inclusion is: You are not alone. You are our community, and we are yours. If we can come together and stick together, then nothing can divide us.
>
> (Avery 2018: 207)

However, historians often imply that social exclusion is endemic, frequently carried down the generations and social inclusion takes years, if not decades, to be achieved (Stedman Jones 1971/2013). While the contributions in this volume do not deny that immense efforts are required to achieve social inclusion which can be sustained over time, they nevertheless challenge assumptions that social exclusion cannot be overturned. The contributions in this volume also provide some examples of initiatives which contribute to the realisation of the United Nations' (2015) *Social Development Goals* (SDGs) which were introduced in chapter 1, and which seek to 'leave no one behind'. The *SDGs* are themselves an action plan for moving toward achieving human rights for all as spelt out in the *Universal Declaration of Human Rights* (United Nations 1948). Human rights cannot be achieved without social inclusion. Nor can social inclusion be truly achieved by initiatives which disregard human rights and consider human dignity as an optional extra. Hence, this concluding chapter summarises some key strategies which have emerged from this volume as facilitating sustained social inclusion utilising a human rights framework. These include the construction of knowledge, use of language, promoting dignity, an intersectional lens, multilevel and multisectoral approaches, and resourcing.

Constructing knowledge

Understanding how knowledge is constructed and used to promote and consolidate social exclusion is a starting point to sustain social inclusion. This includes recognition of what knowledges are excluded, including those of Indigenous peoples (chapter 15), women (chapter 4), children (chapter 13), people living with disability (chapters 5, 13, 18, and 20), and refugees (chapter 16), as well as understanding how different philosophical frameworks facilitate the exclusion of the perspectives of many individuals and groups (chapter 14). Not surprisingly, the need to critically reflect and explore possibilities for doing things differently, is raised in several chapters. This includes the need for individual service providers and organisations to critically reflect on their own beliefs and whether or not they are being coerced into neoliberal agendas which do not prioritise social inclusion (chapters 4, 9, 11, and 12). For example, marketisation of care has been promoted by policymakers as being socially inclusive, but the lived experience of those requiring care is that social inclusion is no more than rhetoric unless service delivery systems undergo radical transformation (chapter 14). In some instances, services which have been acclaimed as being high quality have actually isolated those they were designed to serve (chapter 19).

Many of the chapters in this volume discussed the need for consultation in order to really hear the experiences of individuals and groups who experience marginalisation (e.g. chapters 3, 5, 11, 18, and 20). This is essential so that well-meaning individuals and organisations do not assume they know what others require. Rather than assuming that some groups are too difficult to consult, new methodologies might need to be developed or existing methods modified to accommodate the capacities of those whose views are sought. For those whose voices have been historically been overlooked, the opportunity to speak of their experiences might require those conducting consultations to first hear of what has happened in the past before a community is able to explore future options which are more inclusive. Inclusive consultation processes have agendas which seek out the views from potential service users as to what they think would improve their lives rather than only asking about predetermined options. Furthermore, while setting up a process for consultation is important, maintaining community engagement is crucial for sustaining social inclusion.

Enabling the experiences of individuals and groups who experience exclusion to be effectively communicated may, in some circumstances, be best achieved when not confined to conventional modes of communication in the spheres of policy and programme development and delivery. As several chapters in this volume attest, the experiences of social exclusion can be powerfully communicated by utilising the creative arts, including poetry, song, theatre, and film (chapters 13, 17, 18, and 21).

The question of who is best placed to consult with individuals and groups who have excluded needs consideration if the knowledge which is constructed is to be perceived to be valid by different stakeholders. Policymakers and funding bodies may view data as biased when collected by people who directly provide services to marginalised groups, but those being consulted can might find it difficult to trust people they do not know or whom they perceive as being unable to capture their experiences and communicate them to the wider world. Hence, employing people with disability to undertake consultations with people with disability is one approach to consultation which seeks to ensure the construction of knowledge takes account of the views of those consulted (chapter 18). A more radical approach is to ensure that those who have been excluded are not only asked their opinions but collaborate in analysing the data generated in consultative processes, ideally in all aspects of consultative processes as equal partners (e.g. chapters 5 and 20).

The importance of language

When communication of knowledge involves use of words, the need for inclusive language was discussed in several chapters in this volume. For example, chapter 2 noted the need to transform the language pertaining to people who have been injured at work, whom workers' compensation or insurance schemes often treat with disdain and assume claims are to some degree fraudulent. For those organising the community breakfast for the homeless described in chapter 8, referring to participants as 'people' and not as the needs they have, i.e. as 'homeless', demonstrates inclusion rather than exclusion. Similarly, the authors of this chapter commented that 'talking about inclusion promotes the idea of "solidarity with" rather than "charity for" and can draw attention to the exclusion, imbalance in power and silencing of people who are living homeless'.

Even those authors who have not discussed their use of language have carefully considered what is inclusive language in their context. For example, several chapters use the term 'disability', but we recognise that some Indigenous communities in Australia, New Zealand, and North America have no such word in their language and reject the connotations of exclusion, which they consider embedded into this notion (Avery 2018). We also note the emergence of terms such as 'diffability' to refer to 'people who are differently able' (Suharto et al. 2016: 693). The language of diffability challenges the more common conflation of difference with inferiority.

> A corollary of "human capital" is the notion of a "disabled person", an idea that was socially constructed to categorise those people that were perceived to be unable to participate in the market economy, or raw materials in a production process and discarded as not meeting a standard specification.
>
> (Avery 2018: 8)

At times, new language may need to be developed to properly encapsulate experiences of exclusion as a precursor to facilitating inclusion. For example, the term 'apprehended discrimination' has been developed to describe the experiences of people who have come to the realisation that exclusion is a constant in their lives.

> As they become more personally exposed to discrimination, their understanding of discrimination transitions from an intangible judgment to an increasingly rational thought process, in the sense that every incident adds weight to their rational judgment of discrimination. Apprehended discrimination is the

"A-ha" moment when they realise that their perception of discrimination has become their reality, a psychological realisation that involves an unpleasant physiological reaction.

(Avery 2018: 43)

Too often, that 'A-ha' leads to people avoiding situations where they believe they are at risk from further discrimination. Such 'A-ha' moments should be considered a final warning that effective responses which promote and sustain social inclusion are required. This will require service providers and others to work cooperatively in ways which support the aspirations of groups who have been excluded rather than impose their own agendas (Avery 2018). Examples of this can be found at various points in this volume, including chapters 8, 11, and 19.

Promoting dignity

Human rights often feature in discourses about, but are not necessarily reflected in, health and welfare practice (Gilbert and Dako-Gyeke 2018). Programmes which seek to address a lack of social inclusion may in fact reduce individual agency. For example, *The Good Food Box* programmes in Canada have sought to provide fruit and vegetables at a reduced cost to low-income families, but recipients were unable to choose the contents of their box. Moreover, the advice which came with the food, which made assumptions about recipients' lack of knowledge in how to create nutritional meals, was experienced by some participants as paternalistic (Loopstra and Tarasuk 2013). This is in stark contrast with the experience of asylum seekers who shop at the *Food Justice Truck* (chapter 7), which was that they were treated with dignity rather than made to feel shame because they were poor.

The organisers of the community breakfast for the homeless had to fight a proposal to build a service counter which would form a physical barrier between the volunteers who provided the service and the intended recipients. They argued that a barrier created a hierarchy, implied a lack of worth in respect of the recipients, and reinforced a difference between who is included and who is excluded (see chapter 8). The opportunity to meet as equals a wide range of people from the broader community and not just other asylum seekers was one of the attractive features for people who shopped at the *Food Justice Truck*. In particular, the *Food Justice Truck* is an example of an initiative which has been 'designed with empowerment goals in mind, and seek to provide food via mutual support strategies, not just through passive giving and receiving' (see chapter 7).

Building on strengths rather than focusing on addressing deficits is another way of enhancing dignity (chapters 6 and 19). Peer support, such as that offered by members of the *Helpific* community, is offering people who have always been positioned as service recipients the opportunity to make positive contributions to the lives of others in their locale (chapter 19). As was noted in chapter 2:

Peer support operates at a face-to-face level, but its potential to become a sustainable social development depends on peer programs giving voice not only to the suffering experienced by victims of a traumatic event, but also giving voice to the injustices and suffering caused to trauma victims by institutions of care that have failed to meet their needs.

An intersectional lens

Initiatives to challenge social exclusion often consider just one aspect of people's lives. However, people are multifaceted, and an intersectional approach is required if social inclusion is to be sustained (Choo and Ferree 2010; Cho et al. 2013). Yet the emphasis of many international declarations which champion the rights of people with a shared experience or identity as if they are homogenous. As one of the participants in the *Opening Doors* programme commented in chapter 6, people are often not aware of the lived experiences and perspectives of people whose backgrounds are different to their own. Hence, without intentional adoption of an intersectional lens, the diversity of people who share a particular characteristic (such as gender, sexuality, ethnicity, disability, religion, or poverty) is easily disregarded, ignoring the shaping of their experience by interaction with all the other sociodemographic characteristics that they possess.

Almost 50 years after his book *Homosexual: Oppression and Liberation* was published in 1971, author and activist Dennis Altman reflects back on his own experiences of negotiating worlds in which at times he withheld some aspects of his identity in order to experience inclusion.

> the old gay liberation cry to come out; except today it has taken on a psychological rather than a political meaning, and "coming out" means expressing an authentic self, that is assumed to be dormant, waiting for the right moment to declare itself.
>
> "Coming out" is only possible when one's identity is not visible, which is why it rarely applies to racial identities, however complex they are in reality. I have the same choice when it comes to declaring I am Jewish, and there have been times, especially in would-be "progressive" circles, when it's seemed easier to come out as homosexual than as Jewish.
>
> (Altman 2019: 188–9)

Altman's experience demonstrates why social inclusion needs to be considered as 'situated, engaged, relational, ongoing practices rather than end-state orientated' (Keevers and Abuodha 2012: A43). His experience also explains the need to be wary of imposing standardised approaches which do not take into account of the specific needs of individuals and communities in local areas (Chambers 2010).

Multilevel and multisectoral approaches

This book has included approaches to sustaining social inclusion from the very local area (e.g. chapters 6, 7, 8, 11, and 18) to globally (e.g. chapters 14 and 15). As both global and local approaches are required, we should not necessarily think work at one level as superior to the other but as complementary, and as individuals, groups, or organisations, we should be working to promote and sustain social inclusion in ways that best fit with our capacity and the needs of our communities (Brink 2018).

> In order to achieve that end, one must actually go beyond the simplification of an ideal-type community that would warrant a one-size-fits-all approach to participation. Real world rural communities may differ considerably along several important dimensions and, as a consequence, supporting interventions involving the beneficiaries—a praiseworthy end in itself—must be based on a good understanding of the details of context in particular situations. In short, a participatory approach to development is much more complex than is often imagined by donors, and it requires the adoption of a much longer time horizon than they are usually prepared to consider, given the constraint of producing quick results which they typically face.
>
> (Platteau 2008: 128)

Sustaining social inclusion requires a multipronged approach which addresses both the needs of an individual and changes the environmental context (chapter 2). As has been suggested at various points in this volume, this requires dynamic, interdisciplinary, intersectional, and multisectoral strategies to ensure systemic issues are addressed. This will require professionals and organisations going beyond working in their usual silos and intentionally working with those from other professions and organisations who take very different approaches to promoting social inclusion (Schmitz et al. 2012). Siloed approaches lead to thinking that for people who have limited mobility, provision of a wheelchair will enable them to participate in life beyond their home. However, if there are unmade roads and public transport is not wheelchair-accessible, there may be little or no increased capacity to go out independently (Mitra 2018). It was such disconnections between different authorities that resulted in initiatives such as the one described in chapter 20, which brought sought to bring together a wide range of stakeholders with the aim of making a city truly accessible for people with disability.

Although governments provide much of the funding for initiatives to address social exclusion, government agencies cannot do this work alone. In chapter 7, it was proposed that 'social enterprises have emerged in recognition that government provided social support or support provided through charity is limited, and more importantly, is not meeting public need'. The importance of the community sector was noted in chapter 16 in respect of providing services to refugees and in supporting social inclusion initiatives such as *Opening Doors* (chapter 6). Importantly, initiatives developed by community-based organisations often have reach into the community to link both those who benefit from services and volunteers who can provide these (chapters 8 and 19).

Transformations of the magnitude which may be required to sustain social inclusion often require changes to entrenched policies and practices which challenge the interests of social elites (Béné et al. 2012). This includes ensuring policies and practices around professional education which affect both curriculum and student selection contribute to sustaining social inclusion (St Pierre Schneider et al. 2009). As argued in chapters 9 and 10, higher education has a long history of being socially exclusive. Yet in the health and community services, students whose backgrounds have often excluded them from higher education often have the capacity to be effective service providers, particularly to those on the margins of society if they are given the opportunity (Crisp 2018).

Not only is coherence between different policies and practices required (Murphy 2012), but also coherence of policies. In Australia, asylum seekers are able to attend government primary and secondary schools as local students who pay no tuition fees. However, the university system treats asylum seekers as international students who are not only subject to much higher fees than local students but are also denied the option provided to domestic students to defer paying their fees until their income reaches a minimum threshold. Unless a charity is prepared to sponsor their higher education, most asylum seekers are effectively prevented from continuing their education beyond secondary school. In the short term, this restricts participation in Australian society and in the longer term reduces their employability (White 2017). Lack of coherence in policy between different levels of government was also noted in chapter 4, in respect to policy about reproductive health as well as the competing societal expectations of women as mothers and women as workers.

Policy coherence is not only required at a local or national level, but also internationally. Arguably the agendas of international organisations such as the World Bank are often in conflict with the *SDGs* and the *Universal Declaration of Human Rights* (Murphy 2005; Sukarieh and Tannock 2008), and unless this is addressed, initiatives for sustained social inclusion are unlikely to be achieved. Even when World Bank initiatives are seemingly aligned to the *SDGs*, they can be readily undermined by local priorities. For example, World Bank programmes to improve the quality of housing have often had enthusiastic buy-in from governments when it has come to clearing slums, but maintaining replacement housing stock tends not to be a priority. Thus improvements in health and well-being associated with adequate housing are unlikely to be sustained over time, without ensuring that funding for ongoing maintenance is secured (Corburn and Sverdlik 2017). This is not surprising given that neoliberalism, which dominates economic and political decision-making in many countries, tends to prioritise fiscal restraint over social inclusion. This has led to declines in life expectancy and public expenditure on health and education and increases in poverty and health inequalities in many countries (De Vogli et al. 2013).

Resourcing

Promoting and sustaining social inclusion may incur costs which would not accrue if the status quo is maintained (Béné et al. 2012), but these costs may well be recovered over time (Abbott et al. 2017). Therefore, the costs of not investing in promoting and sustaining social inclusion may ultimately prove more costly in the longer term (McDonald and Bertram 2018). In seeking to gain the most benefit from investing in social inclusion, different approaches may need to be considered. For example, with the *Opening Doors* programme discussed in chapter 6, there was a deliberate choice to take a leadership and capacity-building approach rather than fund short-term projects for specific groups. Furthermore:

> During the programme, participants learn how to plan, fund and implement initiatives to promote social inclusion. They also learn about barriers to inclusion, creating consensus and co-designing, managing challenging behaviours, self-care, social media, advocacy, public speaking, effective promotion strategies and sustainability.

Sustainable social inclusion requires thinking in much longer time frames than in short-term policy cycles, particularly when it comes to funding initiatives. Nevertheless, funding can be an effective lever for facilitating sustained social inclusion, provided funding bodies are able to try new ways of working toward social inclusion (chapter 11). For example, an aid project in rural Pakistan recognised the significant role which women had in the agricultural workforce, but at the same time these women often had involvement in decision-making. As a result of capacity-building activities associated with the provision of financial aid, the women became much more involved in a wide range of decisions, including sale and purchase of livestock but also in household expenditure, including education and medical expenses (Chambers et al. 2018). The effects of this are expected to not only have changes for the project participants but may also benefit future generations of girls and women.

Sustainability requires that an initiative not only 'fits' with those organisations which facilitate it, but also that it continues to be perceived as meeting the needs of those it serves. Someone to 'champion' an initiative may be critical to its longevity, as may stakeholders who provide support from other organisations (Scheirer 2005). These champions include policymakers, who seek to ensure social inclusion through policy and legislative developments, but do not necessarily see their visions realised when programmes are designed and delivered (Walsham et al. 2019).

While the role of champions should not be underestimated, equally crucial are the personnel on the ground developing and implementing policy and programme initiatives. The importance of a programme director or leader was raised in various chapters, as was the recruitment and selection of paid staff and volunteers. For example, in chapter 17 about work in Myanmar with the Rohingya and Rakhine communities, the effectiveness of community facilitators was found to be associated with their motivation and personal attributes rather than their education, experience, or status in the community. Nevertheless, training was required as otherwise staff and volunteers can unwittingly create environments which are experienced as exclusionary, even when inclusion was the intention. This was also the experience of the community breakfast team in chapter 8.

> As not all our volunteers come with an understanding of inclusion, that idea needs to be introduced and explored. People are familiar with the idea of

helping, of doing good—they know that they themselves are fortunate and so they can afford to give some of their time and efforts for people who are less so. This is a valid motivation but inclusion can value add to the provision of food, communicating acceptance and acknowledgement of people's intelligence and capabilities and so be somewhat more strengths based in style.

Social inclusion requires commitment from all levels of an organisation. Hence, a need for understanding one's motivations is equally important for those responsible for oversight of programmes and organisations. In chapter 2, it was reported that 'the agency's journey towards sustainable social inclusion for traumatised people began with the board's governance commitment to a self-reflective practice embracing the vulnerability of their personal woundedness.'

Training and support of staff and volunteers does not end with induction processes but needs to be ongoing. The work of social inclusion is often difficult and confronting, particularly for frontline workers, and ongoing support mechanisms are required. Yet many organisations regard the costs associated with ongoing support of staff and volunteers as being too costly. While this can produce short-term budget savings, in chapter 12 it was found that not providing necessary supports ultimately places efforts to promote social inclusion at increased risk of not being able to be sustained.

Conclusion

We recognise that in a single volume, we cannot provide a comprehensive coverage of initiatives which sustain social inclusion. Nevertheless, we are heartened by the fact that 'although, achieving diversity and respect for people is a challenge all over the world, there is also good progress being made in some corners of the world' (Amin 2019: 17). For example, as in chapter 16, it was noted that 'the successful settlement of refugees in Australia is an under acknowledged narrative of social inclusion'. Indeed, when social inclusion is sustained, it can be taken for granted and past experiences of exclusion forgotten.

Social inclusion frameworks tend to have been developed in high-income countries, but this book includes many examples from low- and middle-income countries which could provide valuable learning for high-income countries, which still have much to learn about creating societies in which sustained social inclusion is a realistic expectation (see chapter 7). However, what works in one place does not necessarily work in another, without some adaptation. Furthermore, mistakes will be made by individuals, programmes, and organisations which are well-intentioned (chapter 8). However, rather than being a disincentive to challenging social exclusion, mistakes need to be regarded as opportunities for learning how social inclusion can be sustained and form the blueprint for transformed inclusive societies.

When Raewyn Connell devised her wish list of a good university (see chapter 9), being socially inclusive was one of her priorities. While she notes that wish lists can be fatuous, many of the examples in this volume emerged because one or more people had a dream for social inclusion and set out to work towards this.

All of the authors who have contributed to this volume are very aware of just how difficult it is to achieve and sustain social inclusion, but equally attest that not having sustained social inclusion is no longer an option for civil societies. Moreover, it may be costly not to have sustained social inclusion. For example, it has been proposed that although

> diversity cannot be reduced; however, its effects can be minimized by providing equal opportunities to all the individuals of the society, in order to create a secure and peaceful society through shaping the economic life of a country in a variety of ways and by promoting more cohesiveness.
>
> (Amin 2019: 17)

Finally, sustained social inclusion is now gaining recognition of being one of the attributes of a 'decent society', a characteristic to which many countries aspire but none have yet arrived at the point at which no further improvements are required (Abbott et al. 2017). The 'decent society' is arguably what the *SDGs* are seeking to achieve. At a time when social inclusion has lost favour among policymakers in many countries, hopefully the emergence of the idea of a 'decent society' will once more stimulate a desire to aim for sustained social inclusion.

There are numerous challenges for this decent society. These include policy cultures which privilege the already privileged, such as the Australian Prime Minister Scott Morrison and American President Donald Trump offering 'thoughts and prayers' to those who had lost homes and livelihoods as a result of fires. Sustaining social inclusion requires acknowledging the very real issues associated with climate change and addressing them. This is encapsulated by the international movement of School Strike for the Climate (SS4C) which in Australia is organised around three demands:

1   No new coal, oil and gas projects;
2   100 per cent renewable energy generation and exports by 2030; and
3   Fund a just transition and job creation for all fossil-fuel workers and communities.

> (School Change for the Climate 2019a)

In a letter to Australian coal workers and the communities in which they live, the need for a future which embraces social inclusion principles was spelt out as follows:

> As workers, you and your families' deserve respect, certainty and sustainable employment. As young people, we deserve a safe future and policies that don't hand us more extreme heat, drought, storms, food and water insecurity. None of us deserve to live in fear. We can work together in a fair transition to the industries of the future that protect our climate and livelihoods.
>
> (School Change for the Climate 2019b)

Sustaining social inclusion, in the context of climate change and declining bio-diversity, requires careful attention to all of the issues we have identified in this chapter, including the construction of knowledge, use of language, promotion of dignity, intersectionality, multilevel and multisectoral approaches, and resourc-ing. This is the terrain on which we need to further develop our understanding and practices.

References

Abbott, P., Wallace, C. and Sapsford, R. (2017) 'Socially inclusive development: the foun-dations for decent societies in East and Southern Africa', *Applied Research Quality Life*, 12: 813–39.

Altman, D. (1971) *Homosexual: Oppression and Liberation*, New York: Outerbridge & Dienstfrey.

Altman, D. (2019) *Unrequited Love: Diary of an Accidental Activist*, Clayton, Victoria: Monash University Press.

Amin, S. (2019) 'Diversity enforces social exclusion: does exclusion never cease?' *Journal of Social Inclusion*, 10(1): 4–22.

Avery, S. (2018) *Culture Is Inclusion: A Narrative of Aboriginal and Torres Strait Islander People with Disability*, Sydney: First Peoples Disability Network (Australia).

Béné, C., Godfrey-Wood, R., Newsham, A. and Davies, M. (2012) *Resilience: New Uto-pia or New Tyranny? Reflection About the Potentials and Limits of the Concept of Resilience in Relation to Vulnerability Reduction*, Brighton: Institute of Development Studies, Working Paper 405. Online. Available at https://onlinelibrary.wiley.com/doi/abs/10.1111/j.2040-0209.2012.00405.x (accessed 29 July 2019).

Brink, C. (2018) *The Soul of a University: Why Excellence Is Not Enough*, Bristol: Bristol University Press.

Chambers, B., Spriggs, J., Heaney-Mustafa, S. and Taj, S. (2018) 'Women and marginalised group inclusion in Pakistan smallholder agriculture', *Development Bulletin*, 79: 88–92.

Chambers, R. (2010) *Paradigms, Poverty and Adaptive Pluralism*, Brighton: Institute of Development Studies, Working Paper 344. Online. Available at https://onlinelibrary.wiley.com/doi/abs/10.1111/j.2040-0209.2010.00344_2.x (accessed 29 July 2019).

Cho, S., Crenshaw, K.W. and McCall, L. (2013) 'Towards a field of intersectionality stud-ies: theory, application and praxis', *Signs*, 38: 785–810.

Choo, H.Y. and Ferree, M.M. (2010) 'Practicing intersectionality in sociological research: a critical analysis of inclusions, interactions, and institutions in the study of inequalities', *Sociological Theory*, 28: 129–49.

Corburn, J. and Sverdlik, A. (2017) 'Slum upgrading and health equity', *International Journal of Environmental Research and Public Health*, 14: 342.

Crisp, B.R. (2018) 'From distance to online education: two decades of remaining respon-sive by one university social work programme', *Social Work Education*, 37: 718–30.

De Vogli, R., Schrecker, T. and Labonte, R. (2013) 'Neoliberal globalization and health inequalities', in J. Gabe and L.F. Monaghan (eds) *Key Concepts in Medical Sociology*, 2nd edn, London: Sage.

Gilbert, D.J. and Dako-Gyeke, M. (2018) 'Lack of mental health career interest among Ghanaian social work students: implications for social work education in Ghana', *Social Work Education*, 37(5): 665–76.

Keevers, L. and Abuodha, P. (2012) 'Social inclusion as an unfinished verb: a practice-based approach', *Journal of Academic Language and Learning*, 6(2): A42–59.

Loopstra, R. and Tarasuk, V. (2013) 'Perspectives on community gardens, community kitchens and the good food box program in a community-based sample of low-income families', *Canadian Journal of Public Health*, 104(1): e55–9.

McDonald, S. and Bertram, M. (2018) 'Job creation through income generation: an evaluation of Re-Cover, a decorating project developed with forensic mental health service users', *Journal of Mental Health Training Education and Practice*, 13: 148–56.

Mitra, S. (2018) *Disability, Health and Human Development*, New York: Palgrave Macmillan.

Murphy, J. (2005) 'The world bank, NGOs and civil society: converging agendas? The case of universal basic education in Niger', *Voluntas*, 16: 353–74.

Murphy, K. (2012) 'The social pillar of sustainable development: a literature review and framework for policy analysis', *Sustainability: Science, Practice and Policy*, 8: 15–29.

Platteau, J-P. (2008) 'Pitfalls of participatory development', in *Participatory Governance and the Millennium Development Goals (MDGs)*, New York: United Nations. Online. Available at http://unpan1.un.org/intradoc/groups/public/documents/un/unpan028359.pdf (accessed 29 July 2019).

Scheirer, M.A. (2005) 'Is sustainability possible? A review and commentary on empirical studies of program sustainability', *American Journal of Evaluation*, 26: 320–47.

Schmitz, C.L., Matyók, T., Sloan, L.M. and James, C. (2012) 'The relationship between social work and environmental sustainability: implications for interdisciplinary practice', *International Journal of Social Welfare*, 21: 278–86.

School Strike 4 Climate Change (2019a) 'Our demands'. Online. Available at www.school-strike4climate.com/about (accessed 9 December 2019).

School Strike 4 Climate Change (2019b) 'Dear coal workers & communities: a solidarity message from school strikers across Australia to coal workers and communities'. Online. Available at www.schoolstrike4climate.com/post/dear-coal-workers-communities (accessed 9 December 2019).

Stedman Jones, G. (1971/2013) *Outcast London: A Study of the Relationship Between Classes in Victorian Society*, London: Verso.

St. Pierre Schneider, B., Menzel, N., Clark, M., York, N., Candela, L. and Xu, Y. (2009) 'Nursing's leadership in positioning human health at the core of urban sustainability', *Nursing Outlook*, 57: 281–8.

Suharto, S., Kuipers, P. and Dorsett, P. (2016) 'Disability terminology and the emergence of "diffability" in Indonesia', *Disability and Society*, 31: 693–712.

Sukarieh, M. and Tannock, S. (2008) 'In the best interests of youth or neoliberalism? The world bank and the new global youth empowerment project', *Journal of Youth Studies*, 11: 301–12.

United Nations (1948) 'Universal declaration of human rights'. Online. Available at www.refworld.org/docid/3ae6b3712c.html (accessed 4 November 2019).

United Nations (2015) 'Transforming our world: the 2030 agenda for sustainable development'. Online. Available at https://sustainabledevelopment.un.org/post2015/transformingourworld/publication (accessed 4 November 2019).

Walsham, M., Kuper, H., Morgon Banks, L. and Blanchet, K. (2019) 'Social protection for people with disabilities in Africa and Asia: a review of programmes for low- and middle-income countries', *Oxford Development Studies*, 47: 97–112.

White, J. (2017) 'The banality of exclusion in Australian universities', *International Journal of Inclusive Education*, 21: 1142–55.

Index

2018 Disability Global Summit 265
2030 Agenda for Sustainable Development
  5–7, 204, 265, 281

abortion 11, 66
Afghanistan 306
Africa 3, 7, 219, 222, 263; *see also*
  Kenya; Malawi; Rwanda; South Africa;
  Tanzania; Zambia
African Development Bank 7; *see also*
  High 5 Priority Goals
African National Congress 20
age: children 111, 159, 189–200, 306;
  older people, elderly people 93–102;
  young people and adolescents 238–9
aged care 159, 162–3, 165
agency 23, 38, 70–1, 111, 125–6, 159,
  214, 249–55, 310, 324
anti-oppressive practice 173, 191,
  235, 237
Arab countries 52
Argentina 3
arts 27, 249–57, 322; *see also* theatre-based
  programmes
Asia 9, 219, 232–3, 235, 263; *see also*
  Bangladesh; Cambodia; India; Indonesia;
  Malaysia; Myanmar; Vietnam
assistive technology (AT) 10, 80
asylum seekers 14, 110, 114–15, 231, 233,
  236, 240, 324, 327
Athena Swan 15–16
austerity measures 7
Australia 11, 13, 15, 16–18, 19, 25,
  37–49, 51, 65–75, 108, 120, 147–54,
  171, 207, 211–12, 218–27, 231–41,
  329
autism 79, 94–5, 101
autonomy 139, 158, 207, 266

Bangladesh 9, 247–8
belonging 3, 98–102, 124, 159, 234, 273,
  293–4
Bolivia 142
Bourdieu, P. 173–82, 251; *see also*
  habitus; social capital

Cambodia 7, 198–9
Canada 17, 21, 51, 114, 171, 207, 210,
  218–19, 324
capacity building 25, 60, 93–106, 114,
  192, 239, 265, 268, 273, 312, 328
childcare 10, 67, 272
childless/childlessness 7
child protection 18, 160–1, 179
China 233
citizenship 4, 27, 157–8, 249, 281
climate change 5, 6, 12, 25, 142, 330–1
co-design 79, 94, 165, 169, 310–11, 328
collaboration 16–17, 94–5, 101–4, 128,
  152, 157, 183, 200, 232, 237–41,
  367–70, 282, 305, 323
colonialism 219–21, 248
colonisation 218–27
community: gated 3; inclusive 279; online
  27; 277–88, 311, 324; sense of 291–301
community-based organisation 174–83,
  231–41, 310–11
community development 39, 93–106, 111,
  237, 247–60
community gardens 21–2, 109, 113
compensation schemes 9, 37–49
connectedness 23, 100, 227, 239, 281;
  see also social capital; social cohesion
consultation 11, 21–2, 23, 25, 53–61, 71,
  78–86, 198–9, 225, 239–40, 266, 298,
  306, 322–3
contraception 11; *see also* family planning

Convention on the Elimination of All
Forms of Discrimination Against
Women 68
Convention on the Rights of Persons with
Disabilities 189, 195, 207, 263, 279, 295
Convention on the Rights of the Child 189
co-production 72, 79, 85, 237
criminal justice 46
critical race theory 235
critical reflection 163–8, 171–83,
237, 251
Croatia 27, 283–8
culture 41, 58, 66, 68, 77, 80, 86, 142, 174,
200, 221, 226, 248, 264, 307; culturally
appropriate 21, 109–10, 113, 205, 226;
cultural competence 240; multicultural
101, 104, 144, 232–5; organizational
15, 17–19, 46, 139, 180–1; *see also*
ethnicity

Deafblind/deafblindness 11, 77–86
decision making: community 25–6,
158, 251, 266, 268, 278, 291–5;
consultative 11, 21–3, 157–69, 210,
237; organisational 21, 139, 144,
153–4, 157, 167–69, 182–3; policy 27,
51–60, 65–75, 305, 327–8; *see also*
participatory approach/process
Declaration on the Rights of Disabled
Persons 9, 69
Declaration on the Rights of Indigenous
Peoples 9, 218, 227
deprivation 3, 77
disability: 153, 210, 291–301, 307–8;
intellectual 4; learning 23; physical 4,
211–14; sensory 4, 11, 77–86
disadvantage 12, 67, 95, 127, 152, 179,
213, 218, 234, 280; *see also* equality;
equity; inequality
discrimination 4, 10, 68, 72–3, 158, 190,
256, 279, 304, 312, 323–4; *see also*
rights
displaced persons 306
diversity 307, 312, 329; *see also* culture;
disability; ethnicity; gender; religion;
sexuality
domestic violence 7, 52, 161

economic development 263–6, 273
education: access to 3, 4, 140–1, 143,
147–54, 197, 238, 263, 292; higher
education 15–16, 135–44, 147–54,
327; school 54, 57–8, 111, 113, 140,
143, 147–9, 196–7, 219, 236, 262,

309–15, 327; university 10, 18, 19,
135–44, 329; vocational 143, 226–7
employment: access to 3, 4, 10, 65–75,
238, 263, 292; foreign workers 10, 17;
maternity leave provisions 10, 72–3;
policies 10, 67–73; short term 10;
unemployment 12; *see also* income;
welfare
empowerment 6, 100, 102, 112, 121, 237,
247–51, 259, 301, 307, 324
England 12–13
environment: attitudinal 20; built 14, 20,
25–7, 291–301; inclusive 22, 291–301;
learning, 19; living 26–7; unpolluted 4,
26; workplace 16–18, 135–44, 171–83
equality 5–6, 66–74
equity 4, 24, 310; gender, 15–16, 67,
70–1, 73, 307
Estonia 27, 279, 280–8
ethics 17, 23, 149, 293; conscience clauses
11; frameworks 203–15; professional,
204–6; research 53, 82, 194, 268, 301
Ethiopia 198–9
ethnicity, 52, 308; *see also* indigenous
people; race
evaluation 12–14, 16–17, 46, 53–60,
93–106, 159–69, 172, 196–8,
237–9, 300
Europe 232–3; *see also* Croatia; Estonia;
Germany; Hungary; Ireland; Italy;
Malta; Netherlands; Spain; United
Kingdom
European Union 10, 51
experts by experience 126
exploitation 47, 61, 143,
220, 305

faith, faith-based organization, faith
leaders: *see* religion
fake news 3
family planning 66
feminism 71–2
film 192–7; *see also* video
food: nutrition 4, 21–2; security 7, 8, 14,
108–15, 119–30, 239, 324
Food and Agriculture Association 109
Freire, P. 251
Funding 10, 11, 12–14, 106, 292;
charitable 110–11, 128; corporate, 12,
13, 20, 137; fees 139, 147; government
7, 12, 210; international aid and
development 20–1, 25, 189–200;
military 137; philanthropic 12; research
15–16; short-term 4, 12–13, 20–1

gender: discrimination on basis of 4,
15–16, 52; female 19, 67, 152, 262,
272; heteronormative expectations 7;
male 67, 306, 312; roles 65–75, 312;
transgender 311–15; *see also* equity;
men; women
Georgia 199
Germany 26, 38, 120, 232
Global North 51, 52, 60, 136, 142
Global South 61, 190, 193, 263–4,
266–7, 314
governance 25, 26, 39–40, 45, 58, 159,
211, 224, 249, 266–8, 280–1, 292,
297, 329
Greece 232

habitus 173, 175–7
Haiti 25
health: inequities 114; outcomes 7, 51,
158, 271; social determinants of 52, 93,
223; *see also* health care; mental health
health care: access to 9; medication 4;
policy 52–3; services 17
health promotion 95, 111, 113, 236, 239,
304–11
High 5 Priority Goals 7
homelessness, 111, 113, 119–30, 159–64,
293, 323–4
housing 4, 24, 238, 271, 280, 287, 327;
access to 8, 226, 291–3; estates 26–7;
policy 231, 296–7; services 124, 159,
165, 288
human rights *see* rights
Hungary 27, 279, 283–8

identity 253, 264; community, 226, 232,
248, 254; group 161–6, 264, 273, 294,
325; individual 39, 41–2, 121, 161,
171–83, 254, 281, 310, 325
inclusive research 4, 11, 54–61, 190–200,
240, 262–74, 294–301, 322–3
income: high-income countries 6, 9,
109–10, 120, 134, 329; individuals and
families 21, 93, 108, 112–15, 210, 239,
264, 267, 270–2, 287, 324, 327; low and
middle-income countries 3, 21, 52, 236,
306, 314, 329; *see also* employment;
livelihood; social protection; welfare
India 24–5, 140
indigenous peoples/knowledges 21,
142, 144; Aboriginal and Torres Strait
Islander Australians (ATSI) 120, 149,
150, 152, 218–27, 233, 235; Maori
142, 181

Indonesia 25, 27, 219, 233, 262–74
industrialisation 5–7, 9, 38, 48, 221
inequality 7, 24, 108, 119–20, 140, 173–4,
204, 224, 235, 239
information technology/information and
communication technology (IT/ICT) 27,
277–88
International Covenant on Economic,
Social and Cultural Rights 109
International Labour Organization (ILO)
8–9
Intersectional/intersectionality 69–70,
72, 74–5, 104–5, 234, 237, 268, 321,
325–7
Ireland (Eire) 15, 19, 232
Italy 120, 232

Kenya 25–6
Knowledge translation 53

language 77–86, 199, 162, 193–7, 204,
220–6, 238, 269, 321, 323–4; of social
exclusion 3–4, 22–3, 122–3, 160
Latin America 3, 143, 235; *see also*
Argentina; Bolivia; South America
leadership 17, 93–106, 119, 125, 127–8,
150, 152–3, 159, 166–7, 180, 251,
206, 328
Lebanon 11, 51–61
legislation 4, 11, 27, 38, 41–2, 44, 53, 71,
266, 292
life course 7, 72
literacy 250–3; financial 270–2;
health 239
livelihood 26, 249, 259, 262–74, 330
loneliness 99, 102; *see also* social isolation

marginalisation: addressing 10, 121;
economic 3, 52, 153, 262–74; social
4, 77, 82, 241, 262–74, 293; *see also*
disadvantage; oppression
Malawi 9
Malaysia 9, 233
Malta 232
medicine 205, 281; *see also* psychiatry
mental health: policy 4; service provision
237, 283, 307; service users 23–4, 41
migration: forced 7, 231, 247
Millennium Development Goals
5–6, 272
mobility 4, 77–86, 211–12, 272, 279,
293, 326
Mozambique 21
Myanmar 25, 27, 247–60, 328

National Disability Insurance Agency
(NDIA) 211–12
National Disability Insurance Scheme
(NDIS) 207, 210–12, 297
National Health Service (NHS) 17,
210, 214
neoliberal/neoliberalism 70, 136–40, 143,
144, 171–83, 322, 327
Netherlands 279–80
network society 277–88
New Zealand 17, 142, 171–83,
218–19, 233
non-government organisation (NGO)
157–69, 189–200; *see also* community-
based organisation
nurses/nursing 18, 205, 313

occupational health and safety 37, 46
occupational therapy/therapists 212
oppression 69, 77, 82, 172, 174, 180,
190, 209, 251, 293, 310; *see also*
marginalisation
Organisation for Economic Co-operation
and Devleopment (OECD) 51, 68, 71
Othering 123, 220, 235–6, 254
Ottawa Charter for Health Promotion 236

Pacific region 189–200
Pakistan 314, 328
Papua New Guinea 21, 190–200
parents 10, 42, 160–1, 196–7; support for
23, 27, 65–75, 100–1
participatory approach/process 80–6,
237; 249, 265–70, 291–301; to policy
development 11, 51–61, 71–2, 224, 263
peer support 40–6, 94, 282–8, 324–5;
worker 40–6
Peru 199
physiotherapy 204
Poland 140
Post-traumatic stress disorder (PTSD)
41, 236
poverty: 3, 213, 247–8, 279, 325, 327;
intergenerational 7, 12, 67; reduction 5,
10, 12, 24–5, 115, 121, 249–50, 264–6,
272; *see also* disadvantage; income;
welfare
privilege 11, 18–19, 136, 143–4, 163,
179, 330
professional associations 18
professional development 18, 172, 176
professional education 224, 327
professional supervision 18, 171–83

psychiatry 41
psychology 206
public health 53

quality of life 7, 26, 282

race 4, 20–1; *see also* ethnicity
reciprocity 252, 264, 277–88, 294
refugees 22, 198, 231–41, 329; *see also*
asylum seekers; forced migration
religion: Buddhism 247, 258–9;
Catholicism 7; Christianity 22;
discrimination on basis of 4, 52; Islam
22, 142, 247, 258–9, 271; Judaism
325; religious beliefs 218–27; religious
communities 22; religious leaders 306;
religious organisations 37–49; *see also*
spirituality
resilience 5, 22–3, 176, 209, 224,
236–9, 281
restorative justice 45–9, 235
rights: civil 4; cultural 4; economic 4;
human rights 4, 65, 209, 231, 235,
249, 321; of persons with disabilities
262–74; political 4, 51; reproductive
65–75; social 4; to vote 23–4, 125–6,
308–9, 314
rights-based approach 157–69
Rwanda 9
rural 7, 9, 13, 121–9, 147–8, 262–74, 326

Scotland 7
self-esteem 100
self help 42–3
Senegal 199
service design 4, 11, 72, 123–9, 148–50,
157–69
sexuality: bisexuality 307; gay 305, 307,
325; heterosexuality 305; homosexuality
325; lesbian 307; sexual minorities 7,
307; transgender, 307, 311–14; *see also*
gender; identity; rights
sex work 7
silencing 4, 14, 47–8, 67, 77, 82, 123, 158,
164–7, 323
social capital 22, 174, 180–1, 240,
264, 277
social cohesion 24, 113, 203, 298, 232,
234–5, 250, 256–7, 279, 306; *see also*
connectedness
social development 24–7, 52, 245–315
social enterprise 14, 114–15, 285–8, 326
social isolation 39, 93, 95, 100–1, 111–12

social justice 4, 47–8, 235
social media 3, 284–8, 311–12, 314
social policy 4, 65–75, 231–41; coherence 9, 327
social protection: floor 8–9; programmes 265
social seclusion 3
social work 171–83, 205, 210
South Africa 3, 19–20
South America 142; *see also* Argentina; Bolivia; Latin America
Spain 10
spirituality 43, 223–7; *see also* religion
Sri Lanka 199
stigma 94, 100–1, 110, 115, 124, 239, 279
strengths-based approaches 94, 97, 103, 123, 173
substance abuse/misuse/use 127–9
suicide 44–5, 179, 226
sustainable development 24–7, 251, 263
Sustainable Development Goals (SDGs) 5–7, 24, 51, 85, 272, 321, 327, 330

Tanzania 4
theatre-based programmes 27, 269–70, 304–15
Timor-Leste 197, 314
trade unions 18, 38
transport 284–5; public 9, 285, 297, 326
trauma 37–49, 99, 127, 227, 231, 235–40, 253, 325, 329
trust 51, 58, 60–1, 82, 125–6, 136, 177, 179, 196, 205, 250, 255, 258, 270, 277–8, 283, 295, 294, 322

Ukraine 27, 283–8
United Arab Emirates10

United Kingdom (UK) 7, 9, 11, 12, 15–16, 23, 26, 120, 213–14; *see also* England; Scotland
United Nations (UN) 4, 5–7, 9, 109, 192–3, 197, 199, 209, 281
United Nations Development Program (UNDP) 25
United Nations High Commissioner for Refugees (UNHCR) 231, 233
United Nations International Children's Emergency Fund (UNICEF) 198
United States of America (USA) 17, 23, 112–13, 120, 143, 208, 213, 218–19, 277, 307–9
universal access 8, 262, 266, 291–301
Universal Declaration of Human Rights 4, 6, 9, 69, 141, 207, 209, 236, 254, 321, 327
universal design 26
urban 291–301

Vanuatu 21, 190–200
video 306; *see also* film
Vietnam 233
volunteers 13, 40, 42–3, 110, 119–30, 213, 249

water 4–6, 8, 24, 248–9, 330
welfare 67, 112–13, 120, 213
women 15–19, 24–5, 42, 65–75, 95, 258–9, 272, 327–8; *see also* gender, female
World Bank 248, 327
World Café 80–6
World Health Organization (WHO) 51, 236

Zambia 306

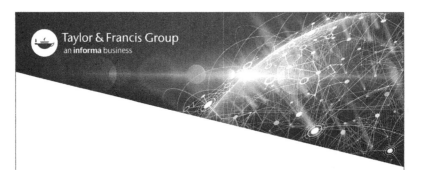

Printed in the United States
by Baker & Taylor Publisher Services